Surgery and Arthroscopy of the Knee

First European Congress
of Knee Surgery and Arthroscopy
Berlin, 9–14. 4. 1984

Edited by E. L. Trickey and P. Hertel

With 215 Figures and 58 Tables

Springer-Verlag Berlin Heidelberg New York
London Paris Tokyo

E. L. Trickey, FRCS

Institute of Orthopaedics
Royal National Orthopaedic Hospital
Brockley Hill
Stanmore, Middlesex, HA7 4LP, U. K.

Professor Dr. Peter Hertel

Rudolph-Virchow-Krankenhaus
Augustenburger Platz 1, 1000 Berlin, FRG

ISBN-13: 978-3-642-71024-7 e-ISBN-13: 978-3-642-71022-3
DOI: 10.1007/978-3-642-71022-3

Library of Congress Cataloging-in-Publication Data. Surgery and arthroscopy of the knee. 1. Knee – Surgery. 2. Arthroscopy. 3. Artificial knee. 4. Knee – Surgery – Patients – Rehabilitation. I. Trickey, E. L. (Edward Lorden), 1920– . II. Hertel, Peter. [DNLM: 1. Arthroscopy. 2. Cartilage, Articular – surgery. 3. Knee Injuries – surgery. 4. Knee Joint – physiology. 5. Knee Prosthesis. 6. Ligaments, Articular – surgery. We 870 S9608] RD561.S85 1986 617'.582059
86-13745 ISBN-13: 978-3-642-71024-7

Typesetting: Brühlsche Universitätsdruckerei, Giessen
Offsetprinting: Saladruck, Berlin. Bookbinding: Lüderitz & Bauer, Berlin
2124/3020-543210

Preface

This book is a record of the papers read at the first meeting of the European Society of Knee Surgery and Arthroscopy (ESKA). This was held in the magnificent International Congress Centre (ICC) in West Berlin.

Planning for the inaugural meeting of a proposed large society is inevitably fraught with problems and doubts. However, thanks to the tremendous assistance given by the ICC organization and to the participation of so many orthopaedic surgeons from Europe and all over the world the society had a very successful meeting, and it is fitting that the papers are collected together in this book as a permanent record.

Various factors combined to delay the appearance of the book until now, shortly before the second ESKA meeting (1986) in Basle. We should like to take this opportunity of thanking Springer-Verlag for all the hard work involved in ensuring that the book was finished before this occasion and while the subject matter is still so topical.

The knee joint is exceptionally important in various ways. This joint connecting the long bones of femur and tibia is particularly prone to injury, but at the same time it is vital for it to be in good working order, and not only for athletes. It is essential for balance and mobility, which in turn are fundamental to financial and social independence in older people and all working people. This is also reflected in the considerable sums expended by our social security and health insurance systems on the treatment of knee injuries and on disability pensions payable as a result of knee injuries.

It is therefore incumbent upon us to coordinate our scientific endeavours without allowing ourselves to be restricted to our own national societies; such international congresses in Europe allow us to pool our knowledge so that information on the advances made can be disseminated more quickly, to the ultimate benefit of the patients.

August 1986

E. L. Trickey, Stanmore
We. Müller, Basle
P. Hertel, Berlin

Name List of Authors

Abbink EP
Ackroyd CE
Aglietti P
Aigner R
Albrektsson B
Alho A
Ali MS
Arms S
Arvidsson-Johansson I
Aubaniac JM
Aubriot JH
de Baere GAJ
Baily RAJ
Bandi W
Bannister GC
Bauer M
Baumgartner R
Behfar AS
Benazet JP
v.d. Berg A
Blankevoort L
Blauth W
Boe S
Bopp P
Borg G
Braun W
Bühlmann H
Burri C
Buzzi R
Canata GL
Cardoso T
Casolo F
Cerulli G
Chaix C
Giuccarelli
Claes L
Constantinides C
Contzen H
Crawford RJ
Cusimano S
De Santis E
Dive JM
Drobny TK
Dupont JY
Dumont P
Ecke H
Edixhoven Ph
Eickhoff W
Engesaeter L
Eriksson E
Feagin
Fabbriciani C
Feldkamp G
Fonda G
Franceschi JP
Franke K
Freeman MAR
Gaechter A
Gallai V
Galanis J
Gaudernak T
Geesinck RGT
Georgoulis A
Giebel G
Gillquist J
Gorecki A
Gradinger R
Graf HJ
Gschwend N
Hackenbruch W
Häggmark T
Hager D
Hahn M
Hamberg P
Hardinger K
Hassenpflug J
Hauspal
Hehne HF
Heinert K
Hempfling H
Hepp WR
Herberts P
Hertel P
Hillen B
Holzheimer R
Hoogland T
Hörterer H
Huiskes R
Hungerford DS
v. Hussen FAJ
Hutton P
Iusim M
Jackson A
Jackson RW
Jäger M
Janssen G
Jensen J
Johnson R
Johnson DP
Junger CH
Junker
Kalbe P
Karpf PM
Kayser M
de Keizer G
Kemp HBS
Kieser CH
Klein W
Klemann T
Knutsson E
Kölzer D
Kolb M
Korisek G
Krackow K
Kramer FJK
Kus W
Kuyper W
Lais E
de Lange A
Lauritzen J
Legre G
Lerat JL
Leyshon A

Lim TE
Lindberg U
van den Linden AJ
Livingstone B
Lysholm J
Mailaender C
Mang W
Mann M
Maquet P
Mariani PP
Marti R
Mason J
Mazotta G
Menachem A
Menche DS
Mendes DG
Meyrat R
Meystre JL
Milachowski KA
Miremad Ch
Mitsou A
Mockwitz J
Molster AO
Motta F
Mukherjee SK
Müller KH
Müller W
Müller-Färber J
Münch EO
Munzinger U
Murphy JC
Neugebauer R
Niedermann B
Noesberger B
Nordin M
Odensten M
Oestern HJ
Ogilvie-Harris D
Older J
Oransky M
Panni Schiavone P
Papadelis P
Parker J
Passl R
Paul B
Perren SM
Perugia L
Peterson L
Pförringer W
Pieper
Pietrogrande V
Pisaneschi A
Piscopakis N
Pitman MI
Pokorny V
Pope M
Poster
Pozo JL
Prahl R
Pudden
Raugstadt TS
Recanatini L
Refior HJ
Regan J
Rehder U
Rehm K
van Rens Th JG
Rether JR
Robinson MP
Rodriguez M
Rofman R
Roffman M
Rogge DH
Roy-Camille R
Rubak JM
Rüter A
Sächler A
Sagstetter C
Saillant G
Salomon Z
Samuelson KM
Sandt A
Savoldi E
Schabus R
Scharf W
Scheier H
Schmid R
Schmidt JM
Schmidt MA
Schmiebusch H
Schreiber A
Schulitz Kp
Schultheis KH
Seiler H
Shatwell M
Siegel A
Simonsen
Skredderstuen A
Skorpik G
Sloof TJJH
Soudry M
Steiger U
Strand T
Tarquini C
Tegner Y
Tosca L
Trickey EL
Tscherne H
Tsemanis V
Ulivi M
Vallatta A
Wagner M
Weber J
Weh L
Weigert M
Weinel P
Weismeier K
Wentzensen
Werhahn
Wirth CJ
Wyss U
Zander C
Zeegers FJB
Zifko B

Table of Contents

Biomechanics

Articular Cartilage

Arthroscopy

Menisci

Anterior Cruciate Ligaments

Posterior Cruciate Ligament

Synthetic Ligaments

Patello-femoral Joints

Osteotomy

Knee-joint Replacement

Rehabilitation

Biomechanics

Epidemiology of knee joint injuries

K. Franke

Dept. Surgery, Municipal Hospital Berlin-Pankow
DDR-1100 Berlin
German Dem. Rep.

Sequelae of single impact and recurrent microtrauma may not be separated either in all cases of knee joint lesion, mainly concerning those of menisci and hyaline cartilage. The missed early treatment of cartilage and ligamentous lesion leads to a degenerative damage of the joint.

As the latter appears with others separately from the trauma accidents in the ICD, ninth revision, this WHO-document does not cover in all respects the practical necessities of trauma statistics. It causes therefore also difficulties in real information about epidemiology of trauma accidents. An additional difficulty occurs from regional differences in trauma expostion and also by the profile of hospitals.

Among all accident traumas, the knee joint region is injured with about 5% – mainly located into capsule, ligaments, and menisci. There occur less than one percent joint fractures. But among all sports accidents the knee joint is injured from 15 to 30%.

This is, of course, different to the pattern we have found among 2 600 operations in our specialized department. There were 51,1% meniscus lesions, 33,8% ligamentous injuries, and 4,7% joint fractures.

In the etiology of knee joint lesions traffic and home accidents predominantly cause joint fractures, and sports and working accidents cause lesions of ligaments and menisci.

An increasing consideration should be paid to the chondromalacia, which is important for the functional prognosis of the joint. Therefore the diagnosis is more often. This is also proved by our figures. Among the knee joints operated on because of injuries, between 1971 and 1980 we found as an average 65% cartilage destructions – but 1981/1982 it were already 77,4%.

Primary operation of joint fractures is acknowledged everywhere as a rule, but this is not recognized for ligamentous lesions. An international survey shows that only 10% are treated by early operation, which should take place as optimum within 72 hours after injury.

Reflections about epidemiology of accidents should never end in itself. They should help to organize prevention, medical care, and the qualification of doctors.

The biomechanics of anterior cruciate ligament rehabilitation and reconstruction

I. Arvidsson, S. Arms, E. Eriksson, R. J. Johnson and M. Pope

Section of Trauma, Dept of Surgery, Karolinska Hospital
Stockholm
Sweden

The rehabiliation of knee injuries involving the anterior cruciate ligament (ACL) is controversial. This paper describes strain in the normal and reconstructed ACL during a series of passive and active tests of knee flexion with and without varus, valgus and axial rotation torques on the tibia.

Material and methods
Twenty-one knee from 19 cadavers were tested using a Hall effect transducer attached to the midportion of the anteriomedial fibre bundles of the ACL. A goniometer was strapped to the medialside of the knee. In nine specimen the strain in a patellar tendon reconstruction placed in the assumed ideal position was measured. In two knees the reconstructions were placed one centimeter anteriorly to the ideal postion and the same experiments were repeated.

Results
Simulated isometric quadriceps contractions increased ACL strain significantly through the first 45° of knee flextion ($p < 0.005$). Isometric contractions at flexion angles greater than 60° decreases ACL strain. In the reconstructions there was significant difference between the strain in passive motion and in eccentric quadriceps contraction similar to the normal ACL. The strain in the anteriorly placed graft was significantly greater than both the normal ACL and the posteriorly placed graft in full flexion. No other tests were possible since the suture cut through these reconstructions at full flexion.

Discussion
From our studies it is evident that if ACL is repaired or reconstructed it is important that the structure is placed in the proper position far posteriorly. The graft or ligament should be sutured at a flexion angle of 35° followed by a passive range of motion from full extension to 90° to control that the ligament has not loosened. If motion or quadriceps activity are utilized angles greater than 60° are safe.

Summary
Strain in the human knee ACL is significantly different depending on whether the knee flexion angle is changed passively or via simulated quadriceps contraction. This latter motion increases ACL strain in the range from 0° – 45°. Varus and internal rotation increases ACL strain. The capsule is an important aspect of strain protection of the ACL. ACL reconstructions anatomically placed exhibit strain patterns similar to normal ACL. Lachman and anterior drawer tests create potentially high strains in the ACL. Those who elect to use motion or quadriceps activity following ACL repair or reconstruction should understand that strains are produced in the ACL.

In vitro measurement of stress and strain in knee ligaments under various load and position conditions

L. Claes and R. Schmid

Department of Traumatology, University of Ulm
7900 Ulm
Federal Republic of Germany

For the post-operative treatment of acute ligamentous injuries as well as for prosthetic ligament reconstruction the knowledge of knee ligament biomechanics is necessary. Conflicting results have been published on the biomechanical properties of knee ligaments under different load and position conditions. To determine the stress and strain in knee ligaments special measuring cells and a knee simulator were developed.

Material and methods

Measurements of stress and strain were obtained in the collateral ligaments of 20 cadaver knees using the newly designed measuring cells. Additionally, experiments on both collateral ligaments and both cruciate ligaments were performed on 4 knees with intact capsule and then repeated following resection of the capsule. The knees were fixed in the simulator and then flexed cyclically between 0° and 130°. Rotation, valgus, varus and quadriceps muscle forces were applied either singly or in combination by the simulator. For each of these loads the stress and strain in each ligament were plotted as a function of the angle of flexion of the knee.

Results

All ligaments showed their maximum stress and strain between 0° and 30° flexion. The strain in the collateral ligaments was about 5 times that of the strain in the cruciate ligaments. When the capsule was resected the strain increases in all ligaments to about 300%. The ventral and dorsal parts of the broad MCL showed contrary behaviour. In extension the ventral part was under minimum strain whereas the dorsal part was under maximum strain. Stress and strain were not proportional, i.e. the largest strain but the lowest tensile forces were measured at the dorsal part of the MCL. The highest strain under pure flexion was 5% and the largest tensile force was about 20 N. Valgus, varus and rotation loads increased the stress and strain in specific ligaments. From the 24 different load combinations which were measured two significant results were:

1) increased strain in the ACL with internal rotation and valgus and
2) increased strain in the LCL with external rotation and varus. In both the ACL and LCL a quadriceps muscle force of 50 N resulted in a decrease in the strain and stress in the loaded ligaments.

Discussion

These results demonstrate that stress and strain in the four main knee ligaments were small when flexion is limited to 30° – 120° and when there are no valgus, varus or rotation loads. Clinically this can be achieved with a limited motion cast. Furthermore, the measurements point out the importance of the quadriceps muscle force and the surrounding joint capsule for the stabilization of the knee.

The functional anatomy of the knee joint – kinematics of the ligaments

U. Rehder

Orthopädische Klinik, Universität Hamburg
2000 Hamburg
Federal Republic of Germany

Material and methods

The ligaments of 32 knees from 20 cadavers were prepared and morphometrically measured. The attachment areas were related to the geometry of the femoral condyles. In a previous paper the shape of the condyles was described as an involute of a circle. Based on this model the kinematics of the attachment points of the ligaments were calculated by mathematical methods and compared with two-dimensional models of the knee joint.

Results

The polhodies of gliding motion of the femoral condyles is a circle rolling on a line perdendicular to the tibial plateau. During gliding motion different points of the femoral condyles describe different curves in the space-fixed coordinate system of the tibia. In general these curves are cycloid.

Discussion

Cycloid movement of the attachment points of the ligaments of the knee implies that at different angles of flexion different fibres of the ligaments are stretched. Stretching of a fibre occurs, when the fibre crosses the instant axis of rotation.

Summary

The curvature of the femoral condyles can be described as an involute of a circle. Based on this mathematical model the movement of the attachment points of the ligaments was calculated. In general these points described cycloid in the space fixed coordinate system. Fibres of the ligaments were under tension, when they crossed the instant centre of rotation of the knee joint.

The three-dimensional freedom-of-motion characteristics of the human knee joint

R. Huiskes, A. de Lange and L. Blankevoort

Lab. Experimental Orthopaedics
University of Nijmegen
The Netherlands

Introduction

The present study attempts to quantify the three-dimensional freedom-of-motion characteristics of the knee-joint in vitro, and their dependence on external forces, knee ligaments and menisci. This information provides descriptions of knee-joint kinematic behaviour in general, which can be applied to the development of improved diagnostic tools and operative procedures.

Methods

A test apparatus is used in which all three-dimensional motions in the knee-joint can be simulated and in which axial forces, AP-forces and exo-endorotation couples can be applied. The changes in spatial positions of tiba with respect to femur are very accurately determined using a Roentgen-stereo-photogrammetric measuring system described earlier (1). These motions are represented by anatomical rotation angles (flexion-extension, ab-adduction and exo-endorotation) and translations, and by so-called helical axes (compare instant-centres-of rotation in plane motion). In addition, the cruciate and collateral ligament fibre length patterns during the knee motions can be reconstructed, using a technique described previously (1).

The present experiments were performed on four post-mortem specimens, of which two bilateral ones. Each joint was moved from extension to 90 degrees of flexion in approximately 10 steps, while several combinations of the aforementioned loads were applied. Each test was repeated after meniscectomy.

Results and discussion

An example of results is shown in Figure 1: exo-endorotation curves as functions of flexion for several combinations of external loads (left) and before/after meniscectomy (right) in one of the specimes. Evidently, freedom-of-motion was mostly found in the flexion and exo-endorotation motions, the limits of the latter depending on the flexion angle and the rotation couple specified. These limits are hardly influenced by axial forces, but these forces do have an effect on the neutral motion pathway, where no exo-endorotation couples are applied. The application of an AP-force shifts the neutral curves to either endo- or exorotation, but again the limits of the latter freedom-of-motion remain unaltered. Meniscectomy results in slightly increased exo-endorotation limits, but in general has very little influence on the joint kinematic characteristics, nor on the ligament length patterns. Although the results in the four specimen differ to some extent, their trends are comparable.

The helical axis representation proves to be very sensitive to slight differences in motions, although attractive for visualizing movement patterns.

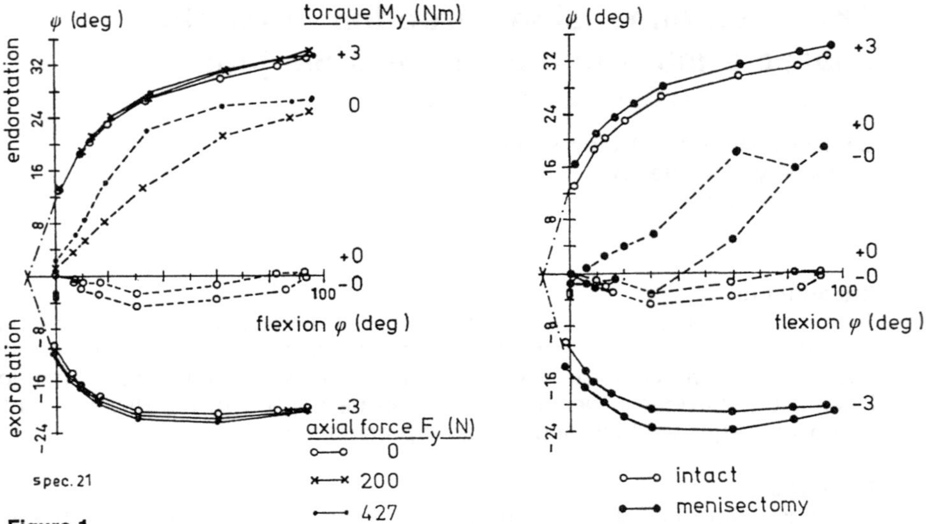

Figure 1.

Acknowledgement

Partly sponsored by Grant 90-90 of the Netherlands Organization for the Advancement of Pure Research (ZWO).

Reference:

(1) Dijk, R. van, Huiskes, R. and Selvik, G. (1979) J. Biomechanics 12, pp. 727 – 731.

An instrument for quantitative clinical evaluation of the AP-drawer in the knee joint

P. Edixhoven, R. Huiskes, T. J. G. van Rens and T. J. J. H. Slooff

Lab. Experimental Orthopaedics
University of Nijmegen
The Netherlands

For diagnostic and post-operative patient evaluation purposes in relation with knee-joint trauma and instability, the clinical AP-drawer test fulfils an important function. However versatile this test may be in the hands of experienced clinicians, it does not produce reproducible, quantitative information and as such hampers objective comparisons of pre- and post-operative patient data. Although several devices for objective in vivo knee-laxity measurements were presented in the recent literature, they all suffer, to our opinion, from one ot two shortcomings: they are either inaccurate, or so complicated that routine applications in the clinic are infeasible.

The apparatus presented in this paper is, to our opinion, an excellent compromise in this respect. Its principle is schematically drawn in Figure 1. The patient is seated in relaxed position and the leg fixed in 20-30 degrees of flexion. The foot is fixed in neutral endo-exorotation position, and the thigh is clamped (but not rigidly fixed) above the knee, as shown in the figure. Anterior and posterior forces, respectively, are administered manually with a spindle, and registered electronically. While the forces gradually increase to maximal values of 250 Newtons, the displacements of the tuberositas and the patella are monitored electronically as well. The difference between the two displacement signals is representative for the actual AP-shift. The essential feature of this method is, that a (quite impossible) rigid fixation of the bones is not necessary, in view of the differential displacement registration.

The three signals (force and two displacements) are fed into a micro-computer, which executes the required calculations and continuously produces the actual

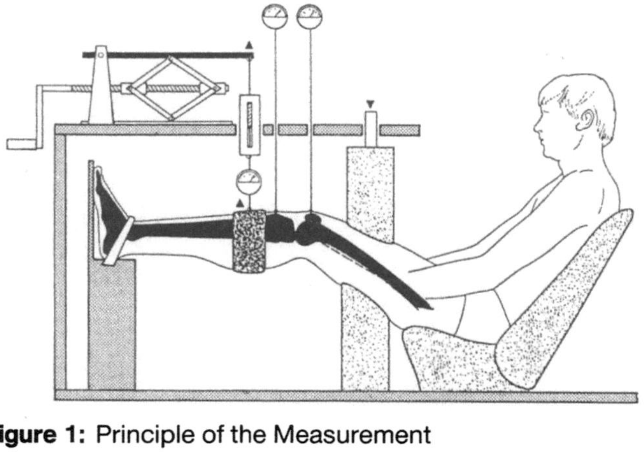

Figure 1: Principle of the Measurement

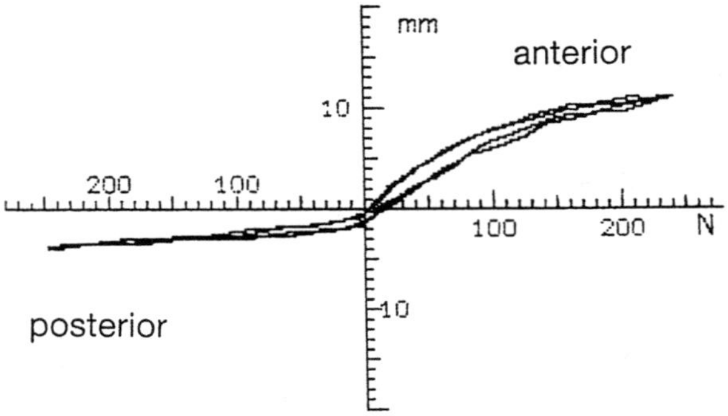

Figure 2: Monitor Display of (repeated) force-shift curves

force-shift graphs on a TV-monitor (Figure 2), which can be copied and stored in the patient file. Additional copies on floppy-discs warrant possibilities for statistical patient series evaluations later.

Systematic and random errors in the measurements were evaluated, using postmortem specimen, volunteers and patients in normal condition and under local anaesthesia. The reproducibility proved to be better than 10% in a number of repeated tests. The applicability of the method was tested on 150 normal individuals, 60 patients with chronic instabilities, and 7 pre-operative patients with hemarthrosis and assumed ligament tears. The test predicted ACL ruptures in three of the latter patients, a PCL rupture in one, and no cruciate ruptures in three patients, all of which were confirmed in the operation.

Radiological assessment of tibial torsion in relation to knee instability

J. L. Meystre

Service Universitaire d'Orthopédie et de Traumatologie
Lausanne
Switzerland

The fragility of ligaments of the knee, the prognosis of the lesions of these ligaments, and the difficulty of their treatment are in direct relationship to the complexity of the dynamic forces, expecially rotation, which effect the stability of the knee.
The symptoms of instability are first seen when the knee is subjected to a movement of rotation because it is in rotation that the kinematic modifications consecutive to lesions have the highest influence on the leverage of muscles and remaining ligaments.
The assessment of the tibial torsion is essential in this context.
Actually the CT scan is the only reliable method of studying this problem. We have tried to develop a radiological method based on a trigonometrical study of the trochleas of condyles and of talus, using two orthogonal X-rays made simultaneously of knee and ankle.

Material
Forty knees were X-rayed and then submitted to CT scan. The results of the measurement were compared.

Results
After a trial period, the radiological method proved to be reliable. The average difference between the two methods was 4°, the maximum was 8°.

Discussion
The causes of error were studied. The precision of this radiological method proved to be sufficient for the evaluation of mechanical problems of the knee.

Summary
The assessment of the tibial torsion is an essential element in the study of:
1) Traumatic lesions of the ligaments of the knee
2) Their treatment
3) Their prognosis
The radiological method described in this paper measures with adequate precision tibial torsion.

Pes anserinus transfer according to Slocum: new biomechanical concepts and indications for surgery

A. Vallatta[1], *F. Casolo*[1], *V. Pietrogrande*[2] *and F. Motta*[2]

[1] **Department of Mechanics, Politecnico, Milano, Italy**
[2] **Institute of Clinical Orthopaedics, University, Milano, Italy**

Introduction
The purposes of this study are to investigate the effect of Slocum's operation on the mechanics of the knee joint in its globality, using a mathematical model, and obtain useful information for the surgeon.

In 1968, Slocum conceived and was the first to perform the pes anserinus transfer to compensate actively the rotatory instability of the anteromedial capsular ligament in the knee. Slocum's operation consists of almost fully disinserting the pes anserinus and in a proximal upturning of its distal end (Figure 1). Hereafter, this operation is referred to as Slocum's operation of the first type.

At present, several surgeons adopt a variant consisting of fully disinserting the pes anserinus and suturing it proximally and anteriorly without upturning it (Figure 2). This procedure is known as Slocum's operation of the second type. In this case, the surgeon has some leeway in selecting the position of the new insertion.

This study considers both types of operation.

Methodology
For the biomechanical investigation of the effects of Slocum's operation we used a model consisting of a tibia and a femur. On these bones we made sev-

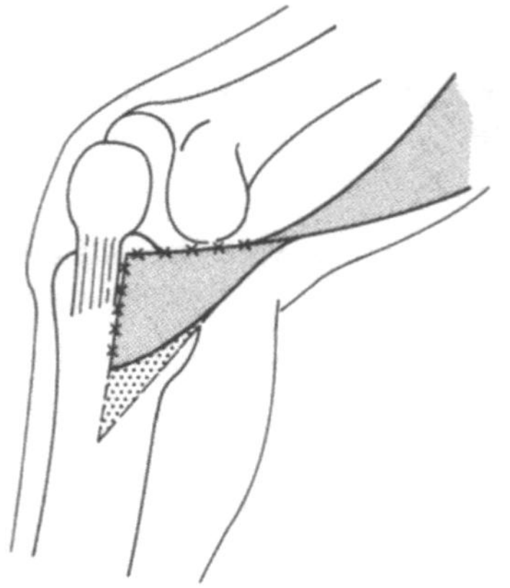

Figure 1. Pes anserinus transfer according to Slocums' operation of the first type

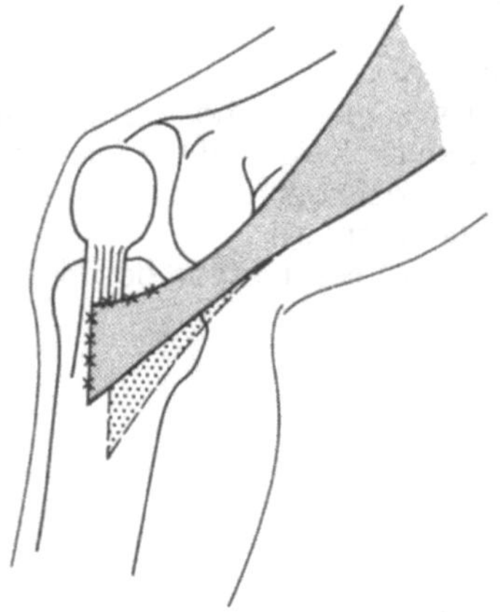

Figure 2. Pes anserinum transfer according to Slocums' operation of the second type

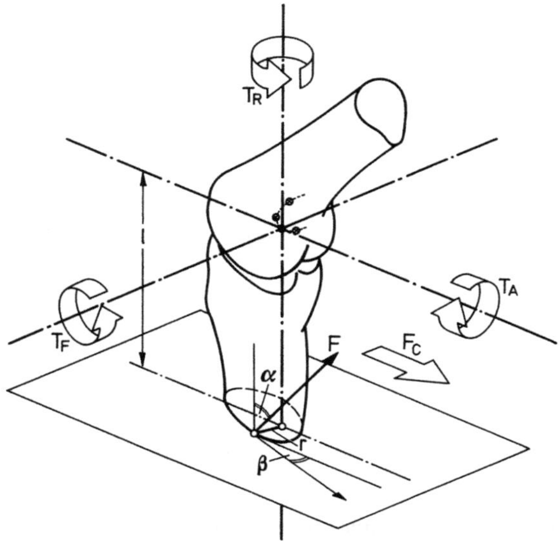

Figure 3. Measurements taken for the sartorius, gracilis and semitendinosus muscles (see text)

eral measurements and some considerations, to determine the parameters needed to calculate the flexion and intrarotation actions and the control of valgus condition and anterior drawer performed on the knee by the pes anserinus muscles.

We adopted the following procedure:

We located the physiological position of insertion of the pes anserinus muscles on the tibia and its insertion after Slocum's operation of the first and second type. We then measured and evaluated the following quantities for each of the three muscles (sartorius, gracilis, semitendinous) in their different insertion positions, before and after either type of operation (Figure 3): *l*, distance of the muscle from the flexion axis of the knee; *r*, distance of the muscle from the anatomical (mechanical) tibial axis; α, angle between the muscle and the anatomical tibial axis; and β, angle between the muscle and the anteroposterior axis of the knee.

Our measurements and readings are not rigorous and refer to the specimen under examination. However, the considerations that ensue are in general qualitatively valid. Data approximation and the quantitative differences from subject to subject do not significantly affect the results.

Results

The gracilis, sartorius and semitendinous muscles exert multiple actions. They contribute in different measure to: (a) knee flexion, (b) tibial intrarotation, (c) valgus condition control, and (d) anterior drawer control.

Let T_F be the flexural moment with respect to the knee axis, T_R the moment with respect to the tibial anatomical axis, T_A the moment with respect to the anteroposterior axis of the knee (valgus condition control) and F_C the antero-

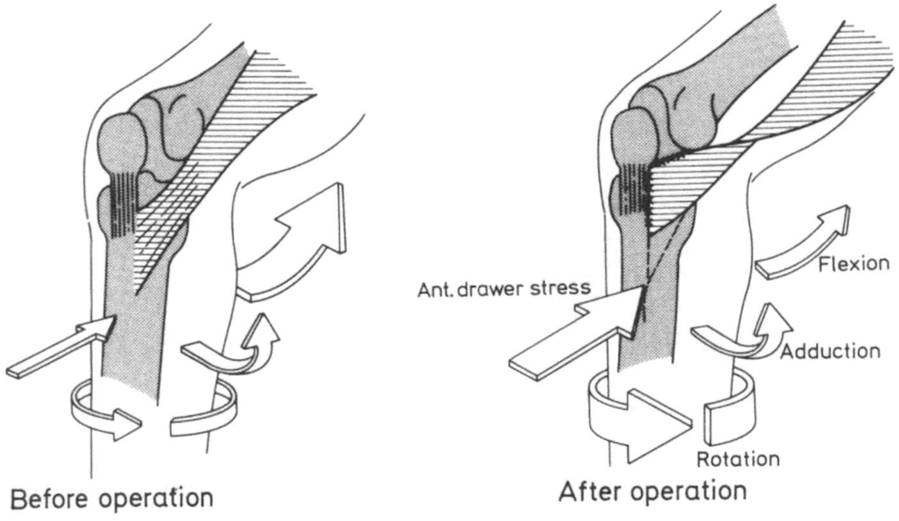

Figure 4. Actions of the pes anserinus before and after Slocum's operation: rotation increases, flexion decreases and anterior drawer stress increases compared with flexion

posterior component of the force (anterior drawer control). Let index *g* be used for the gracilis, *s* for the sartorius and *t* for the semitendinous muscle.

Figure 4 illustrates the above actions. From the geometrical data, we calculated the magnitude of these actions for various knee flexion angles, unit muscle force and various muscle insertion locations: physiological, after Slocum "first type" and after Slocum "second type".

Index 0 is used for the physiological location, 1 for that after Slocum first type, and 2 for that after Slocum second type.

We then calculated the ratios $a = T_R/T_C$, $b = T_A/T_F$ and $c = F_C/T_F$ for the various situations and for each muscle.

To assess the effect of the operation, we calculated the ratios $u_1 = a_1/a_0$, $u_2 = a_2/a_0$, $v_1 = b_1/b_0$, $v_2 = b_2/b_0$, $z_1 = c_1/c_0$ and $z_2 = c_2/c_0$.

The results are summarized in Figure 5: it can be seen that both Slocum's operations yield *u* and *z* values greater than the unit; *v* was not entered as it closely approximates the unit and is scarcely significant.

Actually, the value of *u*, the ratio of valgus condition control action with respect to the knee's flexural moment only depends on the angle β, the values of which do not swing widely and are in any case difficult to measure and hardly controllable by the surgeon.

This means that, for a given flexion action, both the intrarotating effect and anterior drawer control increase, while valgus condition control remains nearly unchanged. Since a certain flexural moment is needed to obtain a

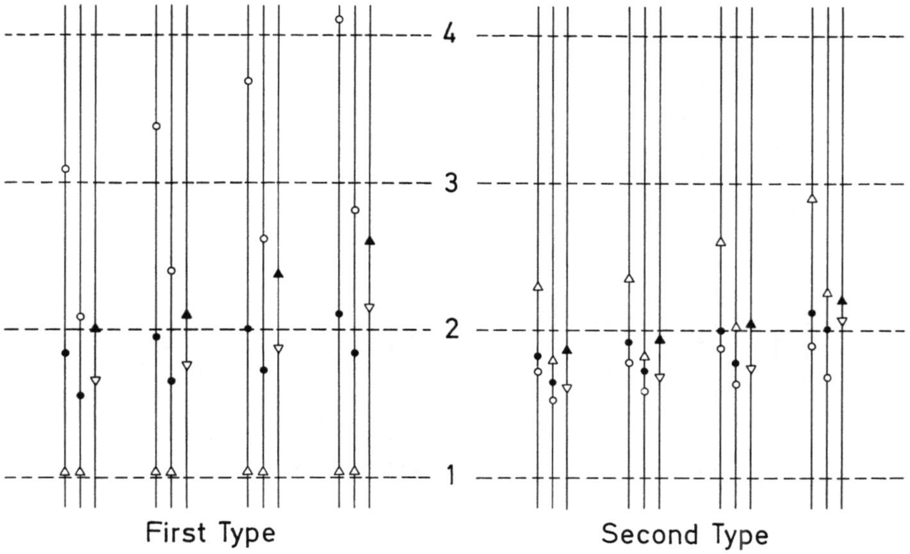

Figure 5. Increases in rotation (*first line*) and the anterior drawer stress (*second line*) compared with flexion. Our data. ○ sartorius; □ gracilis; △ semitendinosus; ∗ total rotation; ★ total anterior drawer stress

given flexion under certain conditions, the above is tantamount to saying that, for any flexion effect, Slocum's operation of either type causes the intrarotating effect to increase and drawer control by the three pes anserinus muscles to improve.

We believe an evaluation of the global effect of the pes anserinus to be of interest. To do this, the magnitude of the action of each muscle with respect to the others should be determined: in other words, the relationship among the respective forces should be assessed.

The most suitable index of a muscle's force is its cross-sectional area.

The gracilis and sartorius muscles have roughly the same area; this confirms that they exert approximately equal forces.

The cross-sectional area of the semitendinous muscle is roughly twice that of the others, and its force too should be double. Let us then assign the value 1 to both the gracilis and sartorius muscles, and a value of 2 to the semitendinous muscle. The global flexion effect T_{Fc} thus becomes: $T_{Fc} = T_{Fg} + T_{Fs} + 2\,T_{Ft}$ and the others: $T_{Ac} = T_{Ag} + T_{As} + 2\,T_{At}$ and $F_{Cc} = F_{Cg} + F_{Cs} + 2\,F_{Ct}$.

As previously, let us calculate the ratios: $a_C = T_{Rc}/T_{Fc}$, $b_C = T_{Ac}/T_{Fc}$, $c_C = F_{Cc}/T_{Fc}$, and ratios u_c, v_c, z_c; u_c and z_c appear in Figure 5.

It is interesting to make the above calculations with the data supplied by Noyes (2); these calculations are in part in his work.

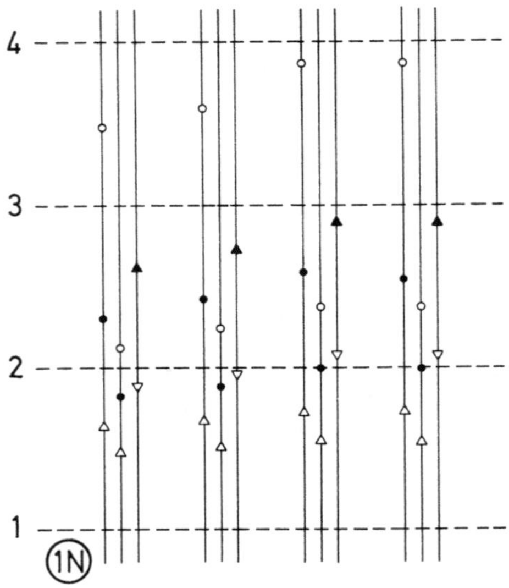

Figure 6. Increases in rotation (*first line*) and the anterior drawer stress (*second line*) compared with flexion. Noyes (1973). ● sartorius; ■ gracilis; ▲ semitendinosus; ∗ total rotation; ★ total anterior drawer stress

The results are plotted in Figure 6.

Discussion

Our calculations show that Slocum's operation, either of the first or second type, has a twofold effect. It is effective as concerns both the intrarotating action on the tibia (this being the operation's primary purpose) and the knee's anterior drawer control. The intrarotating action on the tibia is increased because the reinsertion is made where the cross-section of the tibia is greater (greater r). It increases in advance compared with the flexion moment, because the muscles are inserted closer to the knee axis (lower l).

Since the strongest muscle of the pes anserinus is the semitendinous muscle, the shift of its insertion point is especially relevant.

The ratio $a = T_R / T_F$ is also affected by the value of β, which should be as small as possible after the operation. The value of β does not vary much with the point of insertion and tends to increase with knee flexion while this point moves forward. As mentioned before, however, one cannot rely on the values taken by β, which in any case has no bearing on the actions considered here.

Drawer control is more effective than flexion moment because the muscles are closer to the knee axis; actually, this control effect is inversely proportional to l.

Valgus condition control is not significantly affected by Slocum's operation. Indeed, a more proximal reinsertion of the muscles does not cause the ratio $b = T_A / T_F$ to change.

Strong muscle action is needed to control adequately tibial extrarotation with respect to the femur and for anterior drawer control. This can be achieved with suitable, specific postoperative rehabilitation cures. Strengthening the muscles becomes useful, or rather necessary, to reinstate the knee's flexion, which is impaired owing to the more proximal reinsertion of the pes anserinus.

Conclusion

A full biomechanical analysis of the action exerted by the pes anserinus before and after Slocum's operation clearly shows that this operation is decidedly advantageous are concerns tibial extrarotation control and anterior drawer control, while better valgus condition control cannot be expected.

The operation is the more effective the more anterior and proximal is the pes anserinus transfer. The best results are obtained by moving the semitendinous muscle forward in a proximal direction.

Whether to perform the first or second type of operation essentially depends on the physiological location of the pes anserinus. As a rule, the first type of operation should be more advantageous. Only when the pes anserinus physiologically lies in a rather distal position may the second type of Slocum's operation be suitable. An interesting variant could be to perform Slocum's operation of the second type, while upturning the pes anserinus as in the first type.

References

1. Hallen LG (1965) The lateral stability of the knee joint. Acta Orthop Scand 36:400–407
2. Slocum DB (1968) Pes anserinus transplantation. A surgical procedure for control of rotatory instability of the knee. J Bone Joint Surg [Am] 50:226–242
3. Noyes FR (1973) Biomechanical function of the pes anserinus at the knee and the effect of its transplantation. J Bone Joint Surg [Am] 55:1225–1241
4. Slocum DB (1974) Pes anserinus transplant: impressions after a decade of experience. Am J Sports Med 2(3):123–136
5. Warren LF (1974) The prime static stabilizer of the medial side of the knee. J Bone Joint Surg [Am] 56:665–674
6. Di Stefano V (1976) Pes anserinus transfer: an in vivo biomechanical analysis. J Bone Joint Surg [Am] 58:285
7. Fox JM (1976) The patient's view of the pes anserinus transfer operation for rotatory instability of the knee. Am J Sports Med 4(4):131–135
8. D'Arcy J (1978) Pes anserinus transposition for chronic anteromedial rotation instability of the knee. J Bone Joint Surg [Br] 60:66–70
9. Ostering LR (1978) Rotatory mechanism after pes anserinus transplant. A method for dynamic assessment. Am J Sports Med 6(4):173–179
10. Perry J (1980) Functional evaluation of the pes anserinus transfer by electromyography and gait analysis. J Bone Joint Surg [Am] 62:973–980
11. Chick RP (1981) The pes anserinus transfer. J Bone Joint Surg [Am] 63
12. Pietrograndi V, Motta F, Vallatta A, Casolo F. Considerazioni biomeccanichi sull-intervento di trasposizione della zampa d'oca secondo Slocum. Communication of the 68th Congress, Italian Society of Orthopaedics

Biomechanics of the patello-femoral joint under normal conditions and after transfers of the tuberositas tibiae

H. J. Hehne

Section of Orthopaedics, Dep of Surg., University of Freiburg
Freiburg
Federal Republic of Germany

Biomechanic conceptions have been based on osseous patella cross sections and vector analysis using the rope-roll-model. Frequent dysplasies and operative procedures were thus justified. Our present result do not agree with this.

Methods
Contact areas (CA), pressing forces (PF), pressure (P) and pressure distributions (PD) at facets and segments were measured simultaneously as a function of the quadriceps force and the knee flexion with 22 cadaver knees. Using a thin flexible foil the values are optically recorded. Electronic equidensitometry allows quantitative evaluation. Supporting arthrografies by 250 patients and 30 cadavers evaluated the motions and the form of bone and cartilage. The bone density was demonstrated using thin cuts of bone. Vectorial analysis were made taking into account the patella as a rigid body, the CA, the insertion height of the tendons into the patella and the wrapping of the quadriceps tendon around the femur. The Maquet-Bandi and Roux-Hauser procedures were performed with 16 cadaver joints and measured with the foil. CA variation due to Morscher's osteotomy was measured.

Results
For all Wiberg types the form of bone and cartilage is found to be adapted to the abutment, in particular by the cartilage ridge subdividing the medial facet. The side of the CA depends on pulling force and flexion, its position varies with flexion. The border segment contacts under strong flexion only. The PF increases with pulling force and flexion, but is limited by the wrapping of the tendon. Both CA and PF of the lateral and medial facet have a constant ratio of 1.6. The same ratio is obtained for the cartilage areas. The P is highest in the center of CA's. It only depends on the pulling force in increases more slowly because the CA becomes larger. The average pressure on all segments is equal. The wrapping of the quadriceps tendon produces the same pressure. The CA's are narrow in such way that the rigid patella acts as lever arm and contributes to the vector force diagram. The different height of the quadriceps and the patellar tendon merging into the patella results in different forces in these tendons. The force ratio is equal to that of their cross sections. Due to its vectors the retinacula contribute insignificantly to the PF. CA, PF, P and PD are found to be equal before and after the Maquet-Bandi operation, as can we see by the new vectorial analysis. The Roux-Hauser operation produces incongruence, reduces CA and thus increases the pressure by 25%. Similar effects are generated by the Morscher operation.

Discussion

The patella is well adapted to its abutments trochlea and condyles. CA, PF and P correspond to biomechanical functions and are evenly distributed. The stress applied to the patella is thus minimized. Patella dysplasias are rare. Even the Wiberg types III and IV and the hunter's hat are normal and adapted to the particular form of their abutments in agreement with Pauwels theories. The investigated operations cannot be longer recommended.

Chondromalacia of the knee joint – principles of medical and surgical treatment

K. Franke

Dept. of Surgery, Municipal Hospital Berlin-Pankow
DDR-1100 Berlin
German Dem. Rep.

Among 2 500 knee joint arthrotomies within 12 years (1971..82) we found in 65% of all cases a chondromalacia (CHM) with a different stage of severity. The exogenous etiology is predominant to the endogenous one.
Aims and methods of medical CHM-treatment are:

1. stabilizing cartilage structure by optimazing metabolism of chondrocytes with intraarticular injections of Arteparon (R) and glucose 5,4%;

2. blocking enzymatic feed-back reaction by enzyme-inhibtion (Arteparon (R), Salicyl etc.);

3. treating synovialitis and pain;

4. starting measures of rehabilitation.

In 450 patients the good results from intraarticular injections of Arteparon (R) ± glucose were ranging from 70 to 85%.
Electron microscopy revealed thereafter an improved cartilage structure with collagen fibers again straightened out, reduced extracellular products of degeneration (Lipofuscine), and no more hint to a lack of mucopolysaccharides.

If a surgical CHM-treatment cannot be avoided, its aims and methods should be:

1. reducing enzymatic feed-back reaction by removing destroyed cartilage, osteophytes, and synovial pannus;

2. inducing cartilage substitution, e.g. by drilling the subchondral bone layer;

3. improving or normalizing disturbed biomechanics of the knee joint.

Results of both medical and surgical CHM-treatment are to be controlled by arthroscopy and additional biopsy.

Articular Cartilage

Stress response of articular cartilage

R. G. T. Geesink

Department of Orthopaedic Surgery, State University of Limburg
Maastricht
The Netherlands

Introduction

As part of a more profound study in the field of osteoarthrosis I will present the results of an experimental investigation into differences in response of articular cartilage to different situations of stress. The aim was to clear up underlying pathogenetic mechanisms.

Methods

Eighty mature rabbits were divided into four groups and subjected to medial meniscectomy, anterior cruciate section, immobilization for 6 weeks or intra-articular injections with autologous blood for 2 weeks to simulate haemarthrosis. After successive intervals the animals were killed and biopsies were taken at standardized localizations all over the knee joint. Histological grading of cartilage abnormalities was carried out according to the Mankin score, which ranges from 0 for normal to 14 for maximal damage to the cartilage. Additionally, geometric measurements were carried out on whole joints.

Results

Changes occurred, generally speaking, in three regions, with transition from one type of tissue to another: (1) cartilage surface, (2) tidemark with the region of the calcified cartilage and (3) region of the subchondral bone.

Early changes were seen within the first few weeks: nuclear pyknosis occurred in the superficial layer of articular cartilage, progressing to necrosis of many chondrocytes. We saw chondrocytes with fatty degeneration, losing their vitality. Later on clustering of chondrocytes was visible, caused by proliferation of the remaining vital chondrocytes. Sometimes lesions progressed to fissuring and total erosion, but more often the cartilage remained vital in part. Secondarily abnormalities of calcification near the tidemark were seen, with funnel-shaped canals of uncalcified cartilage within the area of calcified cartilage. The thickness of the cartilage was increased or decreased, depending upon local remodelling forces from the subchondral bone. Increased osteoclastic activity in the subchondral bone was seen under these circumstances.

After medial meniscectomy and anterior cruciate section there were high osteoarthrotic scores in the region of the medial femoral condyle, with low scores in the patellofemoral joint and intermediate scores in the tibial part of the joint. After medial meniscectomy these alterations occurred mainly in the central region of the medial femoral condyle overlying the former border of the medial meniscus. After anterior cruciate section alterations were more apparent in the anterocentral region of the medial femoral condyle. Frequently there were secondary degenerative ruptures of the medial meniscus. In contrast, with immobilization and haemarthrosis we see a more even distribution of changes over the joint, although the two groups have different degrees of damage to the cartilage. Changes after haemarthrosis appeared to be largely reversible. At 3 months stabilization occurred, after which reparative phenomena became more prominent. Changes in the synovia were seen at a later stage, as against changes in the cartilage, which were seen quite early. Geometric measurements, demonstrated here in the case of meniscectomy, showed an early increase in thickness of articular cartilage at the medial margin of the medial femoral and tibial condyles formerly in contact with the medial meniscus. This process was followed by remodelling of the subchondral bone. Sometimes the speed of remodelling of bone was such that the overlying avascular cartilage could not keep pace with it and erosions subsequently developed. After anterior cruciate section remodelling was more prominent in the anterocentral region of the medial femoral condyle, whereas after immobilization intense flattening of both femoral condyles occurred. After haemarthrosis no remodelling was seen.

Discussion

It seems important that the early response of cartilage is predominantly adaptive, but when these adaptations must occur in too short a period the chondrocytes in the upper layer of the cartilage cannot keep pace with this process of remodelling in the lower part of the cartilage and subchondral bone. At the same time they must divide into new cells *and* increase their synthesis rate of collagen and matrix proteins. This is frequently impossible, probably due to their lower rate of metabolic supply. With insufficient synthesis of collagen and matrix proteins, deposition of these only occurs in the direct circumference of the chondrocyte cells and clusters. Mechanical and biochemical insufficiency of the matrix collagen architecture is the result, and total disintegration of the remaining cartilage follows, leaving only aspecific fibrous and bony repair processes; although this sometimes may be adequate, as is visible by tangential orientation of the fibrocytes along the joint space, more often it is not.

The results show that joint cartilage has a specific pattern of response, depending on the rate and kind of stress exerted upon it. Changes in joint loading certainly play a role in the induction and differentiation of remodelling. As long as intensity or time of exposure to stress do not exceed a certain limit, articular cartilage seems to have in-built capabilities for regeneration and adaptation, limited mainly by the low metabolic supply of articular cartilage. This healing process can probably be stimulated by appropriate medical or other treatment of the affected joints. Studies are still in progress in our institution to find whether it is possible to ameliorate the response of cartilage, for instance with Arteparon, which inhibits proteolytic degradation of the matrix proteins, or with glucosamine phosphate, which acts as a substituent for glucose in the metabolism of the chondrocyte.

A better understanding of pathogenetic mechanisms would certainly ameliorate our response to patients with osteoarthrotic joint lesions.

Diagnosis and therapy of acute articular cartilage injuries

D. H. Rogge and J. R. Rether

Unfallchirurgische Klinik der Medizinischen Hochschule Hannover
Federal Republic of Germany

Even though modern medicine offers a variety of diagnostic and therapeutic procedures, the acute articular cartilage injury still seems to be a problem, especially when associated with the trivial trauma of daily life or minor sports accidents.
Above all, to achieve adequate treatment, it is of course necessary, that the injury will be diagnosed at all! It is therefore of eminent importance, that the surgeon is ready to take the possibility of such a lesion into consideration. Only then the probable high diagnostic failure rate can be diminished and an efficient therapy performed.

Diagnosis
X-ray evaluation in different planes, if necessary including tomography, is essential. In certain cases arthrography may be helpful. Arthroscopy has to be performed in case of any acute haemorrhagic joint effusion, if not an open exploration will be done anyway.

Therapy
The following surgical principles have to be carefully observed:
The main goal has to be the exact reconstruction of the articular surface. This is not advisable or possible, when fragments are too small, irreversibly damaged, or lost. In these cases defect healing with a fibrocartilaginous scar has to be achieved. To facilitate this process, access to the surrounding vascularized bone should be established by drill holes or abrasion.
The use of concentrated fibrinogen adhesive is of great value, when small or mere chondral fragments have to be replanted.
Metal implants should be as small as possible and allow later removal without reopening the joint. Kirschner wires therefore are preferable to intraarticular screws.
Fragment fixation has to be stable enough to allow early functional aftertreatment.
Direct postoperative continuous passive motion helps avoid joint adhesions and improves cartilage metabolism.

Material
At the Trauma Department of Hanover Medical School 132 acute articular cartilage lesions have been operatively treated from 1971 to 1982. Nine operations have been performed on the elbow joint, 7 on the hip joint, 93 on the knee, and 23 on the ankle joint. 50 % of the cartilage lesions of the knee were associated with acute or recurrent dislocations of the patella.
Since the diagnostic and therapeutic procedures vary with different joint anatomy and function, they are demonstrated in detail for each joint.
Only in 68 of 110 joints the lesion was found on X-ray. 24 fragments were replanted, the rest removed. K-wires were used in 9 cases, screws in 6, K-wires combined with screws in 3, K-wires and fibrinogen adhesive in 3, the adhesive alone in 2 cases. One fragment needed support by a cancellous bone graft.

Results

According to the different types of injury, location and treatment it is not possible to report comparable results. All fragment replantations were successful. One case with joint infection was successfully treated with early synovectomy. Five patients developed a significant arthrosis. Follow up was 9 months to 11 years, in average 4.8 years.

Repair of articular cartilage

A. J. van der Linden

Department of Orthopaedic Surgery, State University of Limburg
Maastricht
The Netherlands

Numerous experiments in animals have been performed to develop an optimal scheme for repairing minor articular defects. The defects in question are those encountered mostly in cases of osteochondritis dissecans of the knee joint, but the cartilage defects are also seen as a result of osteonecrosis and osteoarthritis in elderly people. As a rule, for surgical repair of these foci, it is possible to use the available cartilage present as a completely or partially loose body.

If the local cartilage is not suitable for use in restoration of continuity of the articular surface, some other material has to be found for the purpose.

Three factors are important in transplantation: (1) nutrition, (2) local reactions, and (3) preservation.

1. As regards nutrition, there are good reasons to suppose that the complete nutritional supply, especially in adults, originates from the synovial fluid. This is in favour of a transplantation.
2. Insofar as the reactions of the host organism are concerned, allografts of cartilage also seem possible. The occurrence of a defence mechanism appears to be linked to the cells in the graft, and we may perhaps compare the matrix to the wall of a diffusion chamber that screens the cells in the graft; as a consequence host reactions are prevented.
3. In practice it is not easily possible to transplant fresh allografts. Much has been written about the most favourable temperature to preserve the material. As you will see we have chosen a temperature of -45 °C.

To study the results of different types of transplantation in animals a number of young adult rabbits were operated on under general anaesthesia. A hollow trephine 6 mm in diameter was used to bore holes in the anterior surface of the femoral condyles of young adult rabbits down into the cancellous bone (Figure 1).

These defects were repaired by six different methods and after 1 year the animals were killed to study the end results. Because of the same size of all the defects and all the transplants there were no fixation problems and the transplant was held in place by the patella.

Three different types of autografts were used:

1. Cancellous bone ($\times 4$)
2. Cortical bone plate from the tibia ($\times 10$)
3. Cartilage with subchondral bone plate from one knee to the other in the same animal ($\times 16$)

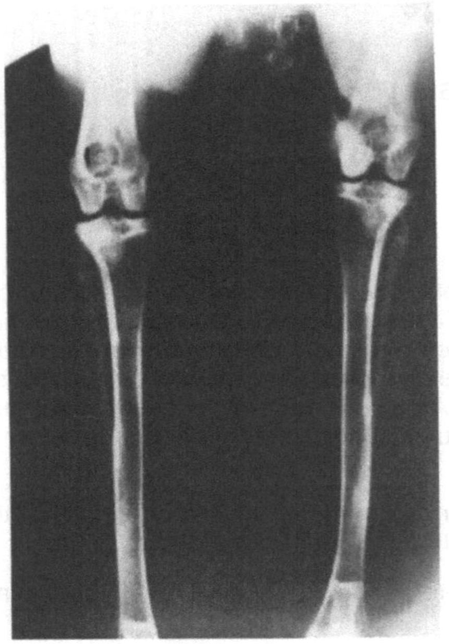

Figure 1.

Three different types of non-autografts were used:

1. Homografts (× 10) (− 45 °C)
2. Mixed (× 10)
3. Xenografts (× 20) (− 45 °C)

When the defect was filled with an intact cylinder of bone and cartilage from the same species of animals it was named a homograft. When the defect was filled with autologous cancellous bone and covered with a refrigerated homograft it was named a mixed graft. The xenografts were derived from a calf joint.

After 1 year the knees were opened and the macroscopic and microscopic results evaluated.

Macroscopic

1. Excellent: The cartilage looks normal
2. Good: The cartilage is slightly discoloured and irregular
3. Fair: Some small superficial defects are present
4. Poor: There are real craters

Microscopic

5. Excellent: Normal hyaline cartilage sometimes of varying height
6. Good: The cartilage layer is distinctly thinner with moderate fibrillary changes (Figure 2). A thin part of the cartilage may alternate with a layer markedly thicker than normal
7. Fair: A thin fibrillary layer of cartilage (Figure 3)
8. Bad: Large defects with necrosis and infiltration (Figure 4)

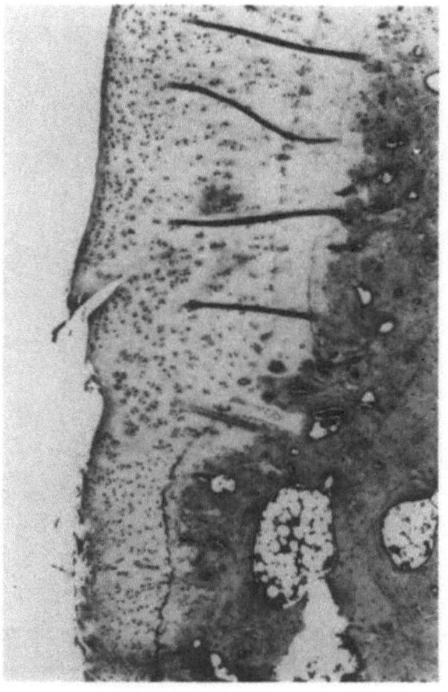

Figure 2. Moderate fibrillary changes in the cartilage layer

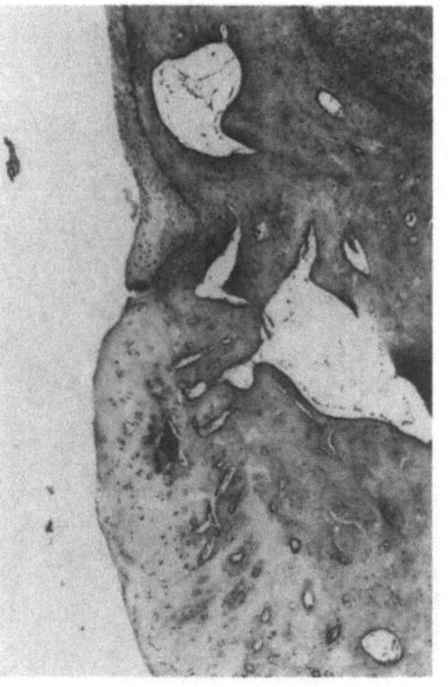

Figure 3. Thin fibrillary layer of cartilage

Table 1. Macroscopic and microscopic results with autografts

	Macroscopic			Microscopic		
	Autografts		Allografts	Autografts		Allografts
	Bo	Ca		Bo	Ca	
Excellent	6	5	1	2	1	0
Good	3	6	4	7	8	4
Fair	1	5	11	0	6	10
Poor	0	0	4	1	1	6
	10	16	20	10	16	20

The macroscopic and microscopic results with autografts were evidently better than those with allografts, while it is remarkable that the results with bone plates seemed to be the best (Table 1). Perhaps it is important to mention that the periosteum was stripped from the bone. The results with xenografts were poor.

Our clinical experience with the cortical bone plate extends to only a small number of patients. There are six patients, with a follow-up of 2–6 years.

Figure 5 shows the knee of a man of 63 years. There was a cartilage defect on the surface of the medial condyle and the entirely loose body of cartilage

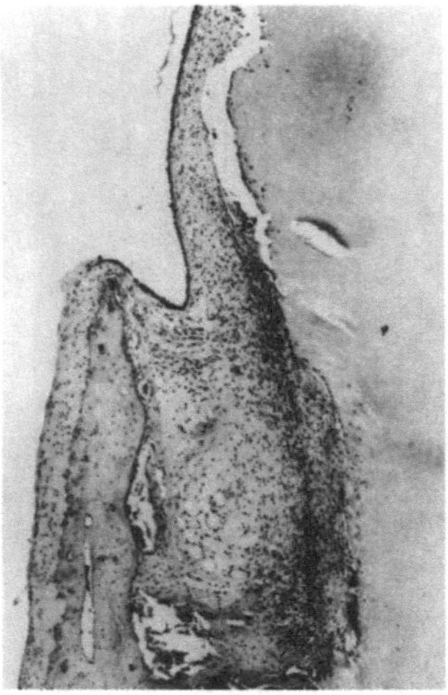

Figure 4. Large defects with necrosis and infiltration

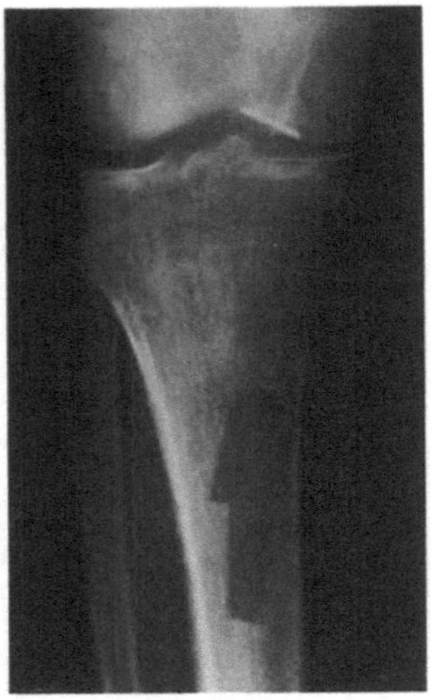

Figure 5. Knee of a 63-year-old man

showed such severe degeneration that it appeared to be unsuitable for repair. The defect was therefore scratched out, then filled up with cancellous bone and covered with a bone plate from the tibia. Fixation was achieved with bone pegs, also derived from the tibia. So far the clinical results are good in all six patients.

Articular cartilage lesions of the femoral condyles

M. Bauer[1], *R. W. Jackson*[2] *and D. Ogilvie-Harris*[2]

[1] **Department of Orthopaedic Surgery, Lund University, Malmö General Hospital, S-21401 Malmö, Sweden**
[2] **Department of Orthopaedic Surgery, University of Toronto, Toronto Western Hospital, 25 Leonard Avenue, Toronto, Ontario, M5T 2R2, Canada**

Introduction

This paper presents a classification of chondral lesions based on their arthroscopic appearance, analyses the results of their treatment and discusses the usefulness of the classification.

Material

In a retrospective study, 167 chondral lesions were studied in 140 patients with a mean age of 37 years. There were 105 men and 35 women in the material, with an equal number of right and left knees affected. Patients who had obvious arthritic changes on X-ray were excluded. Symptoms bringing the patient to an examination were the usual ones for a knee problem. Most patients had two of these, pain and swelling being the most common.

Classification

Looking specifically at the chondral lesions, these could be differentiated in to six types.

The *linear crack type* represents a fissure or a linear crack, which is usually partial thickness but can reach the subchondral bone (Figure 1). This is an uncommon injury; only 6 of the 167 lesions were of this type. Five of these were found within the weight-bearing areas.

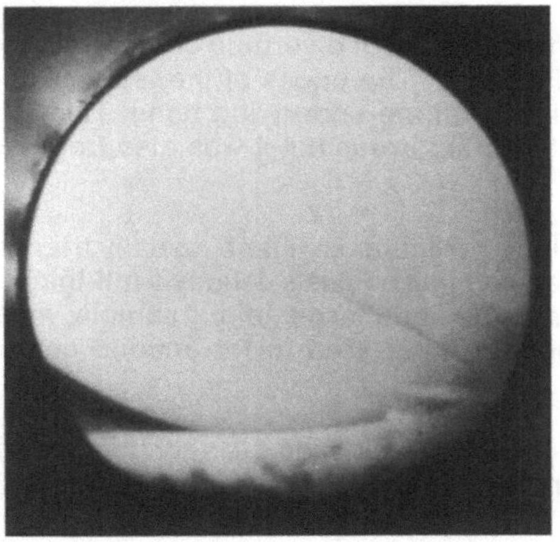

Figure 1. Type 1: the linear crack type

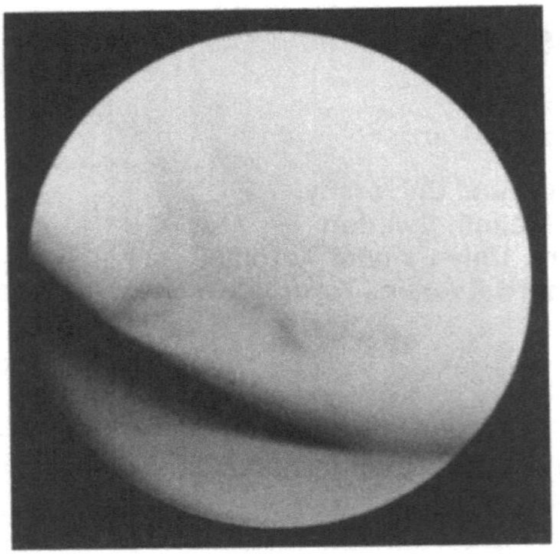

Figure 2. Type 2: the stellate fracture type

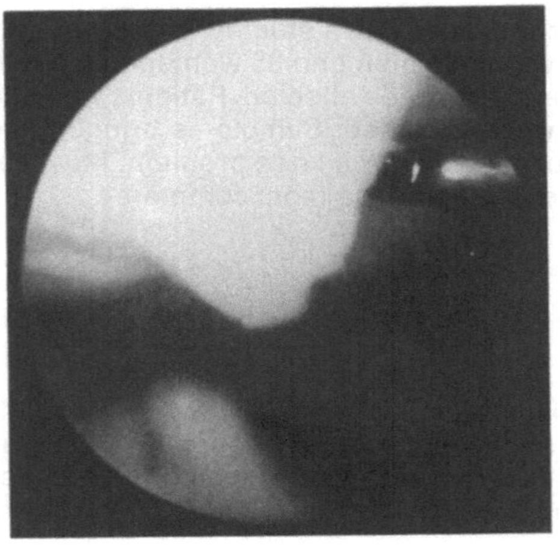

Figure 3. Type 3: the flap type

The *stellate fracture type* represents a system of diverging cracks, often with a central area of desquamation (Figure 2). The edges of the lesion are frequently slightly undermined and lifting off the underlying bone. This lesion is most common within the weight-bearing areas but it was also frequent in the intercondylar region.

The *flap type* presents as a loose flap of articular cartilage, usually triangular in shape with a detachment at the apex (Figure 3). It is usually a full-thickness lesion, where the flap can sometimes be quite large. In our sample, most of these were found within the weight-bearing area in the medial compartment.

The *crater type* represents a loss of cartilage down to the subchondral bone, but with no evidence of a bony injury (Figure 4). This injury is thus a little

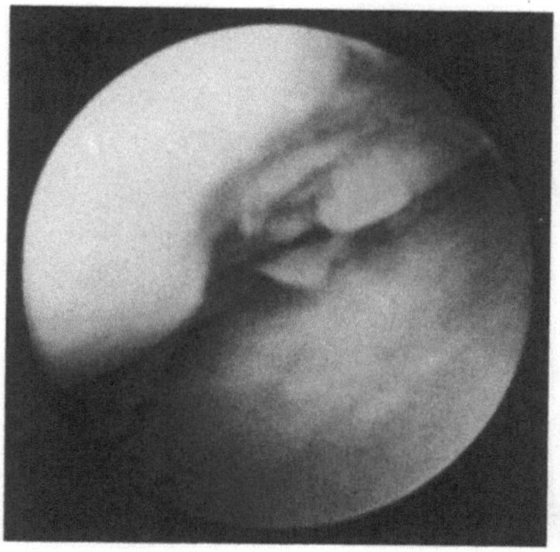

Figure 4. Type 4: the crater type

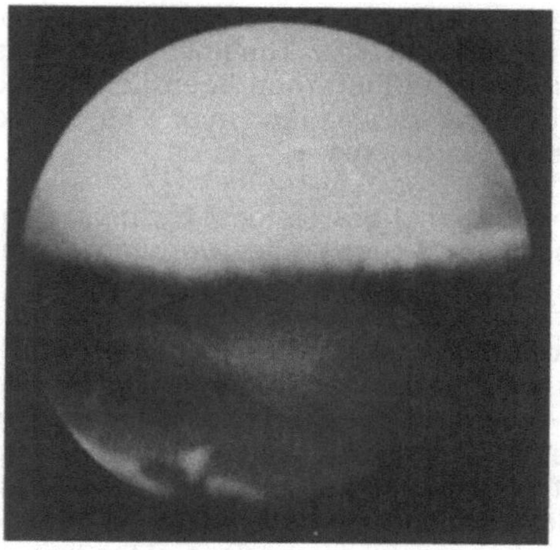

Figure 5. Type 5: the fibrillation type

more superficial than an osteochondral fracture. The edges are usually quite sharp and well defined. As for most cartilaginous lesions, they are most frequent within weight-bearing areas in the medial compartment.

The *fibrillation type* shows a finely fibrillated appearance, and from tangential views the normal curvature of the condyle may look slightly flattened or abraded (Figure 5). This seems to be a partial-thickness injury; it was also the type with the highest proportion of its lesions in the lateral compartment.

The *degrading type* features a breaking-up of the surface into major and minor pieces (Figure 6). It is soft on palpation and shows coarse fibrillation. Except for one lesion, it was only found in weight-bearing areas.

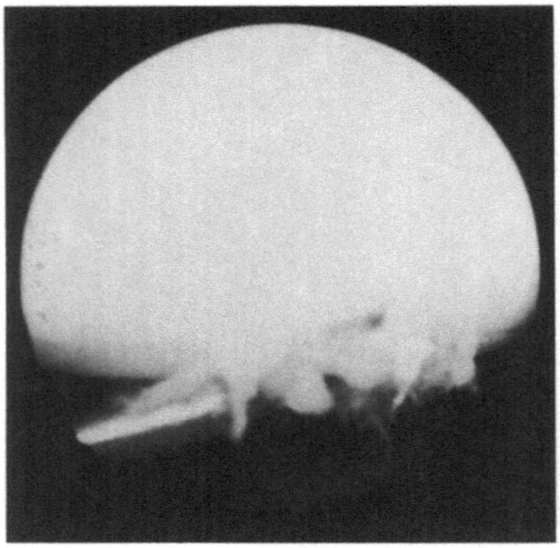

Figure 6. Type 6: the degrading type

The stellate fracture pattern was the most common, accounting for 28% of the lesions, followed by the degrading type with 20%. The linear crack was an uncommon finding. In 26% of the patients there had been no specific preceding trauma. One-third had a rotational trauma, and in one-fifth of the cases a direct blow to the knee started the problems.

Concomitant pathology is very frequent with chondral lesions. The most common concomitant injury was a meniscal tear. Loose bodies were most common with crater-type lesions.

There is a statistically higher incidence of trauma in the first four types, which we thus think represent true chondral fractures, than in the fibrillating and degrading types, which might then represent degenerative changes. The rather high incidence of trauma, even in those types, was often found to be due to rotational trauma and it might, of course, be possible that there is already a degenerative process present, which only becomes symptomatic after an additional trauma. However, after careful comparison of the type of trauma and the type of chondral lesion, we believe these may be interpreted in this way.

The linear crack is caused by a shearing force in the plane of the articular cartilage, which causes a linear crack in this.

The stellate fracture results from a direct blow to the condyle, either with a flexed knee or with blunt impact. The tibial spine can also abut on the intercondylar region, causing stellate fractures here.

The flap-type lesion is most commonly seen following a rotational injury.

The crater type is equivalent to an osteochondral fracture but occurs in a more superficial plane in the tide zone of the articular cartilage. The fibrillating type might represent early degenerative changes, and the degrading type is macroscopically the same as is seen in degenerative arthritis, although here it can sometimes be quite localized. It is also the type in which there has most frequently been no trauma preceding the presenting problem.

Experimental studies in progress lend some support to these theories, although the results are still preliminary.

Prospective series

In a prospective series this classification has been used on 138 lesions in 104 patients. It was found that 132 lesions fitted very well with the classification while six did not fit. Three of these were old osteochondral fractures which had previously been operated on. One lesion was a localized eburnation to bone, which did not show the well-defined edges typical for a crater lesion. One patient had a cartilaginous lesion in the medial femoral condyle in the form of a deep groove filled with fibrous tissue, which did not really fit with the linear crack type, and in one patient there was a localized softening showing no separation and no fibrillation. Thus, 95% of the lesions were easily classified as belonging to one of the groups specified above.

Why classify then? Differences in the genesis of these lesions have already been discussed. There is also a difference in the outcome of the different types of lesions.

Follow-up

Out of the original group of 140 patients we were able to do a follow-up on 125 after an average of 18.8 months. The treatment of these injuries consisted of resection of flaps, excision of undermined cartilage and treatment of other intra-articular pathology present. An easy way to excise undermined cartilage is to use pituitary rongeurs. It is important, however, to bite off the edges and not to pull or twist, as more articular cartilage might then be taken off and the lesion expanded well beyond its original limits. Two years after a successful chondral debridement a typical appearance is a slight irregularity in the shape of the condyle but with all edges smoothed off and well attached to adjacent tissues.

In summary, the results showed that the pain was less and the swelling was less, but clicking was still frequent, especially soon after surgery. This probably reflects the slight defect in the surface, which is a result of removal of cartilage; as this defect fills in, the clicking tends to diminish. The best results are seen in the stellate fracture type and in the flap type lesions, where good or excellent results can be expected in around 80% of the cases. Patients with the degenerative-type lesions often seem to deteriorate, however, and 35% of these still had significant problems and a number had to be operated on with high tibial osteotomies. However, it often takes 6–8 months to obtain a definite improvement following cartilage debridement.

Conclusions

Damage to the articular cartilage itself is a serious injury. As there seem to be various patterns in these injuries, some of the lesions probably representing true chondral fractures while others are signs of a degenerative process, we recommend that the lesions are classified and the results studied within each type. The classification presented is an easy and accurate way of doing this. True long-term data are not yet available, but at present we think we can recommend debridement of flaps and undermined cartilage at the same time as other significant intra-articular pathology is dealt with. The technique should still be considered as experimental, however, and the patients must be followed up for a long time to give us an accurate impression of the outcome of this approach.

Clinical experiences with the use of fibrin sealant in the treatment of osteochondral fractures in the knee

T. Gaudernak, G. Skorpik and B. Zifko

Lorenz Böhler Accident Hospital
Donaueschinger Straße 13
Vienna 1200, Austria

Since 1977 we have used the fibrin-sealing system for fixation of over 100 osteochondral fractures. Our fibrin-sealing system in comparison with others has excellent compatibility with the tissue together with adhesive power [1].

Since lyophilized fibrin sealant has been available we have used this exclusively. The use of a double syringe has proved to be invaluable.

The condition of the osseous bed is very important – it must be free from blood clots and any fresh bleeding. If the osseous bed is poorly vascularized it must be curetted until sufficient vascularized bone appears. If the subchondral bone of the osteochondral fragment is very small it must be drilled several times to improve the likelihood of bony healing. A partial ossification of the basal layers of the cartilage can be recognized in these cases.

If the fragment fits exactly into the bed a few drops of the fibrin sealant and compression for 3 min are sufficient to achieve stability. Problems arise in the case of a cartilage which is enlarged due to oedema or when the bone fragment which is to be replaced is extensively damaged by contusion, laceration or fracture. In these circumstances the fragment cannot be easily replaced in its bed and the osseous bed should be smoothed. In the case of superficial cartilage fractures it may also be necessary to smooth the cartilage. In comminuted fractures gaps are sealed with a mixture of fibrin and cancellous bone. As a rule, plaster immobilization for 3–6 weeks follows. Weight bearing is allowed but should be limited to 20 kg. Where larger areas of the joint are damaged immobilization for up to 16 weeks can be necessary.

Osteochondral fragments on the medial patella facet

Sixteen patients with an average age of 22 years (12–47 years) were examined in a follow-up study. The average interval between the accident and operation was 5.5 days, although in one case a cartilage fragment was successfully replaced after 17 days. The size of the fragments was between 6 mm × 4 mm and 23 mm × 28 mm. Postoperative cast immobilization was between 4 and 6 weeks.

In relation to the mechanism of injury causing the patellar dislocation, cartilage damage and fractures, which influence the result greatly, were very frequent. Patellar subluxation was corrected by operation on the retinacula –

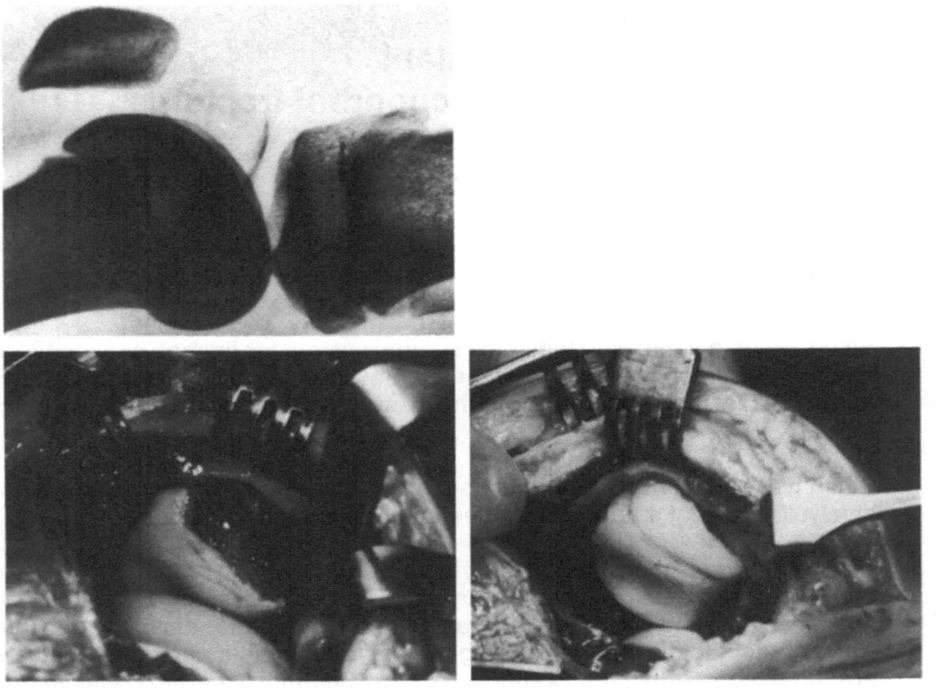

Figure 1. Patellar luxation in a 13-year-old girl. Ideal conditions for replantation of an osteochondral fragment. The cartilage of the flake to be replanted is largely intact and has been torn off together with the adjacent portion of subchondral bone. The cancellous bone of the osseous bed is still bleeding. In this case the fragment can be easily fixed with fibrin sealant; additional osteosynthesis is not necessary. It is essential to correct subluxation of the patella laterally by plication of the medial, and release of the lateral, retinacula

medial plication and lateral release – and in some cases by transfer of the tibial tuberosity. In six cases fragments had to be reshaped in order to replace them. In ten cases healing was complete; in six cases bumps on the reimplanted bone fragments were radiologically definable. Thirteen patients showed no disability of movement, three patients had movement restriction of 10 °, ten patients had no symptoms, three complained of slight symptoms of chondromalacia, and three complained of more severe symptoms, weather susceptibility and problems when climbing stairs (Figures 1 and 2).

Replacement of osteochondral fragments on the lateral femur condyle
The average age of the ten patients in the follow-up study was 17.5 years (11–29 years). The average interval from accident to operation was 13 days.

In five patients the lesion was found on the surface of the condyle and in five cases on the edge of the ocndyle, caused by dislocation of the patella. The smallest fragment was 15 mm × 8 mm, the biggest 30 mm × 20 mm. The open reduction was carried out easily in eight cases; in two it was difficult and in four additional osteosynthesis was necessary. Complete healing occurred in only three cases despite good operative reduction. In four cases the fragment

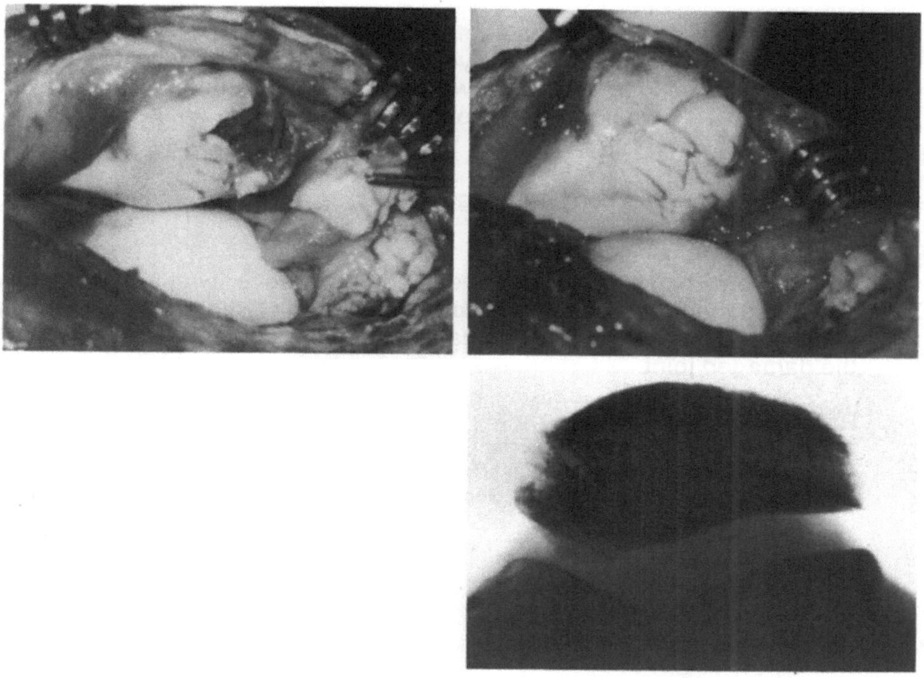

Figure 2. Sixteen-year-old boy with patellar luxation. The patella shows a severe medial conquassation of the cartilage; in addition, an osteochondral fragment has broken out. The fragment was re-implanted with fibrin sealant and the cartilage fractures were also filled. After suturing of the medial retinacula the knee was fixed in a plaster cast for 4 weeks. Four and a half years later the patient is completely symptom-free; the X-ray shows a little ossification on the medial part of the patella. Now the patient can participate in sport again without difficulty

was slightly depressed, in two cases the fragment was raised and in one case it was tilted. Seven patients did not develop arthrosis, while three developed slight arthrosis; nine patients had no symptoms and a full range of motion. In one case reoperation was necessary due to dislocation of the patella, and in two cases osteosynthesis material was removed.

On the *medial femur condyle* we replaced osteochondral fragments in three patients. At the follow-up examination none had any symptoms.

Replantation of osteochondral fragments in comminuted fractures

At the follow-up examination we studied five patients with a comminuted fracture of the lateral tibia condyle. In cases of comminuted fractures the large fragments should first be reduced by osteosynthesis and then the smaller fragments should be fixed with fibrin sealant. Even severe comminuted fractures can be satisfactorily reconstructed in this way.

The patients were aged between 24 and 74 years. The operation was carried out up to 11 days after the accident. Corresponding to the type of injury, the cartilage was affected by multiple fractures and the joint was always involved. Usually additional osteosynthesis was required and in three cases an extensive cancellous bone graft was necessary. Weight bearing was not allowed until 8–16 weeks after the operation, depending on the severity of the fracture.

In three cases the bony healing was ideal; twice we noted a slight depression.

Four patients had symptoms, depending on the severity of the accident, and only two patients were able to practise sport again. A full range of motion was achieved in only one case. Two patients developed generalized arthrosis in the damaged joint.

References

1. Gaudernak T (1982) Klinische Erfahrungen mit dem Fibrinkleber bei der Versorgung von Knorpel-Knochenfragmenten und Dissekaten. In: Cotta H, Braun A (eds) Fibrinkleber in Orthopädie und Traumatologie. Georg Thieme, Stuttgart, pp 158–167 (with detailed review of the literature)

Bone canal drilling in chondropathy

C. Zander

Chirurgische Abteilung, Allgemeines Krankenhaus Ochsenzoll
Hamburg 62
Federal Republic of Germany

The first bone canal drilling was performed in 1845 by Dieffenbach in Berlin and the next in 1929 by Beck in the United States. Both authors carried it out to treat pseudarthrosis. The first instance of bone drilling in chondropathy (osteochondrosis dissecans) was published – as far as we know – in *Bone and Joint Surgery* and referred to a report of Smillie on the occasion of a South West Orthopaedic Club Meeting in November 1954 at the Princess Elizabeth Orthopaedic Hospital, Exeter (Smillie 1955).

At nearly the same time (1954/1955) Pridie (1954) started hole drilling in osteochondritis patellae and I started bone canal drilling to treat different kinds of chondropathy – such as cartilage loss, osteonecrosis (Ahlbäck's disease: Aglietti et al. 1983; Ahlbäck 1968; Ahlbäck et al. 1968; Albers et al. 1985; Subach et al. 1978) and also osteochondritis dissecans – with no knowledge of Smillie's bone drilling. Therefore we called the bone drilling Beck'*sche Bohrungen* (Beck's drilling; Rutscheidt 1959); and we did not drill holes but rather *canals* 4–5 cm in length – on the basis of Roux's theory that shearing stress combined with compression can change immature connective tissue to chondral bone or articular cartilage. Roux stated: "all new formation of chondral tissue depends on the metaplasia ability of the polypotent mesenchymal cell within the meaning of functional adaptation" (Pauwels 1960).

We supposed that once a canal had been drilled into the condylar bone blood cells and fibroblasts would sprout into the canal, fill the canal and finally come up to the condylar surface to protect the area where the articular cartilage is lost. Occasionally we were able to look into a recently damaged knee joint (4 weeks after canal drilling), and we discovered that there was a white cartilage-like tissue around each drilling hole (Figure 1).

We saw what the canals had produced – under orthostatic pressure conditions. It seemed as if the connective tissue – consisting of fibrocytes – had changed to chondroblasts and chondrocytes. That was the mechanically caused metaplasia predicted by Roux (cited in Pauwels 1960).

At that time we did not yet know that the theory of Roux (1912) was not exactly right, and the success we achieved seemed to confirm it.

Chondrology
The primary articular cartilage, the hyaline cartilage, develops from the polypotent mesenchymal cells, influenced by the primary heredity factor and its environment. The multiplication of homogeneous chondrocytes comes from mature chondrocytes only. In this condition the adjacent matrix does not

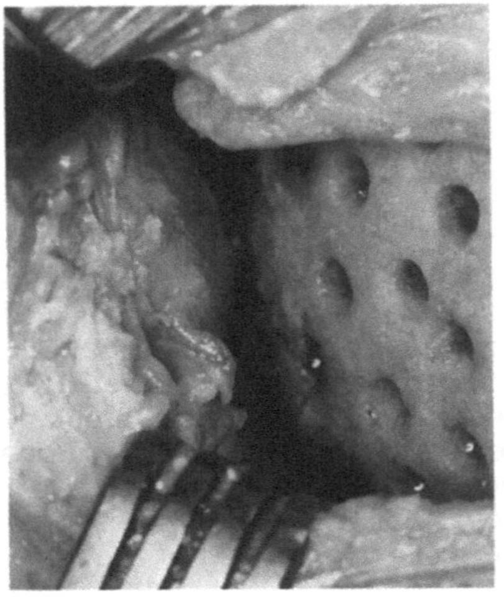

Figure 1. Leg: articular fibrocartilage covering the bone

change. Form variations of the chondrocytes are caused by their changed environment. Otherwise the cytoplasmic metabolism would change – and this change would bring about change of the molecular structures and mutations after all. The effect caused on the chondrocyte by changing its environment is called the "secondary or somatic heredity factor". To summarize: the chondroblast develops from mesenchymal fibroblasts by autonomy of propagation of the species and in their morphological shapes by changing environment and function.

The secondary articular cartilage develops as a result of external pressure on connective tissue (Pauwels 1960; Krompecher 1937) being a form of mechanically caused metaplasia. This theory is only partially correct, for Pauwels (1960) was able to prove that cartilage tissue can originate because of internal pressure – called hydrostatic pressure – i.e. cartilage tissue originates where all-round pressure is generated. The theory of Pauwels was backed by electron microscopical research.

Consequently, we can induce cartilage generation by drilling bone canals where articular cartilage is lost. We started bone canal drilling in 1954 in the St. Georg Krankenhaus, Hamburg, and have continued this procedure in the Allgemeines Krankenhaus Ochsenzoll, Hamburg, since February 1966. Figures 2–5 show the kind of drilling and the results.

In the same way, we treated osteochondrosis dissecans by drilling deeply into the bone. So we had the idea of reconstructing the juvenile pathway of nutrition to the articular cartilage.

Chondroblasts and finally chondrocytes originate from mesenchymal histiocytes in the bony canals due to the internal hydrostatic pressure. It is still unknown why the hydrostatic pressure initiates all this. But the hard walls of the bone canals yield the resistance required to fill the canals with cartilage-like tissue. The growth pressure of the tissue in the canals directs the collagen

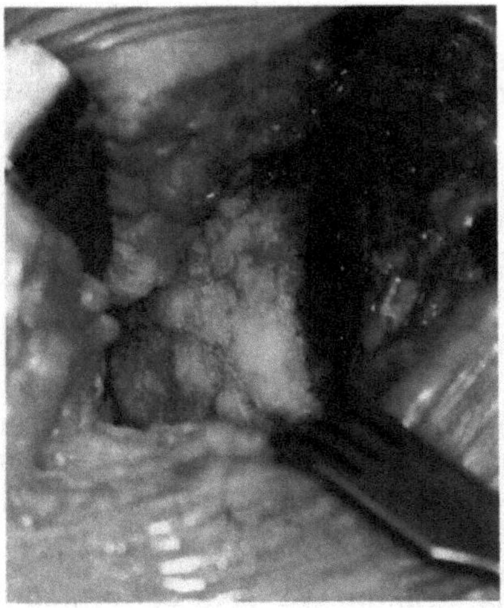

2

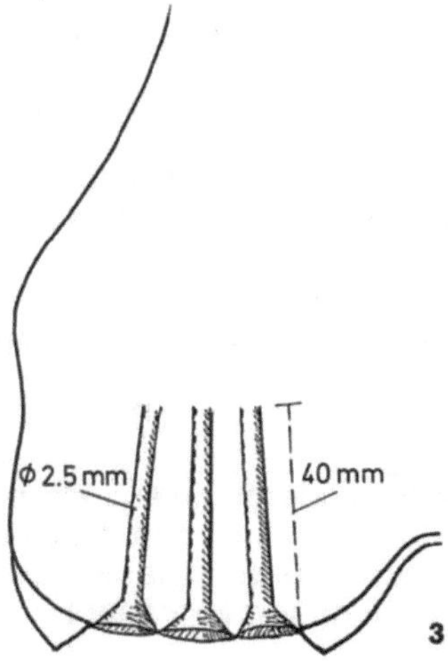

3

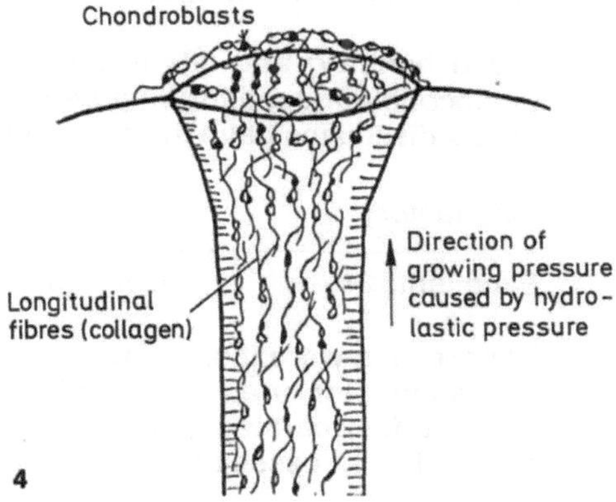

4

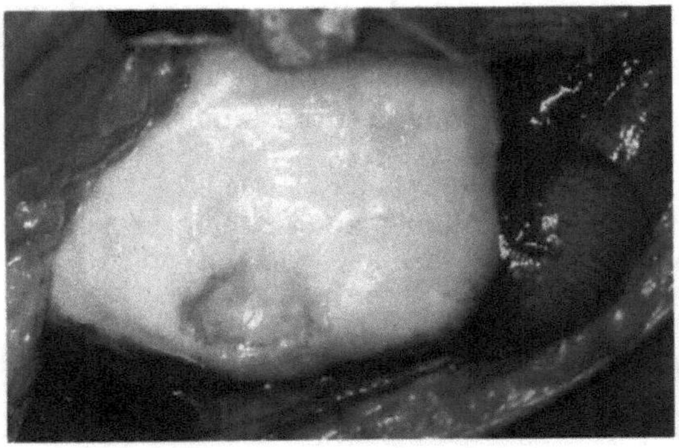

5

Figures 2–5. Bone canal drilling

fibres to the open end of the canal – sprouting around the holes later. The load pressure forms the collagen structures and gives them loading capacity.

The young chondral tissue presents obviously young chondrocytes with a capacity for early division at the base, i.e., near to the bone, and increasingly during maturation or ageing the young chondrocytes are found at the chondral surface. This seems quite contrary to the theory of Otte (1965) about the primary hyaline cartilage. The answer to this seeming contradiction could be as follows:

Ageing and growth of the chondrocytes depends on the prevailing direction of the nutritional flow, i.e. before epiphyseal closing nutrition comes from the bony side and after epiphyseal closing it comes from the synovial fluid side.

That was the theory behind bone canal drilling. We have performed more than 750 operations (canal drilling) and we have been particularly successful in the cases of "dry osteoarthritis" (without effusive synovitis). In these cases the mechanical factor was obviously more significant for the arthritis than the enzymatic and inflammatory factor.

Three hundred and fifty-two follow-up examinations in 500 patients with monocondylar canal drilling because of chondropathy (301) and osteochondrosis dissecans gave the following results:

Satisfactory		Fair	Unsatisfactory
Excellent: 21%	Good: 32%	Fair: 27%	Poor: 20%

Poor results were those where the patient had to undergo an endoprosthetic operation later or an alignment procedure. But all of them had regenerated articular fibrocartilage, independent of sex or age. The condylar surface was covered in all cases but pain had continued for longer than 2 years.

Indications. Entire loss of articular cartilage with sclerosis of the subchondral bone and irrelevant synovitis, osteochondrosis dissecans and osteonecrosis, "Ahlbäck" type.

Contraindications. Pronounced malalignment and rheumatic synovitis and cases where an endoprothesis is justified.

It is worthy of note that some patients older than 50 or 60 years of age were able to achieve tournament-standard fitness in tennis and golf.

References

Aglietti P, Insall JN, Buzzi R, Deschamps G (1983) Idiopathic osteonecrosis of the knee. J Bone Joint Surg [Br] 65(5)

Ahlbäck S (1968) Osteonecrosis of the knee. A radiographic investigation. Acta Radiol (Suppl) 277

Ahlbäck S, Göran, Bauer CH, Bone WH (1967) Spontaneous osteonecrosis of the knee. Arthritis Rheum 11(6)

Albers W, Blümlein H, Süler H (1985) Die spontane Femurcondylennecrose des Kniegelenkes. Zbl Chir 110:607–612

Altmann. Biopolymere and Biomechanik von Bindegewebssystemen. Paper presented at the Seventh Scientific Conference of the Gesellschaft Deutscher Naturforscher und Ärzte

Krompecher ST (1959) Die Knochenbildung. Fischer, Jena

Otte (1965) Über das Wachstum der Gelenkknorpel. Hüttig, Heidelberg

Pauwels F (1960) Eine neue Theorie über den Einfluß mechanischer Reife auf die Differenzierung der Stützgewebe. Z Anat Entwicklungsgesch 121:478–515

Pridie KH (1959) A method of resurfacing osteoarthritic knee joints. J Bone Joint Surg [Br] 41:618

Rutscheidt F (1959) Die operative Behandlung der Osteochondritis dissecans am Knie. Z Orthop 91:180

Smillie JS (1955) Treatment of osteochondritis dissecans. J Bone Joint Surg [Br] 37(4)

Susbach C, Ahuja C, Bullough P (1978) Osteonecrosis of the knee. J Bone Joint Surg [Am] 60(2)

Free periosteal grafts in human knee joints using Fibrinkleber-Human Immuno

B. Niedermann, S. Boe, J. Lauritzen and J. M. Rubak

Department of Orthopaedic Surgery, Aarhus County Hospital
Aarhus
Denmark

Based on animal experiments (J.M. Rubak et al. Acta Orthop Scand 53, 175-191, 1982) articular cartilage lesions in human knee joints have experimentally been repaired by the use of free periosteal grafts.

Material and methods

In clinical cases of osteochondritis dissecans lesion of the medial femoral condyle, not suitable for replacement, a free periosteal graft was transplanted from the tibia to the defect of the articular cartilage. The graft was fixed by use of the two component tissue glue Fibrikleber-Human Immuno®.

Results

The patients were examined after 3, 6 and 12 months clinically, by x-ray and by arthroscopy. The results so far are promising showing the articular cartilage and bone defect filled with bone tissue and covered with cartilage tissue on a level with the normal cartilage.

Summary

In 4 patients with osteochondritis dissecans lesion in the knee joint, not suitable for replacement, free periosteal grafts were transplanted from the tibia to the defect and fixed by Fibrinkleber-Human Immuno®. After one year of observation the results are promising, showing the defect filled with bone and covered with cartilage tissue.

Biomechanical aspects of the pathogenesis of osteochondritis dissecans (Koenig)

W. Bandi

AO International
Balderstr. 30, Berne
Switzerland

Osteochondritis dissecans (Koenig) (OD) denotes the subchondral separation of a bean-shaped, cartilage-coated, partially necrotic bone particle, which arises slowly at typical locations in mostly convex joint parts. This gradual disintegration should be clearly distinguished from chondral or osteochondral fractures.

The usual theories concerning the pathogenesis of OD (aseptic necrosis [1, 3, 8], shear fractures [4, 5, 7, 9], fatigue breaks [2, 6, 10–12]) are not convincing, as they do not explain three facts which are typical of OD, namely:

1. The typical shape and structure of the disintegrated part
2. The predilection locations of OD
3. The fact that the disintegration proceeds within the subchondral bone structure beneath an – initially – macroscopically intact joint cartilage

Rehbein's deductions from his pathogenetic animal experiments [13] approach the true situation, although the shearing forces he employed between the tibia head and the femoral condyle do not occur in nature. In my opinion the pathogenesis must be based on normal, commonly occurring joint mechanisms.

The following exposition is to be thought of as a working hypothesis and is meant to stimulate further experimental work designed to test its theoretical assumptions.

Four facts are of importance for the hypothesis:

1. In most cases the disintegrative process occurs at convex joint structures.
2. Frequently, attacks occur at those joints that lie between long lever arms and which are therefore subject to strong compressive forces (knee joint, elbow joint, astragalotibial joint between the tibia and the lever arm between the trochlea tali and capitula metatarsalia).
3. The disintegration occurs at the point where the radius of curvature of the convex part of the joint changes in magnitude and/or sign:
   - In the knee joint at the point where the long radius of curvature of the inner condylar-trochlea switches over into the short and oppositely directed radius of the fossa intercondyloidea (Figure 1).
   - In the elbow joint at the point where the long radius of curvature of the capitulum humeri reaches the short, inversely directed radius of the groove between the trochlea and the capitulum (Figure 2).
   - In the ankle joint at the medial or lateral edge of the talus where its long radius of curvature in the sagittal plane goes over into the zone of the short frontal radius of the corner of the talus (Figure 3).

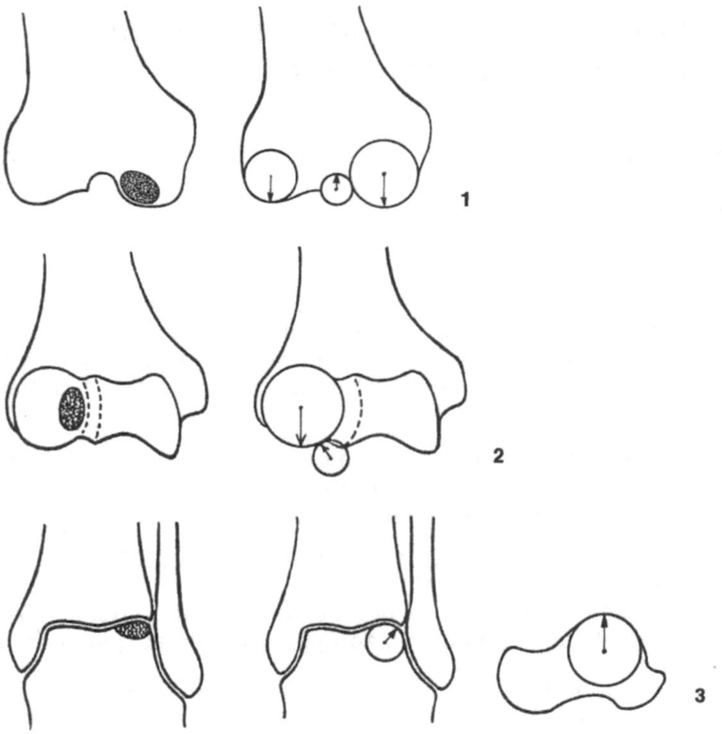

Figures 1–3. Points at which disintegration occurs

4. The viscoelastic compressibility of the joint structures in question has to be taken into account; some specific cases are:
   - The condylar trochlea of the knee joint, which is subject to a convergent pressure of several 100 kp (kiloponds) between the tibial and patellar plateaus.
   - The capitulum humeri, which is subject to the pressure of the radius and – from the medial direction – the pressure of the ulna via the trochlea humeri.
   - The lateral or medial edges of the trochlea tali, which is subject to pressures from the tibia and the lateral or medial malleolus (up to one-sixth of the tibial pressure).

Let me explain the further pathogenetic development using the knee joint as an example.

Under the converging pressure between the patella and tibial plateau the viscoelastic corticocancellous subchondral bone gives way and forms protuberances at all those places where counterpressures are absent in a given joint position (Figure 4).

At a given pressure, this deviation will be larger the larger the radius of curvature of the compressed joint part (similar to the case of the hydraulic press)

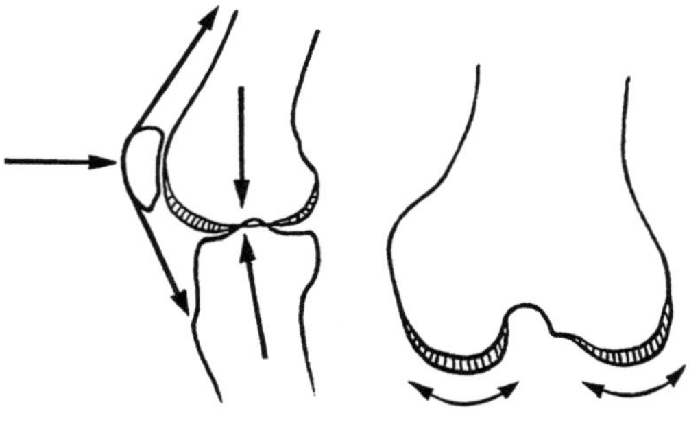

Figure 4. Protuberances at points at which counterpressure is absent

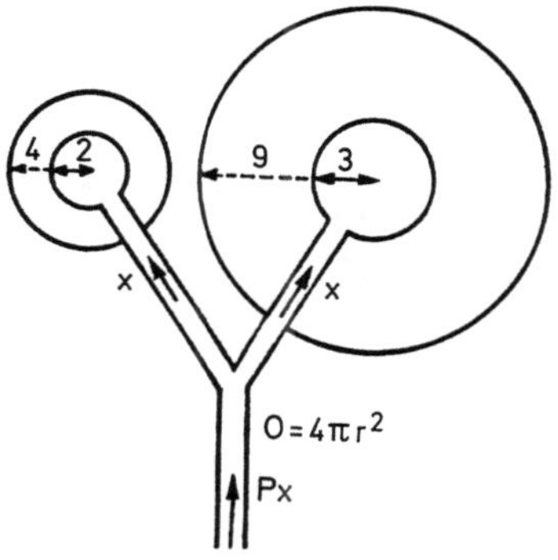

Figure 5. Action of the centrifugally expanding forces

as the surface of the theoretically assumed sphere and thus the sum of the pressure forces grow with the square of the radius ($O=4\pi r^2$). On the other hand the deviation will be small or absent in the region of the fossa intercondyloidea, as the centrifugally expanding forces do not act on a hollow sphere, but on a vault (Figure 5).

As a consequence of the different degrees of deviation of the subchondral bone, its surface is subjected to a tangentially directed deviational elongation, which after many repetitions leads to a distentional fatigue break, which occurs chiefly in the zone between the large elongation, corresponding to the long radius, and the small elongation, corresponding to the short, inverse radius (Figure 6).

This distentional fatigue break determines the localization of the dissected fragment, as it is the first lesion of the convex part of the joint. Under further stress the damaged vault is now subjected alternately to propulsive forces in bending positions between 40 ° and 110 ° and impressive forces between 0 ° and 30 ° (tibial plateau) and 120 ° and 130 ° (patella); i.e. a segment of the vault which was ruptured by the first lesion is forced to oscillate around an axis lying in the subchondral bone and finally undergoes a fatigue break (second lesion) through the repeated bending-stretching stress (Figure 7). Between the first and second lesion the swinging motions induce advancing microfractures in the spongiosa, with a narrow debris zone which is contin-

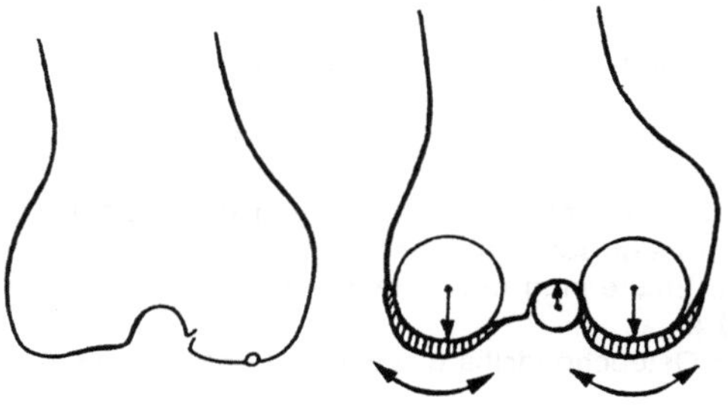

Figure 6. Distentional fatigue break due to tangentially directed deviational elongation

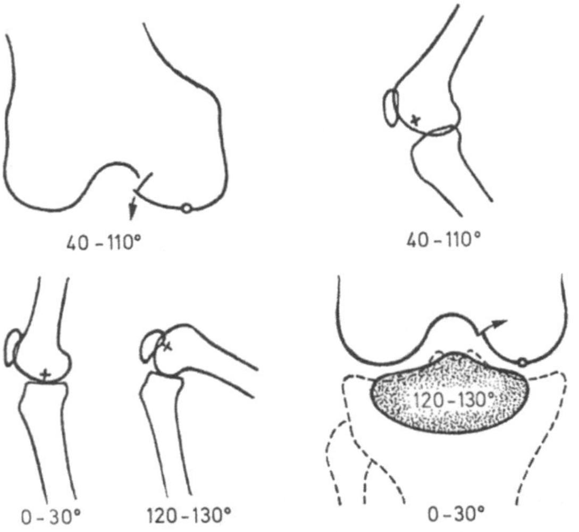

Figure 7. Fatigue break due to repeated bending-stretching stress

ually replaced by fibrous cartilage. Thus the dissected part becomes more and more devascularized and necrotic, resembling an atrophic pseudoarthrosis in its bed of fibrous cartilage. The increasing instability of the dissected parts leads to a final rupture of the surrounding joint cartilage and to the expulsion of the arthrolith by a frequently insignificant trauma, which is then felt to be the causal trauma by the patient as a consequence of the often acute and painful pinching symptoms.

References

1. Axhausen G (1923) Der anatomische Krankheitsverlauf bei der Koehler'schen Krankheit der Metatarsalköpfchen und Perthes'schen Krankheit des Hüftgelenkes. Arch Klin Chir 124:511
2. Bandi W (1951) Über die Aethiologie der Osteochondritis dissecans. Helv Chir Acta 18:221
3. Bandi W (1982) Die retropatellaren Kniegelenksschäden, 2nd edn. Huber, Berne
4. Bergmann E (1927) Theoretisches, Klinisches und Experimentelles zur Frage der aseptischen Knorpelnekrose. Dtsch Z Chir 206:12
5. Baumgartl F (1964) Das Kniegelenk. Springer, Berlin Göttingen Heidelberg New York
6. Büdinger K (1906) Über die Ablösung von Gelenkteilen und verwandte Prozesse. Dtsch Z Chir 84:311
7. Büdinger K (1908) Über traumatische Knorpelrisse im Kniegelenk. Dtsch Z Chir 92:510
8. Burckhardt H (1924) Über die Entstehung der freien Gelenkkörper und Mechanik des Kniegelenks. Bruns Beitr Klin Chir 130:205
9. Bürkl R, Jaeger M (1982) Eine atypische, juvenile Osteochondrose im medialen Femurkondylus. Z Orthop 120:705–707
10. Campell CJ, Ranavat Chitranjan S (1966) Osteochondritis dissecans: the question of etiology. J Trauma 6(2):201
11. Kappis M (1922) Weitere Beiträge zur mechanischen Entstehung der „spontanen" Knorpelablösungen (sog. Osteochondritis dissecans). Dtsch Z Chir 171:13
12. Nagura S (1937) Das Wesen und die Entstehung der Osteochondritis dissecans am wachsenden Knochen. Zbl Chir 35:2049
13. Rehbein F (1950) Die Entstehung der Osteochondritis dissecans. Langenbecks Arch/Dtsch Z Chir 265:69–114

Allogenous cartilage transplantation in the treatment of osteochondrosis dissecans. Technique and results

D. H. Rogge and P. Kalbe

Unfallchirurgische Klinik der Medizinischen Hochschule
3000 Hannover
Federal Republic of Germany

Cartilage transplantation is the adequate therapy for large solitary cartilage defects in otherwise intact joints. An allogenous osteochondral graft has to be used, if due to the extent of the defect an autogenous transplantation is not possible.

Material and methods

During 10 years 25 allogenous cartilage transplantations in knee joints were performed at the Trauma Department of Hanover Medical School. 22 knees suffered from osteochondrosis dissecans, one had a chondromalacia, and two knees posttraumatic defects. 17 defects were located on the medial femoral condyle, 8 on the lateral femoral condyle. The largest transplant diameter was 55 mm.

18 grafts were used fresh. In 6 grafts deep freeze preservation had been used, in 4 cases at -196° C. in liquid nitrogen and in 2 cases at. -30° C. One graft was preserved in CIALIT^{R}.

The surgical technique of WAGNER was used. Fixation was achieved with K-wires, being inserted intraarticular and allowing later extraarticular removal.

Aftertreatment began with continuous passive motion on second day after surgery, walking on 5th day, and partial weight bearing for 3 months. Sports should not be performed for 6 months.

Evaluation was done under strict clinical and roentgenological criteria. Arthroscopy was not permitted by any of the patients, since most of them had nearly no complaints.

Results

Of all 25 cases there was one infection after CIALIT^{R}-perservation.

4 grafts became necrotic. One partial graft necrosis took place after fresh allogenous transplantation. Total graft necrosis resulted once after fresh transplantation, twice after preservation at -30° C., and once after preservation in liquid nitrogen. These complications led twice to a unicondylar prosthesis and in one case of persistent infection to an arthrodesis.

For final evaluation only 20 cases were investigated with a follow up of more than two years, ranging from 3 to 10 years with a mean follow up of 5,9 years.

Correlating with the roentgenologic appearance the clinical evaluation of the fresh transplanted 13 cases showed 8 excellent, 3 good, 1 fair, and 1 poor result. Of the 4 grafts being preserved at −196° C. one was excellent, 2 good, none fair and 2 poor. Both grafts being preserved at – 30° C. were poor due to total necrosis, the same regarding the CIALIT^{R}-preserved graft, leading to persistent infection and total necrosis.

Discussion

According to experimental findings it has to be assumed, that after preservation at −196° C. only part of the graft cells survive. All other methods of preservation seem to lead to total graft necrosis. Only by fresh transplantation the graft can be maintained viable and a good long term result achieved.

Summary

According to the reported good long term results the fresh transplantation of allogenous osteochondral grafts can be regarded as standard procedure for large cartilage defects, especially in osteochondrosis dissecans of the knee.

On the operative treatment of osteochondrosis dissecans – longer term arthroscopic follow up

W. Blauth and M. Mann

Department of Orthopaedic Surgery, University of Kiel
2300 Kiel
Federal Republic of Germany

127 patients suffering from osteochondrosis dissecans of the knee joint have been investigated arthroscopically – some on several occasions – since 1978 in the Orthopaedic University Clinic at Kiel.

The visual and tactile findings in the affected area provided by arthroscopy represent together with X-ray and scintigraphy for us the essential aid in deciding the type of treatment to be chosen – conservative or operative. Furthermore, control arthroscpies during conservative relief therapy (Thomas-splint) should reveal at an early stage a loosening of the fragment, if this should after all occur, and make possible operative intervention at the right time.

After conclusion of the conservative and operative treatment, i.e. after the fragment had healed roentgenologically and also the increased nuclide covering, previously present, had receded scintigraphically, a control arthroscopy was carried out again. The question to be clarified here was whether the complete clinical and roentgenological healing of the fragment is accompanied by an intact cartilage surface. In 38 patients, in whom the fragment was pinned with autlogous bonechips, our follow-up arthroscopic investigations showed that in nearly all cases, in spite of clinical freedom from complaint and in spite of roentgenologically demonstrated healing over of the fragment, the joint cartilage covering the firmly healed bone was changed macroscopically to appear as a chondromalacia.

In the proposed contribution the results of follow-up investigations, not completed at the time of writing, on patients treated conservatively or with subchondral surgery of the spongiosa are compared and discussed in relation to the group mentioned above.

Experimental model for chondrocyte transplantation in rabbits

D. S. Menche, M. I. Pitman and L. Peterson

Hospital for Joint Diseases Orthopaedic Institute
New York N.Y.
U.S.A.

The aims of this research project were to 1) characterize histologically the articular cartilage surface of the rabbit's knee 2) study rabbit chondrocyte cultures using electron microscopy 3) develop an experimental model for the study of chondrocyte transplantation.

The articular surface of the rabbit knee was divided histologically into four distinct layers. Each layer was individually measured in regard to its depth. Articular cartilage specimens obtained from surgery were digested by collaganase, hyaluro nidase and DNAse. Cells obtained were grown in culture. Ultrastructurally, the chondrocytes demonstrated by both scanning and transmission electron microscopy pericellular collagen filaments by day two, and extracellular matrix-like material by day four of culture.

Subsequently, we transplanted autogenous and allogenic cultured chondrocytes into surgically created defects. During the course of these experiments surgical techniques were varied in an attempt to ascertain the most optimal model for cartilage regeneration. Defects varied in 1) size-1mm (13 cases) to 3mm (26 cases) 2) depth-superficial, intermediate and deep 3) location medial femoral condyle (21 cases) vs. patella (39 cases) 4) number-single vs. multiple.

Utilizing our latest animal model, preliminary results have been extremely promising with a total reconstitution of a 3 mm defect with hyaline cartilage. In the rabbit this is the largest defect reconstituted with articular cartilage to date. There was no evidence of cartilage regeneration in the 26 cases of 3 m patella defects or in the 21 cases where the medial femoral condyle was shaved in which no transplants were performed. In the latter group, 28.6% developed osteophytes and 19% had synovitis within a one to three month period.

The implications of our results suggest that in early isolated cartilage lesions of arthritic or traumatic origin hyaline cartilage healing is possible with chondrocyte transplantation.

Total knee replacement using an osteochondral allograft in baboons

M. Roffman

Research Center for Implant Surgery, Haifa Medical Center (Rothschild)
Haifa
Israel

Osteochondral graft was already in clinical use at the beginning of this century but was abandoned for two reasons:

1) No experimental studies were carried out to try and solve problems conerning this method.

2) The excellent progress which was achieved in bioengineering and the understanding of the biomechanical problems in orthopaedics. Recently when we have to solve more and more cases of failed total hip replacement there is a revival in the use of the biological arthroplasty. There are few basic problems concerning this method like the immunogenicity of the osteochondral allograft, the problem of cartilage preservation and the surgical technique of osteochondral graft.

The goal of this study was to investigate the value of ostechondral graft as a biological joint resurfacing, to investigate the hypothesis which was offered that osteochondral graft can be transferred from one animal to another while maintaining the condition for graft survival with good function. For this 2 models in baboons' knee were designed. In 10 baboons, 20 knees were operated on where total knee replacement using osteochondral allografts were performed. On the right side a thin (4-5mm) subchondral bone was transferred and the width of the subchondral bone in the knee was 8–10 mm. The grafts were united within 3 months and good function of the joint was achieved at the same time. All animals were sacrificed at 1 year after transplantation. Clinical results showed failure of 1 knee in the right side and two on the left.

Histological results revealed success in 7 grafts on the right side and only 6 good (thick) knees.

Chondrocyte viability which was assessed by radionuclide studies using S-35 reveales in 80% of the grafted knees normal production of proteoglycans. 7 out of l4 samples showed type II collagen production.

Arthroscopy

Arthroscopy and arthroscopic meniscal surgery in ligament instability

P. P. Mariani, G. Puddu and L. Perugia

Second Department of Orthopaedic Surgery, University of Rome
Rome
Italy

When a young athlete who has previously suffered a knee injury complains of recurrent episodes of giving way during physical activity, a careful history including type of injury, first symptoms of disability and the onset of swelling plus a careful examination including all tests can point to a serious or moderate instability of the knee in a patient at high risk.

There is no doubt about the treatment: meniscal suture when possible, anterior cruciate ligament (ACL) reconstruction and reconstructive capsular medial and lateral plastic.

At the arthroscopy it is seldom possible to see the capsular tear or scar, where some fibres under the meniscus of medial collateral ligament are clear. The arthroscopy can confirm the rupture of the ACL and would only be used to determine the condition of the articular cartilage and the type of meniscal tear. Some authors advocate performing arthroscopic meniscectomy prior to the ligamentous procedure.

But what should be done if the instability is slight or moderate in a patient at low risk? The problem lies in being able to judge which of these cases would require surgical treatment of the chronic ACL lesion in order for healing to take place.

In the past we have tried to resolve this problem by using a clinical rating system based on various parameters, and our results and conclusion will be published in one of the next issues of the *American Journal of Sports Medicine.* But now using arthroscopic surgery, we believe that arthroscopic meniscectomy can be another answer. For this, correct indications and strict selection of patients are necessary.

Many authors have reported their results of arthroscopic meniscectomies with instability of the knee. These results have not always been good since in some cases the functional postoperative score has been low. In many cases these authors have not reported their guidelines for this treatment programme.

In this study, we would like to report the results of 50 arthroscopic meniscectomies performed on selected patients. We selected our patients whose work did not demand particularly heavy physical activity and engaged in sports only at the non-professional level. Most patients were over 25 years old. In conclusion the functional level of demand was low.

History played an important role in our selection. Major complaints had to be pain and locking and the giving way episodes had to be sporadic. Physical examination was also an important factor. We selected only those patients whose jerk test or pivot shift tests were 1+; the anterior drawer test in neutral rotation and in external rotation could be 1 or 2+. If the evaluation under anaesthesia, which allowed us more accurately to determine the type and degree of laxity, showed an increase in score for the dynamic tests such as pivot shift or jerk test, the patients were eliminated from our study. Also the type of meniscal tear was an important deciding factor. If arthroscopic examination revealed a posterior horn tear the patients were eliminated from the study and treated with meniscal suture plus ACL reconstruction.

In the graph the different types of meniscal tears that we have treated are shown. Only in three cases we treated posterior horn tears with partial meniscectomy, this because the patients could not remain inactive for a long period.

Our meniscectomies were performed using the three portal technique described by Gillquist and Hagberg. The type of operation and immediate postoperative evaluations were recorded.

In this associated pathology of the meniscus a careful examination of the meniscus is necessary since it is often possible to see others tear as in this case. After the removal of a flap tear of the medial meniscus, we found a longitudinal tear of the meniscus remnant. The type of operation and immediate postoperative evaluations were recorded.

The average follow-up was 1 year (range 6–24 months). Each patient's functional score results were scored using criteria similar to those described by Lysholm and Gillquist, based on a score of 100 points. Our average score was 89. In only three cases were the results only fair for pain in the contralateral compartment. The distribution of scores is shown.

Forty-six patients reported no episodes of instability and in four cases such episodes were reported as rare. In spite of this, these patients were satisfied and they felt an improvement after the meniscectomy. Only in five cases did the patients give up sports afterwards.

Isokinetic evaluations which were made before the operation and then again 4 and 8 weeks after the operation confirmed full early recovery of muscle function in agreement with the findings of Gillquist and Patel.

In conclusion meniscectomy can be useful in treating irreparable tears of the meniscus in selected patients with specific complaints. We have attempted to show more precisely the guidelines for the selection of patients. Our results are promising. Arthroscopy obviously cannot substitute for careful clinical evaluation but it can work in conjunction with it.

Arthroscopy under local anaesthesia

T. Hoogland, G. A. J. de Baere and F. J. B. Zeegers

Ignatius Hospital
Breda
The Netherlands

Purpose of the study
The study was designed to evaluate the accuracy of arthroscopy under local anaesthesia and the experiences of the patients in regard to pain and discomfort during and after this procedure.

Materials and methods
208 patients underwent 209 arthroscopies of the knee under local anaesthesia with 30 cc. 2% lidocaine with adrenaline. The arthroscopy was performed with a 5 mm Storz arthroscope through the antero-lateral portal.

In the majority of the cases a diagnostic hook was introduced through a second portal for accurate inspection of the structures. 66 Patients had a prior arthrogram. Two months after the arthroscopy a questionnaire regarding the patiens experience during and after the procedure was returned.

Results
At completion of the study it appeared that in 50% of the cases the original diagnosis of the clinical examination including ordinary roentgenograms appeared false. In 42% of the cases the diagnoses of the arthrogram appeared false. In 46% of the cases the arthroscopy has altered the treatment.
110 patients underwent subsequent arthrotomy: in three cases the arthroscopy appeared incorrect, so the accuracy of the arthroscopy was 97%.
83% of the patients had no discomfort during the procedure.
17% had some discomfort.
43% had no discomfort after the arthroscopy.
57% of the patients had moderate discomfort after thre arthroscopy which lasted for an average of 3.3 days.
At an average of 5 days after the arthroscopy the patients could use the knees like before.
88% of the patients would chose for an other arthroscopy under local anaesthesia if the examination had to be repeated.
12% would prefer a general anaesthesia for a repeat arthroscopy.

Conclusions
In this study:
1. Arthroscopy under local anaesthesia was in 97% of the cases accurate.
2. The great majority of the patients did not have significant discomfort during the procedure and was willing to undergo a second arthroscopy if necessary under local anaesthesia.
3. Arthroscopy under local anaesthesia offers a good selection for knee lesions that are suitable for arthroscopic surgical management.

Day case arthroscopy

J. Older and T. Cardoso

**Department of Orthopaedic Surgery, Royal Surrey County Hospital
Guildford, Surrey
Great Britain**

This paper presents the experience of one surgeon using a new day case unit in a district general hospital in a twelve month period. Clinical data and questionnaires were obtained for 130 patients. A third of the 148 knees investigated had more than one pathological lesion, and in 18% the arthroscopic diagnosis differed from the pre-operative diagnosis. Intra-articular arthroscopic surgery was carried out on 59% of knees and only 12% of operations took more than 60 minutes. The time before return to normal everyday activites, work and sport was much shorter than after arthrotomy. An early return to work is of great importance both to the patient and society. The return to full athletic fitness varied according to the individual and the sport, but some of the patients had returned to first class sport in a very short space of time.

Post-anaesthetic sickness or poor communication with staff were the only causes of discontent, and 93% of the patients were pleased with day case treatment. We learnt that the success of ambulatory arthroscopic surgery depends on several crucial factors. Patients must be carefully selected and well informed. There must be sufficient staff of the right calibre to care for the patients in a relaxed and confident manner. Communication with the patient, relatives, general practitioners and community nurses must be thorough and constantly monitored. The incentive for day case surgery in the U.K. has been principally effective use of medical and theatre time being blocked by bed shortage. It is difficult to assess the economic effects of day case surgery on a hospital, but using the day case facilities the number of patients admitted for arthroscopic investigation and treatment of knee disorders has trebled and the waiting list time has been halved.

The place of arthroscopy in sports injuries

S. K. Mukherjee and J. Regan

Department of Orthopaedic Surgery, Monklands District General Hospital
Monkscourt Avenue, Aidrie, ML6 OJS
United Kingdom

Introduction

The place of arthroscopy in sports injuries is not only valuable as a diagnostic aid for an injured knee, but in suitable cases simple surgical procedures through arthroscopy also help in rapid recovery. This paper illustrates the role of arthroscopy as applied to sports injuries following a review of 447 patients seen at the Sports Injuries Clinic during the past 3½ years.

Dehaven et al. reported in 1975 the role of arthroscopy in the diagnosis of internal derangement of the knee and concluded that there can be no doubt that arthroscopy proved to be the most accurate diagnostic tool and played a significant role in his series. The correct diagnosis was made in 94 out of 100 cases and unnecessary operation avoided in 25% of cases. More recently, Northmore-Ball et al. (1983) reported their comparative study of open and closed meniscectomy and concluded that partial meniscectomy carried out by the closed technique under arthroscopic control represents a substantial advance in the treatment of the great majority of symptomatic meniscal tears.

Tregonning reported in 1983 that in suitable cases arthroscopic surgery for meniscal tears helped patients to make rapid recovery and return to work in an average of 12.9 days.

Similar views were published by Casscells (1980), Eriksson and Sebik (1980), Fahmy and Noble (1983), Goodfellow (1983), Hardakar et al. (1980), Ireland et al. (1980), McGinty (1980), Noyes (1980), and Patel (1978) during the past few years.

Material and methods

The Sports Injuries Clinic at Monklands District General Hospital was started on 4 September 1980 with the idea of providing a comprehensive service for all people taking part in various sports requiring medical attention for injuries sustained during sporting pursuits. The total number of new patients seen in the Sports Injuries Clinic up to the end of February 1984 was 447.

Of the 447 patients, 26.8% required surgical treatment. The knee joint was injured in 225 out of 447 cases (which is 50.3% of the total). Surgical procedures were carried out in 105 of these 225 injured knees, i.e. the operation rate on injured knees was, therefore, 44%, compared with the overall rate of 26.8%.

Sites of injuries are as shown in Table 1.

Table 1. Sites if injuries in sports

Spine		29 (6.4%)
Upper limb:	shoulder joint	28 (6.2%)
Elbow joint:	hands and wrists	16 (3.6%)
Lower limb:	hip joint	4 (0.9%)
	knee joint	225 (50.3%)
	ankle joint	39 (8.7%)
	feet	9 (2.1%)
Soft tissue injuries		97 (21.8%)

Arthroscopic examination for diagnostic purposes and arthroscopic surgery in suitable cases were started from 1 December 1981, some 15 months after the beginning of the Sport Injuries Clinic. Most of these procedures were carried out soon after an acute injury to the knee joint.

The total number of arthroscopies of the knee joint between 1 December 1981 and 29 February 1984 was 190 examinations in 183 patients. Of these, 105 arthroscopic examinations were carried out in injured knee joints caused by sporting activities. Analysis of 105 arthroscopic examinations is shown in Table 2.

Table 2. Types of sporting activities causing injuries

Football	51 (48.5%)
Athletics	14 (13.3%)
Rugby	11 (10.5%)
Hockey	6 (5.7%)
Golf	5 (4.8%)
Badminton	3 (2.8%)
Martial arts	3 (2.8%)
Skiing	3 (2.8%)
Weightlifting	3 (2.8%)
Netball	2 (1.9%)
Squash	2 (1.9%)
Swimming	2 (1.9%)
Tennis	1 (0.9%)
Dancing	1 (0.9%)

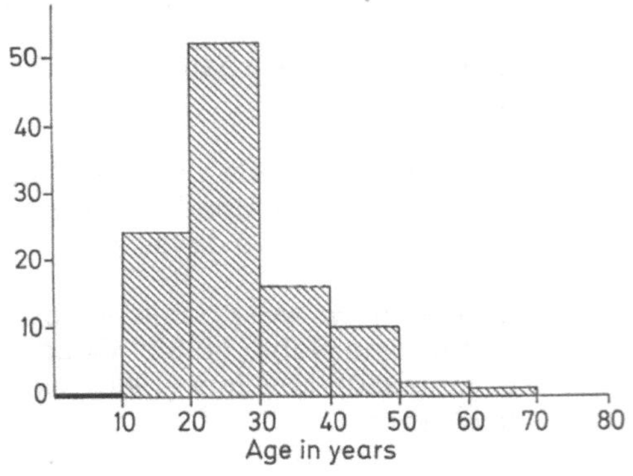

Figure 1. Ages of the patients

The ages of the patients were between 15 and 69 years. The average age was 26.6 years. The vast majority were between 20 and 40 years of age (see Figure 1). There were 87 males and 18 females, a sex ratio of 5:1.

The duration of symptoms at the time of presentation was short (Table 3).

The findings of arthroscopic examinations are summarized in Table 4.

The following two illustrative case reports are presented.

Table 3. Duration of symptoms at the time of presentation following initial injury

Less than 2 weeks	22 patients
Less than 4 weeks	34 patients
Less than 12 weeks	48 patients

Table 4. Findings in 105 arthroscopic examinations

No abnormality seen	20 (21%)
Meniscal lesions	62 (59%)
Anterior cruciate rupture	13 (12%)
Synovial shelf syndrome	6 (6%)
Infrapatellar fat pad lesion	3 (3%)
Osteochondral fracture	3 (3%)
Loose body	5 (5%)
Synovitis	4 (4%)
Abnormal patellar tracking	2 (2%)
Chondromalacia patellae	2 (2%)
Villonodular synovitis	1 (1%)

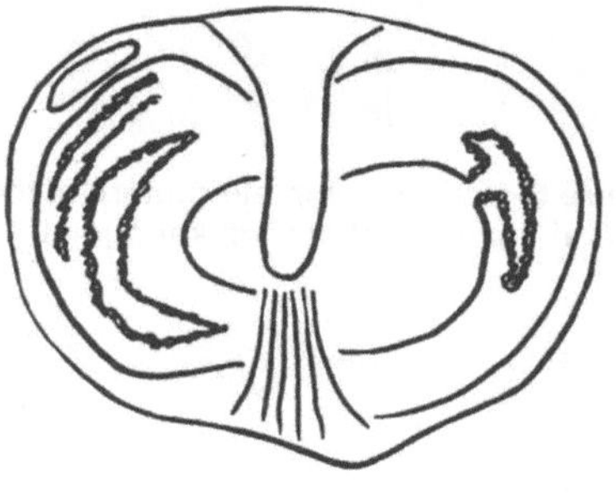

Figure 2. Arthroscopic examination

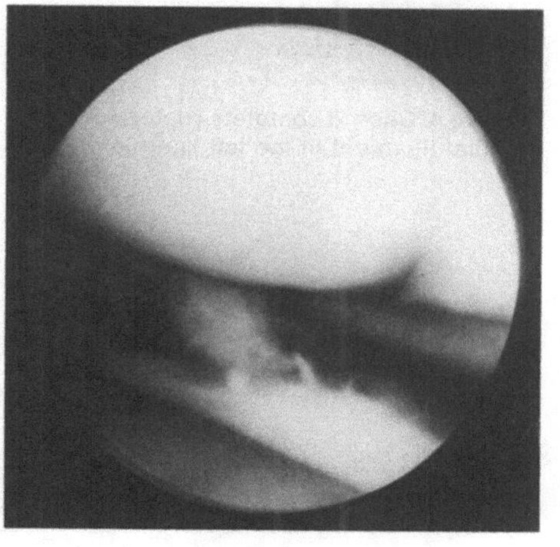

Figure 3. Arthroscopic examination

Case 1

A young man of 23 years presented with an acute episode of injury to his right knee joint while playing football. He also gave a history of two previous injuries to the same knee joint during the previous 2 years. Clinical examination and history suggested the diagnosis of damage to the lateral meniscus of the right knee joint. Arthroscopic examination revealed multiple longitudinal tears of the lateral meniscus and a single longitudinal tear of the medial meniscus (Figures 2, 3).

He was treated with closed partial meniscectomy of the medial meniscus and open total lateral meniscectomy of the lateral meniscus was performed. He made an uneventful recovery and results to date are extremely satisfactory.

Case 2

A 19-year-old footballer sustained a valgus injury to his left knee joint while playing football. Clinical examination and radiological investigations showed

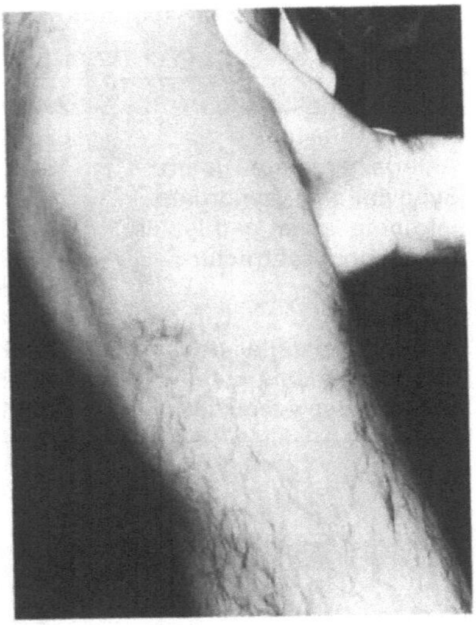

Figure 4. Case 2: complete rupture of the medial ligament of the left knee joint

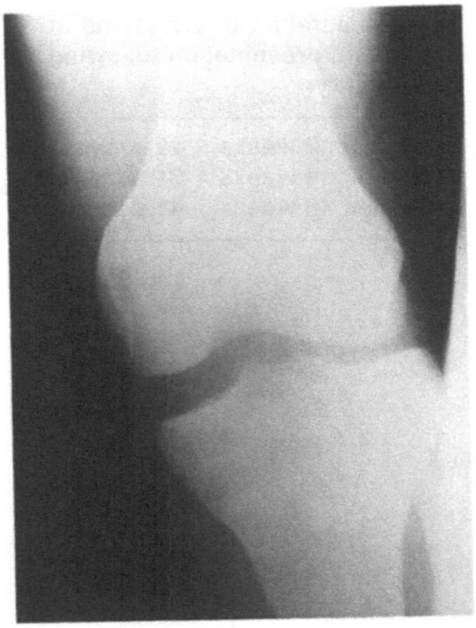

Figure 5. Case 2: complete rupture of the medial ligament of the left knee joint

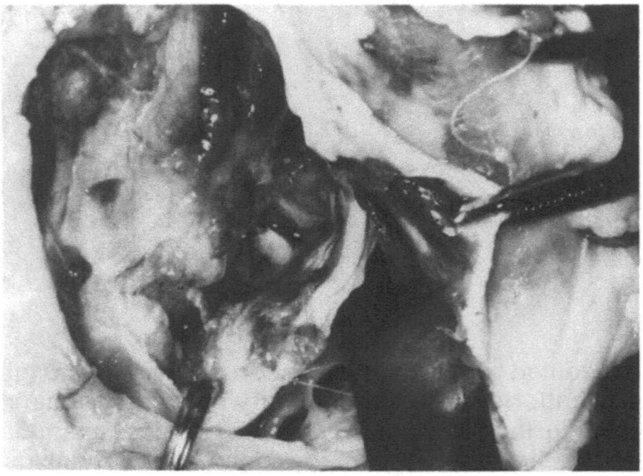

Figure 6. Case 2: open repair of the peripheral meniscal tear and repair of the medial ligament complex

complete rupture of the medial ligament of the left knee joint (see Figures 4, 5). Arthroscopy confirmed the diagnosis of large haemarthrosis, peripheral tear of medial meniscus and partial rupture of the anterior cruciate ligament. He was treated with open repair of the peripheral meniscal tear and repair of the medial ligament complex, 7 days after the injury (Figure 6). At the completion of treatment, an excellent result was obtained. Arthroscopy in this case helped in the planning and management of the injured knee joint. Arthroscopy also helped to save the medial meniscus.

Analysis of 105 arthroscopies confirms that the vast majority of injuries involved menisci, followed by damage to the anterior cruciate element (Table 5).

Table 5. Analysis of 105 arthroscopies of the knee joints

Meniscal lesions:	medial	33
	lateral	29
Anterior cruciate rupture:	partial	10
	complete	3
Synovial shelf syndrome:	lateral	4
	medial	2
Intrapatellar fat pad lesion		3
Osteochondral fracture		3
Loose body		5
Abnormal patellar tracking		2
Chondromalacia patellae		2
Villonodular synovitis		1

Surgical treatments which were carried out on these patients are summarized in Table 6.

Table 6. Surgical treatment of knee joints following 105 arthroscopies

Meniscectomy			52
	Open:	total	33
		partial	7
	Closed:	partial	12
Synovial shelf release:		lateral	4
		medial	2
Excision of infrapatellar fat pad:		open	2
		closed	1
Removal of loose body			5
Synovial biopsy			4
Lateral release of patella			2
Major ligament reconstruction			7

Results

The follow-up period is too short to give any firm results. However, those who have a minimum follow-up of 6 months have had an encouraging outcome to date. Most of the patients have returned to sporting activities in a relatively short period following their injury. The time, naturally, depended on the extent of the injury and the treatment given. However, the time for return to activity was between 2 and 12 weeks for the vast majority of patients, the average time being 6 weeks. However, the time required for athletic prowess to the previous level took longer than the average 6 weeks. The results are classified as follows: (1) good, meaning that the patient had marked improvement in subjective symptomatology, returned to recreational sports, required no medication and returned to full-duty status; (2) fair, meaning that the patient improved subjectively, but objectively has not done well enough to be classified as good; and (3) poor, meaning that the patient continued to have many symptoms, felt that the condition has not improved and does not return to work or sport.

Complications. No major complication was encountered.

Conclusions
The role of arthroscopy of the knee is presented under two headings:

1. Role of arthroscopy in the diagnosis of knee injuries
2. Role of arthroscopy in the management of knee injuries

These are shown in Table 7 and Table 8.

Table 7. The role of arthroscopy in the diagnosis of knee injuries could be summarized as follows:

1. Clinical diagnosis – correct	75 (71%)
2. Clinical diagnosis – incorrect	31 (29%)
3. Unexpected disorders in addition to/or instead of the expected lesions	30 (29%)
4. Unnecessary operations avoided	20 (19%)
5. Repeat arthroscopy helped in making correct diagnosis	3 (3%)
6. Correct diagnosis made with the help of arthroscopy	102 (96%)
7. Prerequisite in cases with appreciable ligamentous injuries	12 (11.4%)

Table 8. The role of arthroscopy in the management of knee injuries could be summarized as follows:

1. Partial meniscectomy (superior to total meniscectomy): open	7 (6.7%)
closed	12 (11.4%)
2. Closed partial meniscectomy gives a better result than open operation	
3. Synovial shelf operations	6 (5.7%)
4. Excision of the infrapatellar fat pad	1 (1%)
5. Removal of a loose body	5 (4.8%)
6. Synovial biopsy	4 (3.8%)
7. Closed lateral release of the patella	2 (2%)
8. Prerequisite to major ligament repair in injured knee: or	7 (6.7%)
conservative treatment of cases with partial ligament injuries	5 (4.8%)

Discussion

The analysis of 447 cases and 191 arthroscopic examinations, which consisted of 105 arthroscopic examinations arising due to sports injuries, confirms that arthroscopy has a place in the management of sports injuries involving the knee joint. Arthroscopy is an excellent diagnostic method for assessing an acutely injured knee joint. In suitable cases, transarthroscopic surgical procedures can be carried out with great benefit to the patient. The role of arthroscopy in the diagnosis of knee injuries is emphasized by incorrect clinical diagnosis in 29% of cases. Over and above this, unnecessary operations were avoided in 19% of cases. It was also gratifying to see that simple surgical procedures carried out by closed technique under arthroscopic control resulted in much reduced morbidity when compared with similar open procedures. Arthroscopy also helped greatly in assessing knee injuries involving damage to the ligaments and planning appropriate treatment for an injury. These included both major ligament reconstruction and also conservative treatment in suitable cases of ligament injuries to the knee joints.

Acknowledgments. We wish to thank the staff of the Records Department and our secretaries for the help in the preparation of the paper. We also wish to thank: Mr. I. Stothers, Consultant Orthopaedic Surgeon, Mr. Irwin and Mr. Milligan of the Department of Medical Illustration, M/S Johnson & Johnson Limited, Farmitalia Carlo Erba Limited, Glaxo Laboratories Limited, Richard Wolf (U.K.) Limited, Syntex Pharmaceuticals Limited, Beecham Research Laboratories Limited and Parke-Davis Research Laboratories for their help in the preparation and presentation of this paper.

References

Casscells SW (1980) The place of arthroscopy in the diagnosis and treatment of internal derangement of the knee; an analysis of 1000 cases. Clin Orthop 151:135–142

Dehaven EK (1980) Diagnosis of acute knee injuries with haemarthrosis. Am J Sports Med 9:9–14

Dehaven EK, Collins HR (1975) Diagnosis of internal derangements of the knee. The role of arthroscopy. J Bone Joint Surg [Am] 57:802–810

Eriksson E, Sebik A (1980) Comparison between transpatellar tendon and lateral approach to the knee during arthroscopy. Am J Sports Med 8:100–105

Fahmy NRM, Noble J (1983) Meniscus pathology and osteoarthritis of the knee. J Bone Joint Surg [Br] 65:24–28

Goodfellow JW (1983) Editorial. Closed meniscectomy. J Bone Joint Surg [Br] 65:373–374

Hardakar TW et al. (1980) Diagnosis and treatment of plica syndrome of the knee. J Bone Joint Surg [Am] 62:221–225

Ireland J, Trickey EL, Stroker DJ (1980) Arthroscopy and arthrography of the knee: critical review. J Bone Joint Surg [Br] 62:3–6

Jackson RW (1976) Partial meniscectomy. J Bone Joint Surg [Br] 58:142–145

McGinty JB (1980) Arthroscopic surgery in sports injuries. Orthop Clin North Am 11(4):787–799

Northmore-Ball MD, Dandy DJ, Jackson RW (1983) Arthroscopic open partial and total meniscectomy. J Bone Joint Surg [Br] 65:400–404

Noyes ER et al. (1980) Arthroscopy in acute traumatic haemarthrosis of the knee: incidence of anterior cruciate tears and other injuries. J Bone Joint Surg [Am] 62:687–695

Patel D (1978) Arthroscopy of the plicae: synovial folds and their significance. Am J Sports Med 6:217–225

Tregonning TAR (1983) Closed partial meniscectomy. Early results for simple tears with mechanical symptoms. J Bone Joint Surg [Br] 65:388–390

Watanabe M, Takeda S, Ilkeuchi H (1969) Atlas of arthroscopy, 2nd edn. Tokyo, Igaku Shoin

Arthroscopy: original experience of a university department which trains young surgeons

J. L. Meystre

Service Universitaire d'Orthopedie et de Traumatologie
Lausanne
Switzerland

The reliability and the technical characteristics of the arthroscopies done in our department were studied.
The particularity of the environment influences the choice of the method of examination; the most reliable method in the hands of inexperienced surgeons is not always the simplest.

Material and methods
Four hundred consecutive arthroscopies, done between 1978 and 1982 by nine different arthroscopists were studied.
In 210 cases, we were able to compare the results with the findings of open knee surgery.

Results
The reliability is generally not very good. 9,4% of the arthroscopies were incomplete. 4% were faulty. The influence of experience is evident. The improvement of the results is continuous, and depends mostly on the choice of the technique.

Discussion
The choice of the optics, of the milieu (liquid or gas), of the anesthesic used, of the premedication, of the position of the patient, the way on introduction of the arthroscope and the palpation are discussed in this particular context.

An adequate method permits an examination which gives good information for diagnosis, even in the hands of inexperienced surgeons.

Knee function after arthroscopic meniscectomy. A prospective study

P. Hamberg and J. Gillquist

Department of Orthopaedic Surgery, University Hospital
S-581 85 Linköping
Sweden

The arthroscopic meniscectomy technique is developing fast thanks to improved instruments, the use of a mechanical leg holder, and the development of endoscopic television. Most studies of arthroscopic meniscectomy have presented a final result without comparison to preoperative knee function. It is important however to relate the results of operation to the preoperative status. This prospective study is concerned with the functional recovery after arthroscopic meniscectomy used as a routine method of treatment.

Material and methods
Operation under arthroscopy was done in 100 consecutive patients, 11 women and 89 men with a lesion of one meniscus. Knee function was assessed before operation and at follow-up with a scoring scale (Lysholm & Gillquist, 1982). A simple printed training programme was given to all patients after operation. In 87 patients follow-up examination was made at hospital. Their muscle strength was measured with a Cybex II isokinetic dynamometer. The remaining 13 patients answered a questionnaire. The mean follow-up time was 10 months (6-17).

Results
Meniscectomy was done in 86 patients with medial meniscus tears (mean age 36 years) and in 14 with lateral tears (mean age 27 years). 67% were treated as out patients and 28% remained in the hospital for only one day. No complications occurred during the follow-up period. There was a highly significant improvement after operation of knee function as measured by the system score in all patients (63 vs. 90 p.). However, in the presence of quadriceps muscle weakness and degenerative joint changes the final score was significantly lower compared to patients not having these changes. After two weeks 85% of the patients were back at work. In elderly patients knee function was generally within the good-excellent group at follow-up and comparable to that in younger patients.

Conclusions
This study supports our opinion that the arthroscopic operating technique facilitates treatment of all meniscus lesions and should whenever possible become the standard method of meniscectomy.

Comparison of the results of open and arthroscopic partial meniscectomy in gas performed by the same surgeons

T. Klemann, M. Hahn and M. Weigert

Dept. of Orthopaedic Surgery, Krankenhaus Am Urban
1000 Berlin
Federal Republic of Germany

Material and methods

Between 1976 and 1983 some 7000 arthroscopies were performed; some 450 of these resulted in an arthroscopic operation. 100 patients suffering from bucket-handle lesions of the medial meniscus who had undergone arthroscopic partial meniscectomy were compared to 100 patients suffering from the same injuries but who had undergone arthrotomy. The same team performed surgery on both patient groups over the same period of time. At least one year went by between the first and the second re-examination. Most of the arthroscopic surgery was performed in gas with N_2O.

Results

Based on the evaluation standards of TAPPER and HOOVER, our findings show that the long-term results of both operation techniques, as far as a partial meniscectomy is concerned, are essentially identical (about 86% excellent and good). The short-term results were significantly more favorable as far as hospitalization, return to work and resumption of sports activities as well as minor subjective discomfort was concerned. Thus, by means of arthroscopic operating techniques, the average hospitalization of two weeks was reduced to three days. On the average patients returned to work within 12 days and and resumed sports activities within 30 days.

Discussion

The results confirm that arthroscopic meniscectomy is as effective as open surgery in view of the long-term results. With regard to rapid convalescence and rehabilitation as well as in the interest of an effective cost reduction, it is considerably superior to open surgery. Arthroscopic partial meniscectomies in gas offer advantages, because over all vision is better and fragments do not float as they do in liquid.

Summary

The results of 100 arthroscopic partial meniscectomies were compared with 100 arthrotomies. The long-term results are essentially identical for both methods. In regard to convalescence, rehabilitation and cost-reduction, arthroscopic surgery is superior. Operations in gas offer advantages.

Arthroscopic failures: complications and prevention. Second time arthroscopic evaluation: A retrospective study

J. L. Mason, Jr.

Associate Professor of Orthopaedic Surgery
Medical University of South Carolina
Florence, SC
USA

A retrospective study was performed on 589 consecutive arthroscopic procedures performed by one surgeon. This encompassed an 18-month period from January 1977 up to and including June 1978. Seventy-four of these patients had a second arthroscopic procedure performed – 12.5% of the total number.

Of these procedures, 17 were planned. Ten of these cases were infectious arthritis and secondary lavage was performed. Seven of the 17 were second-stage synovectomies. The second staging had been planned at the primary procedure. Of these four had rheumatoid arthritis, two had villonodularsynovitis and one had psoriatic arthritis. All were felt to have complete primary procedures.

Therefore, 57 of the 589 or 9.6% had an unplanned secondary arthroscopic procedure. Eleven patients had a secondary injury to the knee that was thought to be the causative agent requiring another arthroscopy. Excluding planned secondary procedures and secondary injuries requiring another arthroscopy, 46 patients or 7.8% had a second arthroscopic procedure without further insult or injury to the involved joint. These were felt to represent operative failures.

During the 18-month period, many of the cases were involved degenerative arthritis and arthroscopic debridement was performed. Judgment of failure of the primary arthroscopic procedures and subsequent total joint replacement, etc. would be the subject of another paper. These cases only involve those knees where a second arthroscopic procedure was performed.

Early failures. Thirty-six patients or 6.1% of the total had a second arthroscopic procedure in less than 6 months. These were felt to represent early failures. The primary cause of failure was felt to be: (a) chondromalacia (20), (b) incomplete or incorrect removal of tears of the medial meniscus (4), (c) incomplete or inadequate removal of tears of the lateral meniscus (5), (d) inadequate partial removal of medial and lateral menisci (3), (e) missed loose body (1), (f) missed meniscal tears (3) and (g) missed medial plica (1).

Late failures. A second arthroscopic procedure was performed in the period from 12 to 18 months and an attempt to discover the primary cause of failure was made. This involved ten patients. All of these patients had degenerative joint disease and had chondromalacia, as well as medial and/or lateral compartment involvement. At the second arthroscopic procedure all of these patients were felt to have either no improvement from the primary procedure or had developed further progression of disease. Six of these ten patients later had total joint replacement. It must be reemphasized that many other of the degenerative knees in the 589 consecutive patients subsequently required total joint replacement as a secondary procedure due to failure of the primary procedure.

Chondromalacia. Twenty out of 36 of the patients requiring second arthroscopy within 6 months had chondromalacia. The primary operative procedure consisted of shaving using the intra-articular shaver and curettes and hand instruments (knives, curettes and punch forceps). The most striking correlation of continued pain was involvement of the degenerative changes in the femoral groove. Reshaving was done at the second procedure. Fourteen of the 20 patients were felt to be unimproved by the second procedure. In the six patients that were significantly improved by the second shave the trimming of the parapatella synovium was felt to correlate with the improvement in their symptoms.

Failed lateral release (5/36). In five of the procedures, the release was performed from the inside out. Three of the patients were felt to have had an inadequate superior release specifically at the superior lateral edge of the patella, i.e. incomplete release of the vastus lateralis at the superior lateral pole and inadequate superior extension of the cut. One patient was found to have an inadequate inferior release of the lateral retinaculum. One patient had a lateral flap impingement or a "pseudoshelf" due to the retinacular incision being too far removed from the patella. All five patients were released using a 25-mm incision 25 mm below the superolateral edge of the patella and release was performed through a semi-open procedure. All five secondary procedures were felt to be successful.

Inadequate removal of torn medial meniscus (4/36). Of these cases one was found to have an unrecognized cruciate tear from what was previously thought to be a double bucket torn meniscus and a third loose fragment was found at the second procedure. Another case had an unrecognized peripheral rim tear in the posterior third. Two of the patients were felt to have had a blunt cut of the middle third of the medial meniscus that proved painful after the first procedure. Both of these cases had triangulation of the remaining middle third rim and balancing of the meniscus and their symptoms were relieved.

Inadequate lateral meniscal removal (5/36). One patient was felt to have a blunt middle third cut and triangulation of the remaining meniscal stump relieved the symptoms. One patient had removal of an inferior flap of the posterior lateral meniscus and superior meniscus was unstable. Removal of the superior flap relieved the patient's symptoms. One patient had inadequate removal of a discoid meniscus; the secondary procedure involved triangulation and creation of a smaller balanced rim. Two of the five patients had inadequate removal of central radial tears of the lateral meniscus. The *T* nature of the meniscal fracture was not appreciated. Subsequent removal of both anterior and posterior portions of the central portion of the lateral meniscus relieved the patient's symptoms. These cases have suggested removal of larger portions of the lateral meniscus in radial tears.

Incomplete removal of both medial and lateral menisci (3/36). Three of the patients had degenerative tears of both menisci with degenerative joint disease. Further removal of the degenerated menisci relieved the symptoms in two of the three; while one got no relief from the second procedure.

Metabolic arthritis (5/36). Three patients with torn menisci had inactive gout. All three developed marked postoperative synovitis. Secondarily lavage and lysis of adhesions were carried out. Secondary lavage was performed in all three and lysis of adhesions in two. All three patients had prolonged convalescence that required intensive physical therapy. Marked haemarthrosis occurred in two other patients, both following synovectomies, one for rheumatoid arthritis and one for villonodularsynovitis. Both responded well to secondary lavage and both patients then resumed a normal postoperative course.

Degenerative joint disease. The primary purpose of this paper is to identify what were felt to be primary causes of failures as seen at the second arthroscopic procedure. A significant number of the 589 cases had marked significant degenerative joint disease. A more detailed study of these cases is being performed and will be the subject of a later paper. However, 18 of the 46 patients that had secondary procedures did afford some general impressions. In isolated chondrolesions associated with meniscal tears, removal of the torn meniscus and trimming of the defect afforded relief of acute pain of sharp catching pain and to a lesser degree relieved some of the aching arthritic pain. Shaving and curettage of smaller localized lesions did afford good healing with fibrocartilage. Generalized degenerative changes of both compartments did not respond well to wide area chondrobrasion in this author's hands. There was significant relief of sharp pain in removal of cartilaginous flaps. Removal of the "mushroom" spur on or near the anterior tibia spine caused significant pain relief. Removal of patella spurs and medially, laterally and inferiorly afforded the same relief as attempts at removal of the corresponding femoral spurs as well. Attempts at removal of femoral peripheral spurs were disappointing with regard to results and to an adequate recovery.

Synovectomies (3/36). Overly aggressive removal of the anterolateral synovium was complicated by creation of an unstable anterior horn of the lateral meniscus. The second procedure of removal of partial anterolateral meniscectomy and balancing of the meniscus afforted good relief. In the author's zeal for removal of the anterior synovium, particularly in the lateral compartment, it is felt that other cases have, also, had the creation of an unstable anterior horn of the lateral meniscus.

Conclusions. Of 589 consecutive arthroscopic procedures, 74 performed during an 18-month period, 74 patients had separate arthroscopic procedures of the same knee. Seventeen procedures were planned as part of the author's protocol. Eleven patients had a second injury to the same knee, which was felt to be the causative agent requiring a second arthroscopy. The remaining 46 patients were felt to represent operative failures. Thirty-six of the 46 required a second arthroscopic procedure within 6 months. Twenty of the 36 had significant chondromalacia, 14 of which twenty received little or no relief from the second procedure. Inadequate lateral release in five patients was corrected by a semi-open secondary release. Incomplete and inadequate removal of tears of the medial meniscus was present in four and inadequate removal of the lateral meniscus was present in five, with three patients having inadequate removal of both menisci.

Of the late failures, all were related to chondromalacia and degenerative joint disease.

Five patients with metabolic arthritis required unplanned secondary procedures. Two had major haemarthrosis following synovectomy and required secondary lavage. Three of the patients had inactive gout that was exacerbated by the primary procedure and required secondary lavage and lysis of adhesions. All three had prolonged disability and required intensive physical therapy. Some knees with moderate to moderately severe degenerative joint disease can benefit from partial removal of torn menisci and removal of spurs.

Over-aggressive removal of the synovium particularly in the anterolateral joint can create peripheral meniscal instability.

Cartilaginous lesions following medial arthroscopic meniscectomy

E. Lais, P. Hertel and A. Georgoulis

Abteilung Unfallchirurgie, Rudolf-Virchow-Krankenhaus
Augustenburger Platz 1, D-1000 Berlin 65
Federal Republic of Germany

Introduction

Arthroscopic resections of menisci are performed in increasing numbers. The advantages of this kind of operation with less morbidity are known. We have carried out an experimental study on iatrogenic cartilaginous lesions due to arthroscopic subtotal meniscectomy. The results were established by macroscopic and microscopic methods.

Material and methods

We have practised subtotal medial meniscectomy using arthroscopy using exclusively small knives, fixing the leg with a simple device. We used the transligamentous access as described by Gillquist. The optical system was initially introduced into the posterior recessus between the medial condylus and the posterior ligamentum cruciatum. After reaching a maximal filling of the knee joint and palpating the optimal perforation point, the knife was introduced dorsomedially into the posterior recessus (Figure 1). We cut the cornu posterius near the capsula. Only in rare cases did we have to recut the end of the cornu posterius in the medial front position. A second incision was made from the anterolateral access in order to loosen the cornu anterius. We continued to mobilize the complete medial meniscus connecting the two initial cuts. In the last step we worked the meniscus into the joint using the forceps we introduced laterally. Finally we extracted the resected meniscus through a widened incision.

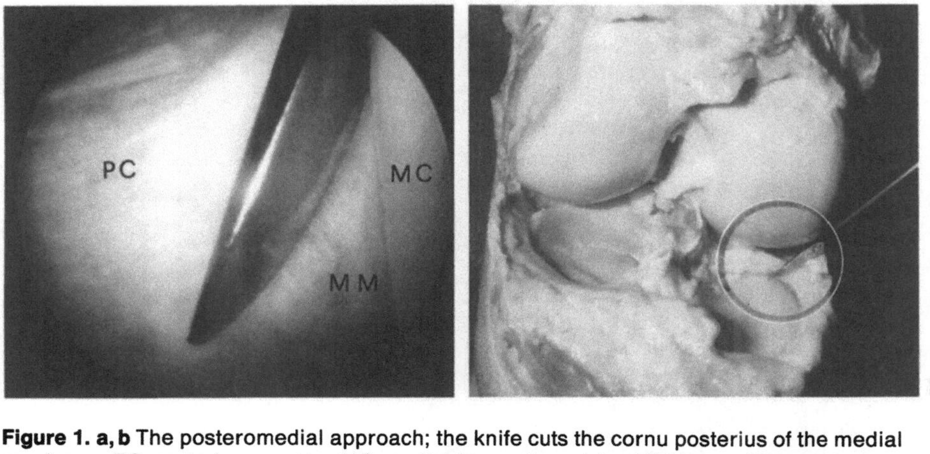

a b

Figure 1. a, b The posteromedial approach; the knife cuts the cornu posterius of the medial meniscus. *PC*, posterior capsule; *MC*, medial femoral condyle; *MM*, base of the cornu posterius of the medial meniscus

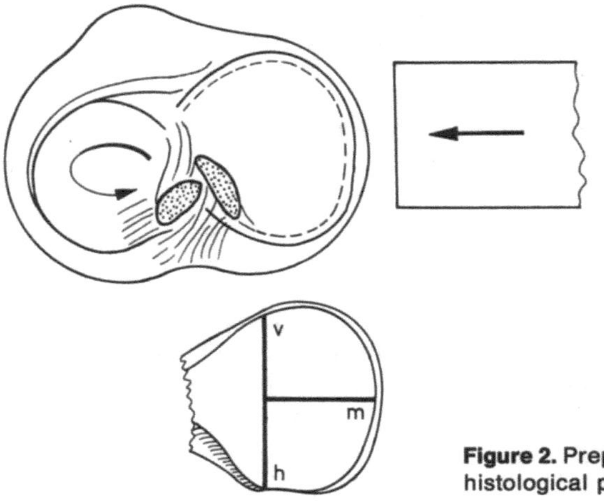

Figure 2. Preparation of the tibial plateau for the histological procedure

In order to evaluate the cartilaginous damage we produced the knee joint was opened and the medial joint surface was examined (Figure 3). The first 11 operations were analyzed from a macroscopic point of view. We only found small cuts which were difficult to see with the exception of one single-edge lesion. To improve the visibility of the damage we coloured the cartilaginous surface blue. By cutting fine slices we were able to evaluate the depth of the injuries. The ten other cases underwent microscopic examination. The tibial plateau was separated and after decalcification the division of the material was made in the form of a *T* and we made microscopic cuts (Figure 2). Using this procedure we were able to demonstrate lesions below all parts of the meniscus (cornu anterius medial part, cornu posterius). Thus we obtained 30 histological series with over ten corpses.

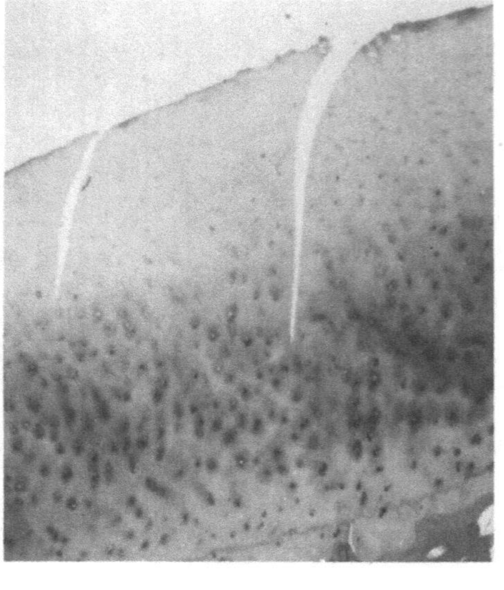

Figure 3. Incision in the cartilage of the tibial plateau

Results
In the first series we found one edge lesion (mentioned above), two injuries of medium depth and five superficial ones. In three cases no injuries at all were found. In the second series using histological methods we found 31 cutting lines of which 23 were limited to the superficialis thirds of the cartilage. Six cuts penetrated half the thickness and only two reached the subchondral bone. The angles of the cuts were almost all perpendicular, varying from 75° to 90° to the basal zone with one exception.

Conclusion
In over 21 cases of arthroscopic subtotal meniscectomy, in 13 cases we found only superficial lesions or no lesions at all. Five times we found damage which was limited to the middle of the chondros and only in three cases did the cuts penetrate to the subchondral bone.

Complications of arthroscopy

G. Saillant, J. P. Benazet and R. Roy-Camille

Sce d'Orthopédie, 83 Boulevard de l'hospital
F-75000 Paris
France

This study refers to a survey concerning 39 French operators who effected 25 433 arthroscopies.
44% were for diagnostic arthroscopy and 56% for operative arthroscopy. Arthroscopy was done with either local, loco-regional or general anesthesia (22 629 cases).

Results
The authors first reviewed the complications due to the type of anesthesia, particularly those, exceptional but severe (10 of 22 629 cases) occurring under general anesthesia and then reviewed the proper complications of arthroscopy: iatrogenic lesions of the cartilage, breaking of instruments (118 cases), vascular injuries, neurologic complications and also 29 cases of hematoma, burn or ligamentary injury reported after setting the leg in a knee support.
Post-operative swelling of variable causes led to a new arthroscopy in 24 cases and to an explorative arthrotomy in 16 cases.
Cutaneous complications: 46 cases of aseptic fistula and 5 of cutaneous necrosis, could be avoided easily.
The septic arthritis observed in 10 cases, always of staphylococcic origin, require strict aseptic measures.

Discussion
This catalogue of complications should not make them appear inexcusable but only point out that the indication of this rather invasive examination must be very carefully established. Although this study has no statistical value because most operators do not readily expose the complications and failures they get, it has the advantage, however, to present a general review of the complications encountered in a series of 25 000 cases.

Arthroscopy of children's knee-joints: its indication and results

A. S. Behfar and H. J. Refior

Orthopädische Klinik der Medizinischen Hochschule
3000 Hannover
Federal Republic of Germany

The arthroscopy of childrens' knee-joints can be termed as an essential method of diagnosis, which nowadays is one of many diagnostic possibilities that cannot be done without.
This report deals with 20 diagnostic arthroscopies of 19 children who at time of investigation were 5 to 14 years of age. The average age being about 12 years.

The arthroscopic investigations were carried out in all cases in a gas medium. For the arthroscopy both 4 mm optics and 2,7 mm optics were used.

The diagnosis in 9 cases was fixed at the moment of hospital entry. 11 further knee-joints were examined due to uncertain knee-joint complaints. The indication for arthroscopy was given in these cases due to other nonproductive measures. Each case will be treated in consideration of the individual indication. In those cases in which the diagnosis was clear at the time of hospital entry, the indication for arthroscopy served to establish further therapeutic measures. For these cases too, the indication will be developed specific to the individual illness.

Concerning the unspecified knee complaints, following diseases could be determined: primary synovitis 4 x, meniscus tear 3 x, osteochondral fracture 2 x, loose bodies 1 x and one tear of synovialis as a result of patellar dislocation.

In those cases with certain diagnosis, it was a matter of osteochondritis dissecans and chondropathia patellae.

Here the operative strategy was determined by using the arthroscopic results

The individual treatment each dependent on the diagnosis will be evaluated individually.

Our arthroscopic indication will be compared with references from the literature, whereby the evaluation of arthroscopy of childrens' knee-joints will be considered particularly.

The medial shelf: an anatomical, clinical and pathological study

J. Older, R. Hanspal and T. Cardoso

Department of Orthopaedic Surgery, Royal Surrey County Hospital
Guildford, Surrey
England

Introduction

It was not widely recognized until arthroscopy became a routine procedure that the medial synovial plica could be a cause of discomfort and disability. Many surgeons still doubt its existence as a pathological entity, and the purpose of this study was to investigate the anatomical, clinical and pathological features of the medial synovial shelf.

Anatomy

Synovial folds, representing embryological remnants in the development of the synovial cavity of the knee, are normal structures. One hundred and fifteen cadaveric knees in a consecutive series of Caucasian adults were dissected to study the anatomy of the four synovial folds best named according to their relationship to the patella (Figure 1).

The suprapatellar plica was found to be the commonest synovial fold, present in 65% of knees. The infrapatellar plica, often known as the ligamentum mucosum, was present in just over half the knees examined. Only one knee was found to have a lateral plica akin to the medial fold (Table 1).

The medial synovial fold lies in the coronal plane on the medial wall of the joint. It arises from the medial fringe of the infrapatellar fat pad (see Figure 2) and runs upwards towards the under surface of the medial end of the superior plica.

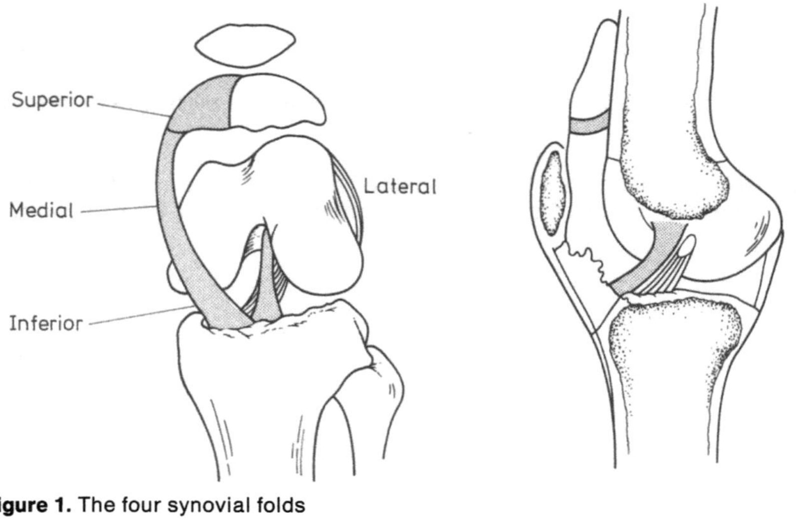

Figure 1. The four synovial folds

Table 1. Incidence of various intra-articular synovial plica in 115 cadaveric knees

Suprapatellar	75	65%
Infrapatellar	60	52%
Medial	47	41%
Lateral	1	1%

Table 2. Incidence of different types of medial plica in 47 cadaveric knees

Type A	10	21%
Type B	29	62%
Type C	8	17%
Type D	–	–

Type A, a cord-like elevation in the synovial wall which can be traced to the inferior fat pad; type B, a shelf-like appearance but not wide enough to cover the articular surface of the medial femoral condyle; type C, a large shelf-like appearance that covers the articular surface of the medial femoral condyle; type D, a special variation in which there is a double insertion in the medial wall

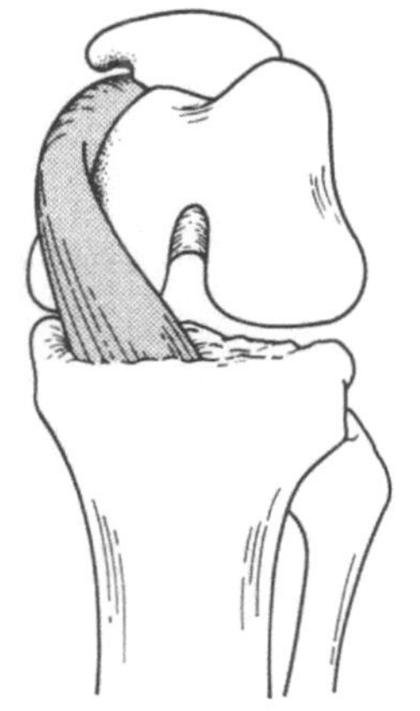

Figure 2. The medial synovial fold

It has had many different names but is commonly known as the "medial shelf" because its arthroscopic appearance is that of a pale, sharp-edged membrane that lies in the horizontal plane. Of the 115 knees dissected, a medial plica was present in 47 knees, an incidence of 41%. It was present bilaterally in 88% of cases and the sex incidence was equal.

Using Iino's [1] classification of the medial plica in our cadaveric dissection, the incidence of the four different types is shown in Table 2. Type A and most of type B should never cause symptoms, but if type C becomes thickened and fibrotic, it may produce symptoms by impinging against the medial femoral condyle.

Clinical study

In a 2-year period starting in 1981, a pathological medial shelf was diagnosed in 65 knees in 50 patients. Thirty-six were in men and 29 in women, between 12 and 57 years with a greater incidence in the younger age group (Figure 3).

By definition, these were patients with anterior joint pain for which no other cause could be diagnosed, and 3–6 months of conservative management had brought no relief. Arthroscopy showed a well-formed, large fibrotic medial shelf which on flexion of the knee was found to impinge against the medial femoral condyle.

The commonest presenting feature was anterior joint pain, with 77% having symptoms worsened by exercise. A history of past injury was present in just

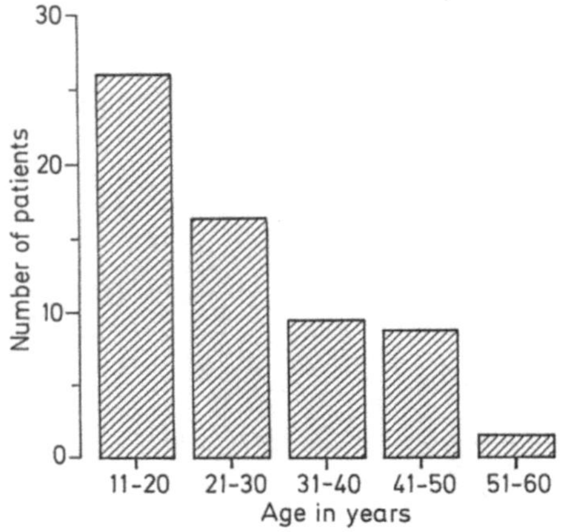

Figure 3. Age incidence of the medial shelf

over a half, and nearly a third complained of a click. In the majority of patients there were few signs on clinical examination, although sometimes medial parapatellar tenderness was present. The commonest prearthroscopic diagnosis was chondromalacia patellae and the pathological medial shelf syndrome was diagnosed in only 13 knees – probably due to the surgeon's own early scepticism.

The pathological medial shelf was treated arthroscopically by either simple division or excision by the same surgeon (J. O.). The arthroscope was introduced through the superolateral approach and the operating instruments through anterolateral and mid-lateral portals.

All patients were independently reviewed by one of the authors (R. H.). The follow-up ranged from 6 to 30 months, with an average follow-up of 16 months. The results are shown in Table 3.

Twenty-six knees were totally asymptomatic and were classed as "excellent". A further 20 knees had marked improvement. Their only symptom was the odd occasional twinge of pain, which was never severe enough to interfere with their work, pastime or sport and the symptoms were often related to changes in the weather. These were classed as "very good". Seventy-one per cent were seen to have an excellent or very good result.

Ten patients had a definite improvement but still had some troublesome symptoms especially on exertion. Five knees remained unchanged. This was

Table 3. Results of arthroscopic surgery for pathological medial shelf

Excellent	Asymptomatic	26
Very good	Great improvement – occasional minimal symptoms	20
Fair	Definite relief – occasional troublesome symptoms	10
Unsatisfactory	Minimal improvement	3
	No change	5
	Worse	1

actually in three patients, two of them with bilateral lesions. Both relapsed after initial improvement. One was a lady of 57 years with considerable damage to the articular cartilage and the second was a 16-year-old boy whose operation was technically difficult. He also had evidence of fibrillation of the articular cartilage. The one patient who was worse after her operation was later diagnosed to have fat pad impingement syndrome that was successfully treated by excision.

Best results were obtained in those cases which showed no damage to the articular cartilage, and the results following excision of the medial shelf were better than those following simple division.

Histology

Thirty-three of the excised specimens that were arthroscopically excised were studied histologically. In two-thirds of them, histological study showed plenty of fibrous tissue containing elastic fibres and dense collagen (Figure 4). Eleven specimens showed evidence of changes much like early osteoarthrosis with villous hypertrophy, subsynovial fibrosis, sometimes even calcification and ossification. Not surprisingly, the former group did better after surgery (Figure 5).

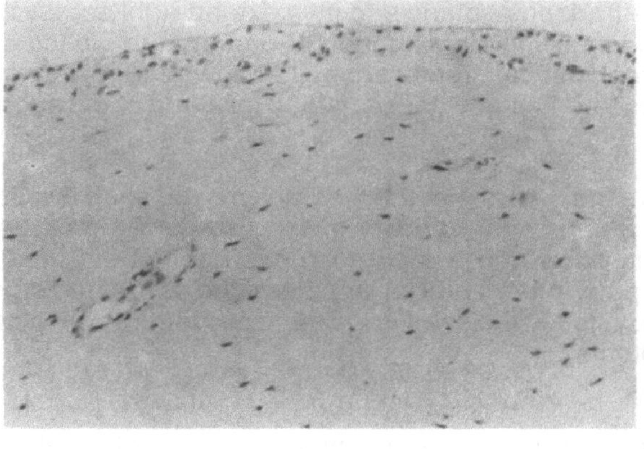

Figure 4. Fibrous tissue containing elastic fibres and dense collagen

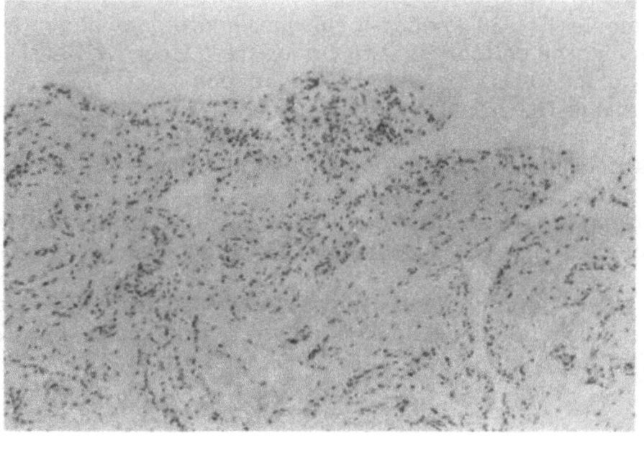

Figure 5. Villous hypertrophy with subsynovial fibrosis

Discussion

The classification of synovial folds of the knee was bedevilled by a confusion of terminology in early publications. Pidhorz [2] gave Morris [3] the credit for the first description of two synovial folds (plica alaris) in 1879. Twenty years later, Testut [2] observed a large semilunar fold between the patella and the medial condyle which he considered different from the plica alaris of Morris, and in 1914 Vallois [4] stressed the frequency of such structures among primates.

It is Iino [1, 5], however, who is usually credited with the first accurate description of the medial synovial shelf, although his description and classification are based on the work of Mayeda [6] in 1918.

In our study, we found some sort of medial shelf in 41% of cadaveric knees, with a complete shelf in 17%. This is identical to the incidence observed by Joyce et al. [7] in their recent anatomical report of an examination of nearly 500 cadaveric knees. We would agree with these workers that in knees with a complete type C medial plica, as flexion of the joint was increased the plica exerted more pressure on the articular surface and usually slid off with a snap to the medial side of the joint.

The medial shelf should not be confused with the suprapatellar plica, which lies above the patella in the horizontal plane and may extend right across the joint to divide it into two compartments. Although at one time this plica did not appear to have any great clinical significance, it is now recognized that it may afford refuge for loose bodies and cause painful swelling of the suprapatellar pouch [8].

The arthroscope has shown the cynics that the medial synovial shelf is a definite anatomical entity. Trauma may convert this remnant of embryonic synovial fold into a fibrotic bowstring, which impinges against the medial femoral condyle, causing pain in the anterior aspect of the joint. This study shows that arthroscopic excision of the shelf is a simple procedure which can dramatically relieve symptoms.

References

1. Sakakibara J (1976) Arthroscopic study on Iino's band (plica synovialis mediopatellaris). J Jpn Orthop Assoc 50:513–522
2. Pidhorz L, Raimbeau G, Laumonier F (1980) Pseudo-menisque fémoro-patellaire interne (ou hypertrophie de l'aileron interne de Morris). Ann Orthop de l'Ouest 12:37–40
3. Morris H (1879) The anatomy of the joints of man. Churchill, London
4. Vallois H (1914) Etude anatomique de l'articulation du genou chez les primates. Thesis, Montpellier
5. Iino S (1939) Normal arthroscopic findings of the knee joint in adult cadavers. J Jpn Orthop Assoc 14:467–523
6. Mayeda T (1918) Über das strangartige Gebilde in der Kniegelenkhöhle (chorda cavi articularis genu). Communications from the Medical Faculty of the Imperial University of Tokyo 21:507–553
7. Joyce J, Harty M, Tetzlaff J (1984) Surgery of the synovial folds. In: Casscells SW (ed) Arthroscopy: diagnosis and surgical practice. Lea and Febiger, Philadelphia, chap 12
8. Ross K, Glasgow M (1984) The supra-patellar plica. J Bone Joint Surg [Br] 66:280

The medial shelf of the knee: a follow-up study

W. Klein

Orthopaedic Department University Clinic Düsseldorf
4000 Düsseldorf
Federal Republic of Germany

After a publication in 1979 on Plica Synovialis Mediopatellaris a review of 1328 arthroscopies from 1978 onwards has been done at the Orthopaedic Department of the University Clinic Düsseldorf. One hundred and eighty knees with medial shelf of the knee were found. Forty three patients were treated by arthroscopic surgery. Plica excision alone was carried out in 17 knees. Twenty nine times multiple intra-articular surgery like patella shaving, lateral release, meniscectomy or local synovectomy have been performed in addition to plica excision. A shelf alone was present in 21.1%. Additional lesion like chondromalacia of the patella occurred in 38.8%. Control of biopsy material and tissue specimen from arthroscopic surgery revealed shelf fibrosis in 15.5% of the 180 knees with plica synovialis mediopatellaris. The best results were obtained in those patients with the medial shelf as the only abnormality in the knee joint. The reason for the relatively high amount of unsatisfactory results in knees with multiple lesion and medial shelf excision in caused by overlap of the other lesions accompanied by the Plica Synovialis Mediopatellaris. Under the impression of the results of the follow-up study a detailed proposal as indication for plica excision is discussed.

Menisci

Classification of meniscal tears: therapeutic implications

J. Y. Dupont

Clinique du Marais
11 bis rue Barbette, F-75003 Paris
France

Both menisci can be so described: two faces, superior and inferior; two horns, anterior and posterior, which are the tibial attachments; two edges, peripheral and central; and three segments, anterior, middle, posterior. Meniscal tears can occur in any part of the meniscal tissue. They can be simple and follow one of the three planes of space: vertical longitudinal, radial and horizontal. Tears can also be complex and combine two or more "simple ruptures". A flap tear can result from the combination of a radial and a horizontal tear.

The vascularized portion of both menisci, according to Arnoczy, represents the peripheral one-fourth of their fibrocartilaginous tissue. It is likely that, in certain conditions, blood vessels can invade the rest of the meniscus, to the free edge.

Clinical research has shown that, 10–30 years after a "traditional" subtotal or total meniscectomy, 20%–40% of the patients suffer from persistent pain, due to cartilaginous problems. The critical factors are:

1. Late diagnosis leading to late treatment
2. Lateral meniscal meniscectomies
3. Associated anterior cruciate ligament (ACL) insufficiency
4. Association of a varus deformity with a medial meniscectomy or a lateral meniscectomy on a valgus deformity
5. Total meniscectomies, compared with partial resection
6. Incomplete meniscectomies with a tear remaining on the portion left in place

Some of these factors were already advocated in 1909 by Jones, and in the late 1800 Anendale attempted to suture menisci. The inability to recognize precisely the type of tears led Smilie and others to promote total meniscectomy as the only treatment.

The end point of all these conditions is a post-traumatic osteoarthrosis, with abnormal X-rays described well by Fairbanks in 1948.

In 1984, diagnostic and therapeutic arthroscopy made possible an entirely different conception of meniscal pathology and treatment. It can be a suture, of a partial or total meniscectomy. Some tears need no treatment. Meniscal preservation is now a goal, with attempts to remove the patients' symptoms without jeopardizing the long-term results with chondral damage. Total meniscectomies are thus performed when they appear to be the only possible treatment.

Meniscal tears can always be separated into five categories:

1. Vertical longitudinal, complete or incomplete; the rupture can pass through the capsule, in the vascular or the avascular portion of the meniscus
2. Radial or oblique (parrot-beak tear)
3. Horizontal
4. Flap tear
5. Complex tear with two or more of the preceding types. Bucket handle tears are part of the vertical ruptures.

We tried to evaluate their span, based upon an arthroscopic prospective study in 300 medial and 212 lateral meniscal tears. All were treated between June 1980 and September 1982, with a follow-up from 18 to 42 months.

We excluded from these patients those who had a complete degenerative meniscus. This means for us an irregular, often yellow meniscus, in which no tear is palpated. The chondral lesions are always important, and the meniscus deserves no treatment at all, because symptoms are related to chondral, but not meniscal, lesions. We also decided to describe the lesions seen without relating them to pathogenesis, which means we avoided the terms "traumatic" and "degenerative" tears.

The 300 medial meniscal lesions were: 48 bucket handle tears; 12 peripheral detachments; 32 incomplete vertical tears, most of which were in the vascular part; 55 complete vertical ruptures, in the same part in two-thirds; 68 complex tears, including 18 bucket handles with a second tear on the peripheral part; 42 flap tears; and 43 horizontal tears and radial tears (23 and 20) placed together because they share the same symptoms and the same pathological conditions.

Vertical and "associated" tears finally represent 60% of the total. In most of the complex tears a vertical component can also be found. If many patients describe a history of trauma, or a knee sprain, 31 advocated a direct impact on the joint, and 88 described a picture of spontaneous and progressive mechanical pain. Pain is the most frequent complaint, involving 93% of the patients. It is the only symptom in 12%, and its location is posterior or lateral in 10%, without any associated lateral lesions. Locking occurred in 23%. Physical examination showed positive meniscal tests in 72%. Cabot's test was the most reliable, positive in 53%; 33% had restricted motion of the knee, flexion limited as often as extension. Varus deformity was met in 43% of males and 23% of females. Valgus deformity was met in 2% of males and 22% of females. Associated intra-articular lesions are important to notice, because of their influence on therapeutic indications. One hundred and six patients had an abnormal ACL, with 62 also having a lateral meniscus tears; 20 had a lateral meniscus tear with a normal ACL; 58 had mild to severe (only 12) chondral damage in the medial compartment. Other lesions were loose bodies, chondromalacia patellae, lateral chondral lesions or noticeable medial plicae.

We tried to correlate these different parameters with the types of tears. There is no strict relationship between the meniscal lesion and its occurrence: 42%

of the radial and horizontal tears are post-traumatic; 29% of the vertical tears are "spontaneous". Traumas and lesions after squatting show more vertical tears. When no trauma is present, radial and horizontal tears are 1.5 times more frequent. In the case of chronic laxity with abnormal ACL, vertical tears are 2.5 times more frequent. They are located in the vascular part of the meniscus in 75%.

The analysis of the lateral meniscus tears shows little difference. Symptoms, physical examination and associated lesions are quite comparable. The main difference is that, when an ACL tear is present, the lateral meniscal tear is symptom less in more than 50%.

The rupture types span is also different, as shown in our 212 cases: 68 complex tears, 55 vertical, 26 flap tears, 25 horizontal and 23 radial, and 15 bucket handle tears only.

Each time a meniscal suture was performed on an instable knee, a ligament reconstruction was also carried out, so as to protect the suture, as advocated by De Haven. Immediate weight-bearing was allowed, and a cylinder cast kept on for 3 weeks.

All our patients were clinically followed, to the disappearance of their symptoms. Those who were not symptom free after a reasonable survey had a control arthroscopy, sometimes an arthrography for whose who were reluctant.

We do not want to discuss here the results of partial meniscectomies or chronic meniscal tear sutures, but only try to evaluate whether the exact recognition of the type of tear is a reliable guide for therapeutic indications. Technical details such as the usefulness of refreshing the capsule in meniscal sutures will thus not be discussed.

Here are our results, in terms of reoperation by arthroscopy. A symptomatic "rupture at second look" means failure of the indication or realization of the treatment, which means an incomplete meniscectomy.

Of the 300 medial meniscal tears: 33 were sutured and 2 sutures failed. These menisci had to be removed after 6 and 14 months. Fifteen received no treatment. One patient had to be reoperated on 4 months later and was healed by a partial meniscectomy. Thirty-six had a total arthroscopic meniscectomy. None was reoperated on. A partial arthroscopic meniscectomy was given to 214. Three needed a further meniscectomy and then healed. All of them had a vertical tear on the posterior part of the meniscus which was not diagnosed during the first procedure. Two of them initially had a bucket handle tear; the last one had a posterior vertical tear.

Of the 212 lateral meniscus tears: 18 were sutured, with no failure; 32 had no treatment and none was reoperated on; 45 had a total meniscectomy of which one needed a second arthroscopy, and a symptomatic meniscal remnant was discovered, which was successfully removed arthroscopically.

Eighteen out of the 51 sutures had a control arthroscopy; four had an arthogram, showing in all cases except the two failures a normal meniscus with perfect healing.

The main difference we met was in the location of these tears, which involve the anterior third of the meniscus in 15% and the popliteus hiatus region in 70%. This is obviously the weakest part of the lateral meniscus and therefore the most frequent site of rupture.

Vertical tears, as for the medial meniscus, are 2.5 times more frequent when the ACL is torn. Less than 50% are reparable.

We excluded from this study tears on a discoid meniscus. Cysts associated with a meniscal tear did not change our indications, because we noticed that after an arthroscopic meniscectomy, the cyst always disappeared without any specific treatment.

Post-traumatic haemarthrosis is frequently related to a torn anterior cruciate, with 65% of associated meniscal tears. They are reparable in 65%, but we found that only 10% are capsular detachments, the remainder being in the vascular part of the menisci.

Our indications can be summarized as follows:

1. Vertical tears were treated by partial meniscectomy, but when a ligamentous problem was associated, the meniscus was sutured as often as possible.
2. Complex and horizontal tears were treated by partial meniscectomy each time a good meniscal remnant could be left in place, but in other cases the meniscus had to be totally removed.
3. Flap tears, radial tears and bucket handle tears were always treated by partial meniscectomy, except two bucket handle tears which were sutured.

Strategics lead to meniscal economy, but tactics in partial meniscectomies vary greatly, according to the type of ruptures. Two or three, sometimes more, portals are used, and there are at least eight or ten different ways of removing a bucket handle tear. The important thing is to be sure at the end of the procedure to have treated the whole lesion and not have left a rupture on the meniscal remnant. When a total meniscectomy is needed, it is better for the final result, and the patient's relief, to perform it by an arthrotomy, than make an arthroscopic attempt, and leave in the joint a symptomatic part of meniscal tissue. The goal is to remove the lesion totally,and the use of the probe is mandatory throughout the procedure.

These results can be considered as satisfying, though our follow-up is too short. The precise description of the meniscal tears seems to be a valuable guide for therapeutic indications. Many questions are still to be answered.

Are ruptures in the avascular part reparable? These lesions are difficult to operate through an arthrotomy, and in most of the cases a partial meniscectomy on such a tear should not lead to osteoarthritis. We have very few cases where such attempts were made, mainly on the lateral meniscus. The peripheral portion of the meniscus is avascular, as stated by microanatomical studies. Arthroscopic controls could show a perfect healing 4 months later, but we need more examples.

Endoscopic sutures are now possible. These techniques are still not mature, and their exact possibilities and limits need to be defined. Their main interest is probably to allow repairs where just meniscectomies were the only treatment up to now.

What are the exact relations between lesions and symptoms? Do we remove too many menisci, just because we now see lesions which were hardly visible through an arthrotomy? The proportion of lateral meniscal tears met in ACL insufficiency is obviously much lower when the joint is checked by medial arthrotomy than by arthroscopy. Most of these tears are symptom free. Which tears can we leave in place, which will not aggravate if the knee is stabilized? The incidence of reoperations for incomplete ruptures that were not treated is very low. Further studies with longer follow-up are needed.

Are cartilage lesions associated with symptomatic meniscal ruptures? Probably not, as long as they do not involve the whole weight-bearing surface, and do not appear on X-rays with a narrowing of the articular space. Do they require an endoscopic treatment? Probably not, except for cartilage flaps which are likely to produce mechanical disorders and symptoms. The decision is often difficult because meniscal and cartilaginous lesions can produce the same symptoms. The indications for cartilage surface surgery are likely to be minimal, anyway.

Finally, we can say that arthroscopy is not only the best way to send a patient back to work or sports after meniscus surgery. It is also a method for preserving the future of joints, and a very useful research tool.

The repair of meniscus lesions by synovial flaps: experimental study

C. Fabbriciani, A. Schiavone-Panni and M. Oransky

Clinica Ortopedica dell'Università Cattolica S. Cuore
Roma
Italy

Introduction

The role played by the meniscus in the mobility of the knee is known to be of the greatest importance: it acts as a shock absorber [6, 16], it helps the joint lubrication [17] and the distribution of the synovial fluid [20] and finally it enhances the knee stability through its action on its complex rotation mechanisms [5, 14].

Furthermore many reports emphasize the high percentage of poor long-term results of both total [12, 13] and partial meniscectomies [4, 18].

Experimental trials [8, 16] confirm these data. On the basis of these principles and experiences the modern trends in the field of meniscal pathology are extremely conservative since there is a general consensus on the advantages of a partial meniscectomy over a total operation [9] and on the long-term positive results of the repair of a torn meniscus [5, 21].

The success of a meniscal suture is certainly closely connected to vascularization problems. In fact the high percentage of success achieved in peripheral lesions is linked to a good vascularization of that portion of the meniscus, whilst attempts to suture the avascular central portion of the meniscus ended in failure.

We proposed to investigate the possibility of repairing injuries within the meniscus by means of an experimental study on dogs, whose meniscal vasculature closely resembles that of man [2, 3, 10].

Materials and methods

Twenty-five adult dogs were employed. The animals were divided into four groups. In group 1 (five dogs) a longitudinal incision was made of approximately 1.5 cm in the avascular portion of the meniscus preserving the integrity of the anterior horn in order to avoid any vascular supply in the area.

In group 2 (five dogs) a transverse incision corresponded to a complete excision of the meniscus up to the peripheral vascularized portion.

In groups 3 and 4 (15 dogs) the same kind of incision was performed as in the two previous groups (longitudinal on 10 dogs, transverse on 5 dogs) but this time a pedicle flap of synovium was included. The limb was immobilized with soft bandaging for 2 weeks and weight bearing was immediately allowed. The incisions were always made in the central portion of the meniscus, which in dogs is completely avascular.

The animals were killed between 45 and 120 days. Before killing the animals 200 ml barium sulphate and Prussian blue was injected through the femoral artery in order to perform an arteriogram. We then removed the menisci, preserving the perimeniscal structures. The specimens were clarified according to the Spalteholz technique and both whole specimens and sections thereof were submitted to microangiographic and photographic examination.

Results

In groups 1 and 2 complete healing was never achieved. Only in the five cases where a transverse incision had been made was a partial penetration (no more than 4 mm) of fibrovascular tissue starting from the peripheral portion observed after the 48th day. In the longitudinal incisions no repair process was observed. In groups 3 and 4, in 11 cases complete healing and in 4 cases a partial repair was observed. The macroscopic morphology of the repaired menisci appeared altered by an abundant scarry fibrovascular tissue that covered the central portion (Figure 1). Microangiographically a rich new vascularization was demonstrated in the repair tissue (Figure 2); there were no substantial differences in the findings obtained between 45 and 80 days. In some cases the newly formed vessels reached the free edge of the meniscus (Figures 3–4). Instead, in the longitudinal lesions managed with a mere suture without including a synovium flap the meniscal tissue remained avascular.

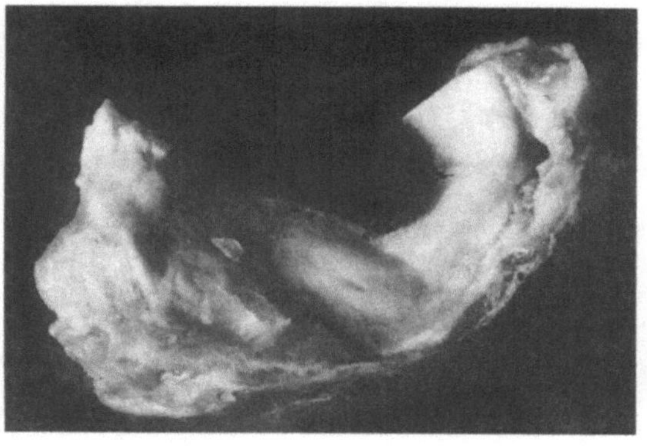

Figure 1. The macroscopic morphology of the repaired meniscus appeared altered by abundant scarry fibrovascular tissue. Transverse lesion at 40 days treated with a pedicle flap of synovium

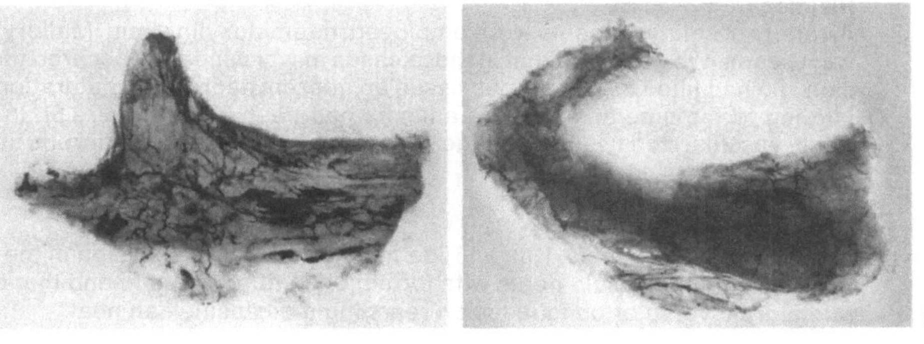

a b

Figure 2 a, b. Microangiography demonstrates a rich new vascularization in the repair tissue of a lesion treated with a pedicle flap of synovium. **a** Longitudinal lesion at 60 days. **b** Sagittal Section in repair tissue of a transverse lesion at 70 days. Spalteholz; **a** ×3; **b** ×10

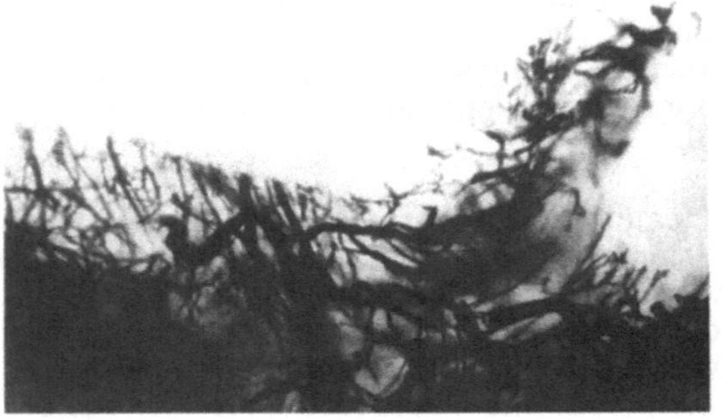

Figure 3. Aspect of newly formed vessels that reaches the free meniscal edge. Spalteholz, × 100

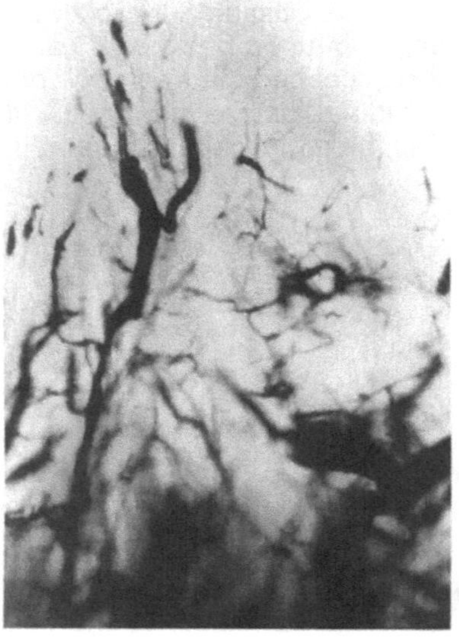

Figure 4. Morphological characters of vessels of scar tissue. Spalteholz, × 100

Histology
A variety of staining agents were employed: haematoxylin eosin, Mallory and van Giesen. We observed that in those cases in which healing occured the lesion site had filled in with fibrous tissue at different degrees of maturation according to the time at which the animals had been killed (Figure 5). In this richly vascularized tissue cartilage cells were found within the fibrous tissue (Figure 5).

Discussion
In previous experiments, King [16] demonstrated that an excision of the meniscus from the capsule heals with formation of fibrous tissue and that even a total transverse or oblique lesion reaching the capsule can heal.

Kim and Moon [15] observed that in rabbits the synovial membrane is essential not only for the healing but also for the regeneration of a meniscus after meniscectomy. However, one of the major limitations to the healing potential

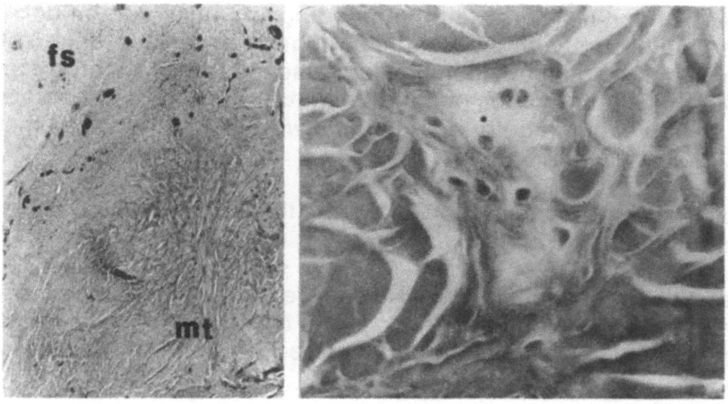

a b

Figure 5. a The lesion site has filled in with fibrous tissue at different degrees of maturation. *fs*, fibrovascular scar; *mt*, meniscal tissue. **b** Sometimes cartilage cells were found within the fibrous tissue. **a** H & E, × 100; **b** Van Gieson, × 320

of synovial cells is due to the fact that they can only invade – and only to a very limited extent – meniscal lesions next to the capsular junction. Therefore, all the longitudinal lesions in the central portion of the meniscus cannot be reached by them. This is the reason why we included a synovium flap in the suture: to make the synovial cells reach the whole extent of the lesion. By this technique a high rate of success (70%) was achieved.

In a recent experimental work Arnoczky [1] performed longitudinal lesions in an avascular portion of the meniscus and secured a vascular supply by means of an additional perpendicular lesion. The technique is certainly intriguing and confirms the principles on which our research work is based, even if an additional lesion to induce healing may appear debatable.

In our cases healing often occurred with a rich formation of fibrous tissue that greatly alters the morphology of the meniscus. Even when this phenomenon is macroscopically less evident, the histological examination still shows a substantial alteration of the meniscal structure with highly vacularized repair fibrous tissue even in advanced stages. Therefore, the inclusion of synovium transforms a fibrocartilaginous tissue into a fibrovascular one in which cartilage cells are only occasionally present.

Microangiographic and histological analysis demonstrate the basic role played by the synovium in the healing process of an injured meniscus for both the rapid proliferation of the synovium fibroblasts and the vascular supply offered by this tissue.

Cabaud et al. [7] report a high rate of success in meniscus sutures without inclusions of synovium flaps. These lesions, however, were made in the anterior horn of the internal portion of the meniscus, an area that in dogs is highly vascularized and richly covered with synovial tissue [19].

The results of this research cannot be totally transferred to a clinical context. In fact, a recent surgical lesion cannot be compared to an old lesion that is the most frequent finding in this kind of pathology. It must also be borne in mind that healing occurs with the formation of more or less vascularized fibrous tissue with a doubtful functional value; also the meniscus morphology is greatly altered. Healing of lesions in the central portion of the meniscus is therefore possible, but in our experiments it was only achieved by including synovial membrane in the suture.

The repair of meniscal lesions depends on both the kind of cells invading the lesion site and the amount of vascular supply.

To conclude, we believe that the results of our research will enable the indications for a meniscal suture to be extended in the future to those cases for which meniscectomy has been so far considered as the only possible solution.

References

1. Arnoczky SP, Rubin RM, Marshall JL (1979) Microvasculature of the cruciate ligaments and its response to injury. J Bone Joint Surg [Am] 61:1221–1229
2. Arnoczky SP, Warren RF (1982) Microvasculature of the human meniscus. Am J Sports Med 10(2):90–95
3. Arnoczky SP, Warren RF (1983) The microvasculature of the meniscus and its response to injury. Am J Sports Med 11(3):131–141
4. Bauer R (1971) Ein Beitrag zur Frage der Total- oder Teilrektion bei traumatischen Meniscusläsionen. Arch Orthop Unfallchir 69:341–350
5. Bousquet G (1981) Les laxités du genou et l'altération du cartilage rotulien. Cahier d'Orthopédie de St. Etienne
6. Brantigan OC, Voshell AF (1941) Mechanics of ligaments and menisci of knee joint. J Bone Joint Surg 23:44–46
7. Cabaud HE, Rodkey WG, Fitzwater JE (1981) Medial meniscus repairs. An experimental and morphologic study. Am J Sports Med 9:129–134
8. Cox JS, Nye CE, Schaeffer WW, Woodstein IJ (1975) The degenerative effects of partial and total resection of the medial meniscus in dogs. Clin Orthop 109:178–183
9. Dandy DJ (1978) Early results of closed partial meniscectomy. Br Med J 1:1099–1100
10. Davies DV, Edwards DAW (1948) The blood supply of the synovial membrane and intraarticular structures. Ann R Coll Surg Engl 2:142–156
11. Fabbriciani C, Schiavone-Panni A, Oransky M (1982) La riparazione chirurgica delle lesioni meniscali: studio sperimentale. Proceeding of the 67th Congress of S.I.O.T, 20–23 October 1982
12. Fahmy NRM, Williams EA, Noble J (1983) Meniscal pathology and osteoarthritis of the knee. J Bone Joint Surg [Br] 65:24–28
13. Fisher V, Matzen K, Bruns H (1976) Arthroseauslösende Faktoren der Meniskektomie. Z Orthop 114:735–737
14. Helfet A (1974) Disorders of the knee. Lippincott, Philadelphia
15. Kim JM, Moon MS (1979) The effects of synoviectomy upon regeneration of meniscus in rabbits. Clin Orthop 141:287–294
16. King D (1936) The healing of the semilunar cartilages. J Bone Joint Surg 18:333–342
17. McConnaill MA (1932) The function of intra-articular fibrocartilages, with special reference to the knee and inferior radio-ulnar joint. J Anat 66:210–214
18. McGinty JB, Guess LF, Marvin RA (1977) Partial or total meniscectomy. J Bone Joint Surg [Am] 59:763–766
19. O'Connor (1977) The histological structure of dog knee menisci with comments on its possible significance. Am J Anat 147(4):407–417
20. Radin EL, Bryan RS (1970) The effect of weight-bearing on regrowth of the medial meniscus after meniscectomy. J Trauma 10:169–175
21. Wirth CR (1981) Meniscus repair. Clin Orthop 157:153–160

Suture of fresh and old meniscal tears – animal experiments and clinical results

C. J. Wirth, K. A. Milachowski and K. Weismeier

Orthopaedic University Hospital Munich
8000 München
Federal Republic of Germany

The important function of the menisci in the biomechanics of the knee joint demands a cautious approach towards meniscectomy. Particularly longitudinal ruptures at the base of the posterior horn of the medial meniscus through the vascularised zone seem amenable to repair by suture. In old longitudinal ruptures the meniscal border has to be freshened.

The possibility to repair fresh and old meniscal tears by suture was examined biomechanically, histologically, and microangiographically in animal experiments. In 22 sheep, a standardized lesion was placed in the posterior horn of the medial meniscus. In 8 animals, a primary suture was performed, in 8 other animals a secondary repair was attempted after 4 weeks, 6 animals served as controls. The evaluation was done after 6 and 12 weeks.

We were able to prove that both after fresh and secondary sutures of meniscal tears at the basis of the posterior horn complete healing takes place.

This is in accordance with clinical results after suture of fresh and old longitudinal tears of the medial meniscus after a control period up to 6 years for fresh and up to 2 1/2 years for secondary meniscus sutures.

Meniscus sutures for old tears – Report on over 100 cases

M. Rodriguez and A. Schreiber

Department of Orthopaedic Surgery of the University of Zurich
CH-8008 Zurich 8
Switzerland

Introduction

The widely recognized fact that arthrosis and accompanying instability are common consequences of meniscectomy, particularly when the entire meniscus is removed, has led us to apply conservative, reconstructive meniscus surgery, i.e., reinsertion in the case of isolated lesions.

Suture of basal tears of the meniscus is not a new idea and is often performed as part of the basic surgical orthopaedic treatment of joint fractures as well as in the treatment of recent and older injuries of the capsule and ligaments. A review of the rather sparse world literature reveals that as early as 1899 Annadale reported excellent results after reinsertion of a meniscus secured with catgut. On the other hand, the first experimental reports date from 1936, when King published favourable results after suturing peripheral meniscal lesions in dogs.

Since the 1970s reports on meniscal sutures and plasties have become a little more common, but mainly in connection with fresh and often complex injuries.

We began suturing old, isolated meniscal lesions succesfully in 1972. For the last 6 years we have done so routinely.

Materials and methods

An arthroscopy is performed in every case to confirm the clinical diagnosis and as a basis for planing of operation itself and for precise information to be relayed to the patient.

The most suitable tears for suturing are those running vertically or diagonally across the vascularized base of the meniscus.

To date we have treated 99 patients with 103 meniscus sutures. Of these lesions of the meniscus, 86 were old and 76 were isolated. Most patients were between 20 and 30 years of age, a 14-year-old girl and a 59-year-old man representing the extremes of the age range (Figure 1).

Suturing was performed between 1 month and 1 year after the injury in nearly three-quarters of the cases, sometimes after 2 and more years and rarely after more than 10 years (Table 1).

Over the years, both surgical technique and postoperative treatment have been gradually simplified. At first lesions were directly approached by ventral, dorsomedial or dorsolateral arthrotomy; today only anteromedial and

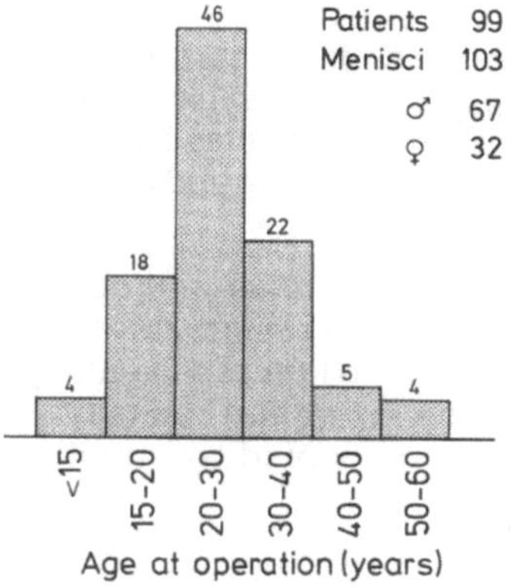

Figure 1. Details of patients. *Figures* at tops of *bars* are numbers of patients in each group

Table 1. Interval between lesion and suture in treatment of old meniscal tears

Interval	No. of cases
Acute	17
< 1 month	9
< ½ year	30
< 1 year	10
> 1 year	21
2–3 years	10
~10 years	2
	99

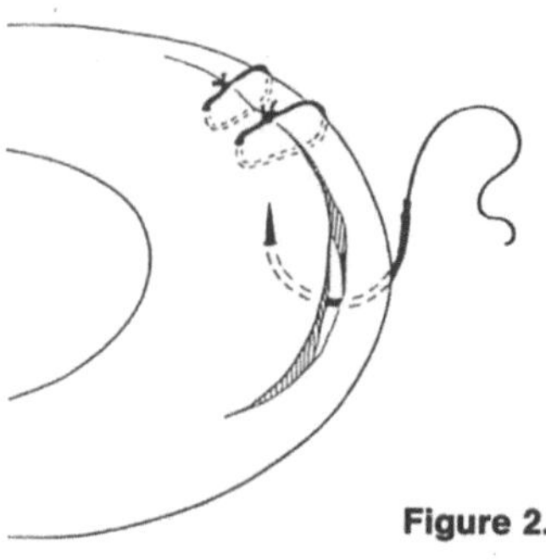

Figure 2. Operative technique

anterolateral approaches are used. This permits complete inspection of the joint, while subcutaneous dissection with the knee in maximal flexion allows additional dorsomedial and dorsolateral exposure and arthrotomy with no problems.

The operative technique is simple: Once the injury is confirmed after entry of the joint, the excess synovium is excised and the lesion carefully freshened by curettage. Depending on the size of the lesion, two to four atraumatic single sutures are placed under direct vision to adapt and join the two parts. After various trials, 2-0 Dexon placed with semicircular needles has proved to be the most suitable material (Figure 2).

After the operation, the knee should be immobilized for 1 week in a full-length plaster splint, fitted before the operation, angled at 30 °. An electric, automatic moving brace should then be used to move the joint actively and passively with increasing force for the next 3 weeks.

Hospitalization averages 2 weeks, while inability to work lies between 3 and 6 weeks, depending on the profession. Sports should not be taken up less than 3 months after the operation.

Results

Of our 99 patients, 91 were followed up clinically, while 66 had an arthrography and 4 underwent arthroscopy. Criteria for judging the results throughout the study were: subjective symptoms, ability to work and pursue sports, objective mobility of the joint, meniscal signs and stability, arthrosis and arthrographic findings.

The majority of patients examined were virtually asymptomatic and could work and engage in sport with no problems (86.6%). These results rated as mediocre (8.9%) or poor (4.3%) were not necessarily due to failure in healing of the meniscus, but were more likely to be due to the instability caused by concomitant ligamentous lesions, and most were accompanied by patellar symptoms (Table 2).

Table 2. Subjective and objective results obtained with meniscal suture for old tears

Subjective			
Very good	47	86.6%	
Good	32		
Moderate	8	8.9%	
Poor	4	4.3%	
Objective			
Very good	35	86.8%	
Good	44		
Moderate	5	5.4%	
Poor	7	7.6%	(arthrography)

Results were assessed objectively by clinical examination in 91 cases, by arthrography in 66, and by arthroscopy in 4.

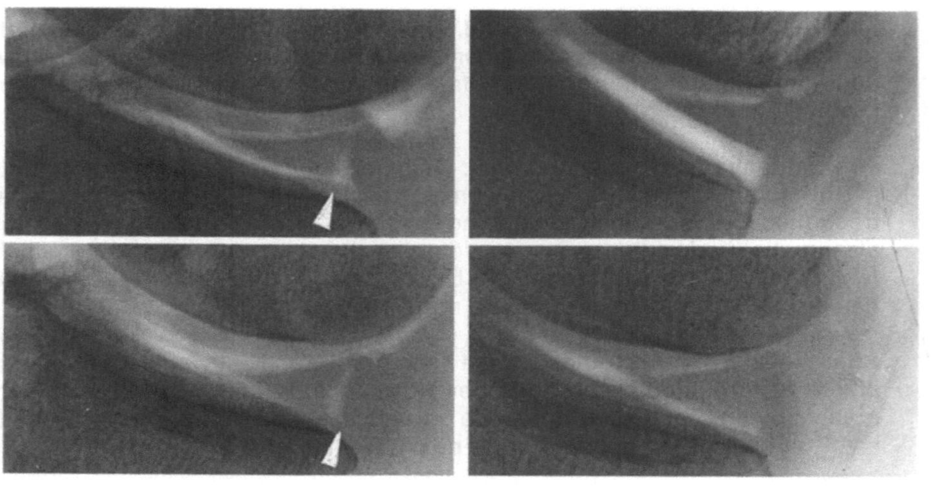

Figure 3. Follow-up arthrograms for patient R.S. 1950 293321. *Left*: 2/83, a 2-year-old lesion of the medial meniscus after a ski-ing accident; *right*: 9/83, at 7 months after meniscus suture; anatomically perfect healing of the meniscus, subjectively and objectively asymptomatic

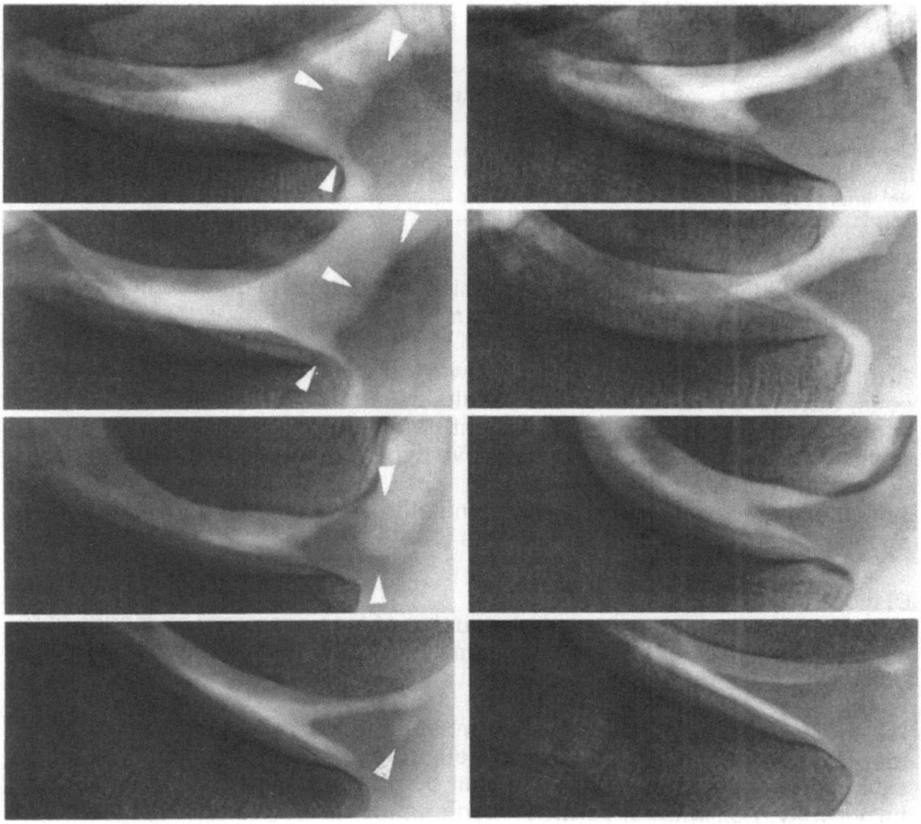

Figure 4. Follow-up arthrograms for patient R.F. 1958 294677, an active footballer. *Left*: 4/83, repeated blocking of the right knee, 3 years after a sports accident. Almost total rupture of the medial meniscus; *right*: 10/83, at 5 months after reinsertion of the meniscus: perfect result, clinical and subject freedom from symptoms. Patient started football again 2 months after the operation

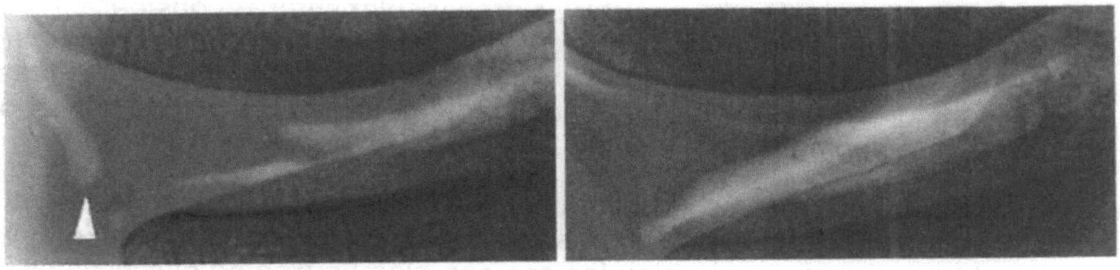

Figure 5. Follow-up arthrograms for patient E.D. 1928 179745. *Left*: 3/84, repeated symptoms and effusions after accident at work 10 years earlier. Clinical and arthrographic examinations revealed lesion of the posterior horn of the medial meniscus; *right*: 10/83, at 7 months after suturing, meniscus had healed well, and patient is completely asymptomatic and working full-time as an elevator mechanic

Table 3. Healing of menisci following suture for old tears in 66 cases examined by arthrography

Result	No.	Percentage
Complete	56	85%
Incomplete	6	9%
Not improved	4	6%

At clinical follow-up after isolated meniscus sutures, no pathologic meniscal signs, instability or arthrosis were found (86.8%).

Arthrographic findings (Figures 3–5) were decisive in evaluation of the results. Objective evaluation of the results as mediocre (5.4%) or poor (7.6%) corresponded to incomplete or absent healing of the meniscus. In contrast to these findings, clinical and subjective symptoms were often absent.

Together with the cases that anatomically were not ideally healed, 93% showed reattachment of the meniscus (Table 3).

Discussion

An attempt to avoid or reduce the sequelae of meniscectomy by means of reconstructive surgery has led us to suture even isolated old meniscal lesions in the last 12 years.

It is widely accepted that the lesion must lie in the vascularized zone of the meniscus to permit healing by revascularization. Such common basal injuries, mainly of the posterior horn, can be shown better by means of air arthrography, i.e., without contrast medium, and enlargement technique than by arthroscopy.

The joint is entered by an anteromedial or anterolateral arthrotomy, which permits easy access to the dorsal compartment by subcutaneous dissection if necessary, after which the lesion is curetted and sutured. In view of our totally uncomplicated early and late results with absorbable material, we can in no way support the common assumption that the sutures must be knotted outside the capsule. On the contrary, extracapsular sutures considerably retard the recovery of extension and flexion of the joint. Our method of placing intra-articular sutures under direct vision has proved simpler and at least equivalent to horizontal, partially transligamentous sutures placed blindly or to other, more complicated, techniques.

Reinsertion of the meniscus is not only recommended for ideal cases with basal lesions. Loose posterior horns with a positive Finochietto sign, meniscal residues and more complex lesions can also be treated successfully in the way described. Trying to place sutures by way of an arthroscope has so far proved time consuming and difficult, but the experience gained is not yet sufficient.

How does a reimplanted meniscus tolerate new traumas? In each of two cases with fresh trauma and complex ligamentous lesions requiring further surgery the previously fixed meniscus had remained uninjured. Two reinserted menisci were partially resected in other hospitals; these patients did not have isolated meniscal lesions, however, but had undergone multiple operations and had residual complex instability.

References

Annandale T (1889) Excision of the internal semilunar cartilage, resulting in perfect restoration of the joint movements. Br Med J 1:291–292

Arnoczky JL et al. (1980) Meniscal nutrition – an experimental study in the dog. Proc Orthop Res Soc 26:127

Boehnel P (1981) Über die Kollagenstruktur, Durchblutung und Innervation der Menisci des menschlichen Kniegelenks. Schweiz Rundsch Med 70:1512–1515

Bracker W, et al. (1982) Zur Frage der Kniebandinstabilität nach Meniskektomie. Z Orthop 120:501

Burri G, Helbling G (1977) Therapie und Ergebnisse nach frischen Verletzungen des Kniebandapparates. Langenbecks Arch Chir 345:451–457

Cabaud HE (1981) Medical meniscus repairs. An experimental and morphologic study. J Sports Med 9:129–134

Cassidy RE, Shaffer AJ (1981) Repair of peripheral meniscus tears. A preliminary report. J Sports Med 9:209–214

Dahn P, et al. (1969) Experimentelle Untersuchungen zur Frage der totalen oder partiellen Meniskusresektion. Arch Orthop Unfallchir 65:209–219

Di Stefano VJ (1980) Function, post-traumatic sequelae and recurrent concepts of management of knee meniscus injuries: a review article. Clin Orthop 151:143–146

Elmer RM, et al. (1977) Meniscal regeneration and postmeniscetomy degenerative joint disease. Clin Orthop 124:304–310

Eriksson E, Palmer I (1983) A great name in the history of cruciate ligament surgery. Clin Orthop 172:4–5

Hamberg P, Gillquist J, Lysholm J (1983) Suture of new and old peripheral meniscus tears. J Bone Joint Surg [Am] 65:193–197

Heatley FW (1980) The meniscus – can it be repaired? J Bone Joint Surg [Br] 62:397–402

Hene HJ, et al. (1981) Tibio-femorale Kontaktflächenmessungen nach experimentellen partiellen und subtotalen Meniskektomien. Z Orthop 119:54–59

Hierholzer, et al. (1975) Reinterventionen nach Schienbeinkopfbrüchen. Chirurg 46:352–358

Ikeuchi H (1976) Surgery under arthroscopie control. Rhumatologie (Paris) H.S. Spec. 33:57–64

Insall JN (1984) Surgery of the knee. Churchill Livingstone, Edinburgh, pp 153–154

King D (1936) The healing of semilunar cartilages. J Bone Joint Surg 18:333–342

Krakow KA, Vetter WL (1980) Surgical reimplantation of the medial meniscus and repair of meniscal lacerations. An experimental study in dogs. Proc Orthop Res Soc 26:128

Meyer ST, et al. (1975) Klinische Ergebnisse mit der Meniskusnaht. Monatsschr Unfallheilkd 78:564–571

Müller W (1975) Die Rotationsinstabilität am Kniegelenk. Hefte Unfallheilkd 125:51–68

Müller W (1982) Das Knie. Springer, Berlin Heidelberg New York, pp 113–124

Price CT, Allen WC (1978) Ligament repair in the knee with preservation of the meniscus. J Bone Joint Surg [Am] 60:61–65

Ricklin P, Ruettimann A, Del Buono MS (1980) Die Meniskusläsion. Thieme, Stuttgart

Rodriguez M, Zollinger H (1983) Die Naht basisnaher Meniskusrisse. Sportverletzungen und Sportschäden. Thieme, Stuttgart

Scapinelli R (1968) Studies on the vasculature of the human knee joint. Acta Anat 70:305–331

Schilling H (1973) Rückblick und Ausblick auf die Meniskuschirurgie. Monatsschr Unfallheilkd 12:549–554

Schreiber A, Dexel M (1979) Gonarthrose nach Meniskektomie und Meniskektomie bei Gonarthrose. Chirurg 50:618–626

Slocum DB, Larson RL (1968) Rotatory instability of the knee. J Bone Joint Surg [Am] 50:211–225
Smillie IS (1978) Injuries of the knee joint, 5th edn. Churchill Livingstone, Edinburgh
Suchardt E (1977) Neue Operationsmethoden zur Rekonstruktion komplexer Bandverletzungen am Kniegelenk. Hefte/Unfallheilkd 129:168–171
Stone RG (1979) Peripheral detachment of the menisci of the knee, a preliminary report. Orthop Clin North Am 10:643–657
Takazawa H, et al. (1969) Surgical experiences in fresh complex injury of the articular meniscus and ligaments of the knee. Orthop Surg 20:1066–1071
Wirth CR (1981) Meniscus repair. Clin Orthop 157:153–160

Meniscus repair

P. M. Karpf, C. Sagstetter and R. Aigner

Orthopädische Klinik rechts der Isar
8000 München
Federal Republic of Germany

The torn meniscus presents a dilemma in regard to treatment. Leaving a torn meniscus in place as well as removing the meniscus, will produce more rapid degenerative changes within the joint. In an attempt to reduce the severity of the degenerative joint disease, repairing peripheral meniscus tears was started.

Material and methods

A study of repaired vertical peripheral tears of the meniscus in sixty patients (twenty-five women and thirty-five men) was carried out from November 1975 to August 1983. There was a total of sixty-two meniscus tears repaired (fifty were medial and twelve were lateral). Forty-three tears were treated within four weeks and nineteen tears were operated on as long as five years after injury. Only six patients had a meniscal tear that was not accompanied by injures of either the anterior cruciate ligament or the collateral ligaments or both.

The surgical technique involved resuturing of the meniscus to the capsule and/or ligaments after debriding the edges of older tears.

Results

Thirty patients had follow-up visits. At a mean follow-up of twenty months (range, six months to six years) all exept one of the patients had clinically apparent healing of the sutured meniscal tear. Fifteen patients had postoperative arthrograms and all except one showed evidence of complete healing. One patient had a second tear at the sutured area after the initial repair.

Discussion

The data of our study support the assumption that repair of peripheral tears of the meniscus is possible. Some new peripheral injuries to the meniscus will probably heal spontaneously with conservative treatment in cast. However these injuries very often occur in combination with ligament tears, which have to be operated.

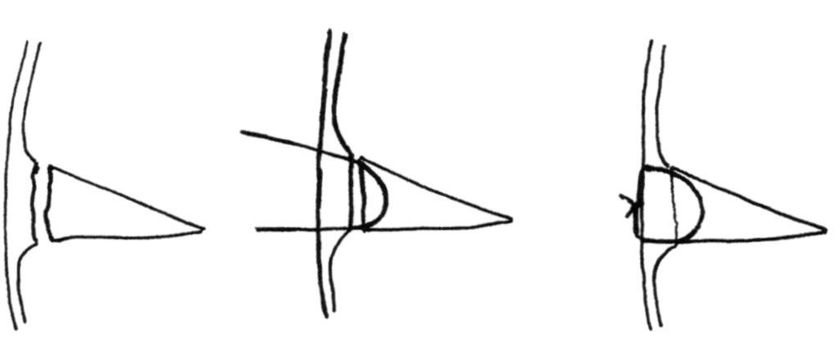

Figure 1. Suture technique

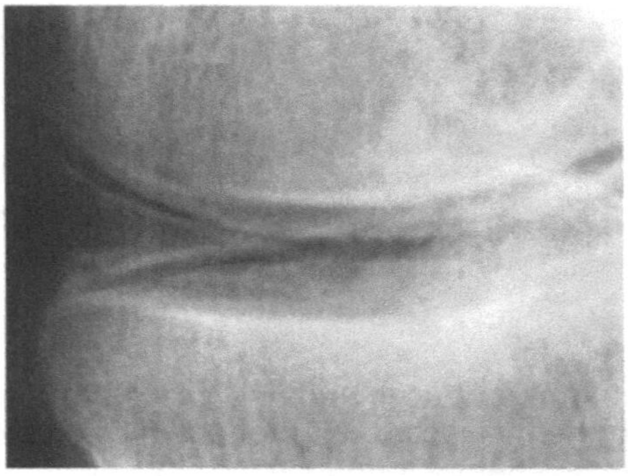

Figure 2. Arthrogram showing irregularities of the meniscus surface after repair

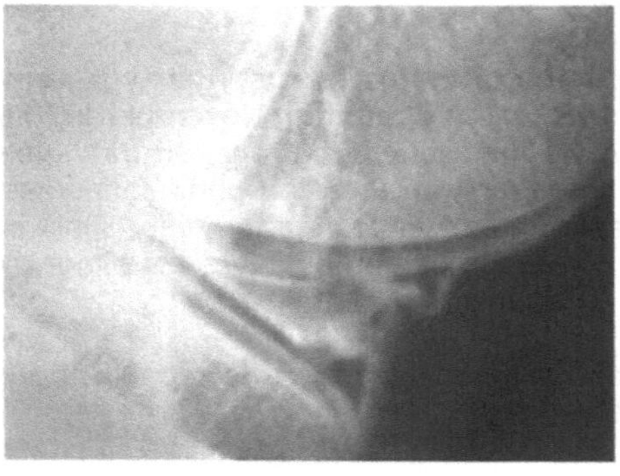

Figure 3. Arthrogram showing a recurrence

Also a significant part of our patients had old meniscal tears that were not expected to heal with conservative treatment.

Summary

Meniscectomy will produce degenerative changes within the knee joint. Therefore we decided in 1975 to start repairing peripheral meniscus tears. Since then sixty-two repairs of peripheral meniscus injuries were performed. Thirty patients had follow-up visits. Fifteen patients underwent a postoperative arthrogram. Only one patient had a second tear at the sutured area.

Partial resection of the discoid meniscus of the knee

P. Papadelis and V. Tsemanis

K A T Hospital and Asclepion Hospital
Athens
Greece

Total surgical resection of the symptomatic discoid meniscus is, in general, the treatment of choice for this pathological condition. The purpose of this paper is to present a new technique, which in effect is a partial resection of the meniscus, that leaves a semi-lunar remnant of the orignal meniscus intact.

Material and methods
Twenty children and young adults between 8 and 20 years were operated for a symptomatic discoid meniscus in the years 1980, 1981 and 1982. In seven of these cases a partial meniscectomy was tried. They all had a small rupture, minimal or early degenerative findings, the thickness of the menisci was moderate and their mobility not remarked (Wrisberg type), with a firm attachment to the capsule of the joint.

Surgical technique
We use the surgical instruments of operative arthroscopy. We start cutting the meniscus from its proximity to the ACL, and we continue in the posterior area in a semilunar way, detaching finally a big frontal part of the discoid matter. We smoothen up the inline surfaces of the cut meniscus as well as we can, using as well the arthroscope to observe more clearly the back of the joint and the posterior parts of the concerned meniscus.

Discussion – results
Partial meniscectomy by an open arthrotomy or closed operative arthroscopy are now common place in the treatment of torn menisci. The original work by Fujikawa helped us to continue on this clinical experimental path. It is obvious that our efforts are linked with the preservation of joint's space, in respect of avoidance of degenerative disease, as well as, the preservation of joint stability, and function. In all our seven cases the clinical, arthrographic and arthroscopic results are considered satisfactory. A case of recurrent effusion, and another one of inexplicable locking sensation – at long intervals – are noted. Time alone will show if the surgical effort to preserve some of the meniscus discoid material is worth the effort.

Recurrent operation on the knee joint – reasons and consequences

K. Franke and B. Paul

Dept. Surgery, Municipal Hospital Berlin-Pankow
DDR-1100 Berlin
German. Dem. Rep.

In all fields of surgery, repeated operations on one region may have a negative influence on the final result. This applies also to recurrent knee joint arthrotomies.

Among 2 254 operations to the knee joint, performed within eleven years from 1971 to 1981 at the Berlin-Pankow Hospital, there were 16% (n= 365) second or third look arthrotomies. One group of patients (54%) had also their first knee joint surgery in our hospital. The other group (46%) underwent preceding arthrotomy in another hospital. Both groups seemed to be of a comparable quantity to analyse the causes of both first and further on operation.

The permanent Pankow patients (n= 197) suffered from

	first op.	second look	
ligamentous injuries	48%	61%	40% due to
chondromalacia	43%	71%	recurrent trauma
meniscus lesion	34%	23%	

In the other group (n= 168) we found

	first op. in another hospital	second look in Pankow hospital	
ligamentous injuries	14,5%	77%	
chondromalacia	6%	80%	mainly due to an
meniscus lesion	78%	50%	insufficient first operation

From our analysis we are drawing the following conclusions:

- by efficient preoperative diagnosis and respective measures during first surgery the rate of recurrent arthrotomies can be reduced significantly;
- in case of not performed arthroscopy the joint incision must be large enough to realize a sufficient inspection of the whole cartilage surface, both menisci, and both cruciate ligaments. No button-hole incision!
- chondromalacia is more frequent than most surgeons believe. It influences to a great extent the functional fate of the joint. Removing destroyed cartilage during an operation is important for an optimal joint rehabilitation;
- blood inside the joint is poison to the cartilage! Therefore we recommend an intra-articular suction drainage for two days;
- immobilizing a joint is poison to the cartilage! Whenever possible we recommend a limited range of motion instead of a plaster cast;
- an optimal rehabilitation is as necessary for achieving a good functional result as an optimal operation.

Meniscectomy by mini-arthrotomy under local anaesthesia

A. Gächter

Orthopädische Universitätsklinik Basel, Orthopädisch-Traumatologische Abteilung
Kantonspital, CH-4055 Basel
Switzerland

Introduction

It is undoubtedly the trend now to perform only partial meniscectomy [1, 3], to diagnose meniscal injuries by arthroscopy and to treat them with arthroscopic visualization [2]. Arthroscopic operations have now been widely performed in North America and Europe for some years, not least because this allows videomonitoring and because athletes demand short rehabilitation times.

The advantages of arthroscopic operation are no longer questioned; it should not, however, be forgotten that it makes heavy demands on the surgeon and on the hospital's organization. In our opinion, the following prerequisites should be satisfied: Adequate time must be allowed for the operation; a hectic pace and the constant knowledge that the next patient is already "out" or that other emergencies are waiting, for example, can be disadvantageous for the surgeon, especially if any technical difficulties do occur during the procedure. Wide experience in arthroscopic diagnosis and in conventional knee surgery is another important condition. Arthroscopic removal of the meniscus can be done as an out-patient procedure, but it is necessary to take account of the organization of the hospital and the insurance company's policy before deciding on this. It would also be desirable for the arthroscopic operation to be performed with local anaesthesia. In this way the general morbidity could be reduced even more significantly. An operation with general or lumbar anesthaesia and with a tourniquet does after all involve surveillance of the patient for several hours. Some preoperative tests are needed, depending on the kind of anaesthesia selected. Lumbar anaesthesia and general anaesthesia also require continuous bed rest for at least a few hours. A tourniquet can cause temporary damage to the quadriceps muscle and make a phlebothrombosis more likely.

Arthroscopic surgery with local anaesthesia does have a few disadvantages. The operation is not very pleasant for the patient, and the operation time is therefore limited. If technical difficulties do occur the operation must be stopped or the patient must have a general anaesthetic administered. The amount of local anaesthetics needed is quite large and POR 8 or adrenaline has to be added because of the bleeding.

Mini-arthrotomy

It was because of above-mentioned disadvantages that we developed a method adapted to our own mixed clinical practice, which involves a large number of emergencies. We must mention that we perform about 1200 arthroscopies a year at the University Hospital in Basel, and that most of them are referred to us by other doctors. Therefore, we cannot plan the arthroscopic output for any one day in advance. The patterns of injuries are quite heterogeneous. Some patients are sent back to the referring doctors for surgery or for conservative therapy. With our own experiments with arthroscopic operations behind us in 1979 we began to perform meniscectomies with a so-called mini-incision. At the beginning, the operation was performed only in in-patients and with lumbar anaesthesia. But since 1981, we apply exactly same technique, the so-called mini-arthrotomy, with local anaesthesia and in out-patients. Self-employed people (e.g., doctors) and athletes are the two groups who have profited most from this method, because of the high motivation to achieve a quick rehabilitation.

Technique of mini-arthrotomy under local anaesthesia

The procedure is as follows: First we perform a diagnostic arthroscopy under local anaesthesia. For this purpose we take 20 ml Carbostesin 0.5% (without adrenaline), 3–5 ml of which is given at the lateral injection site and about 15 ml is used for the intraarticular surface anaesthesia of the synovial membrane. Some of this Carbostesin will be washed out again during the arthroscopy. When the diagnosis has been made and the injury located, we remove the arthroscope and induce infiltration anaesthesia in addition. For the medial meniscus we give an intracutaneous injection at the probable site of the incision's place and a subcutaneous infiltration (Figure 1) "(sausage-shaped)" at the joint line. In addition, 15–20 ml 1% mepivacaine is needed, again without adrenaline. The local anaesthetic is then pressed into the area of the meniscus and the infrapatellar branch of the saphenus nerve with a tampon. We disinfect and drape once more. A leg-holder supports the knee. The incision is horizontally positioned over the anterior horn of the meniscus and about 1.5 cm long (Figure 2). A vertical cut is not so favourable as a horizontal one, because of the possible interference with the R. infrapatellaris.

A meticulous hemostasis is done. The general view of the joint space is surprisingly good despite the small incision. One should make sure to use the narrow Langenbeck hooks to make it possible to swivel the view from the anterior to the posterior horn. Special arthroscopic instruments can be used for

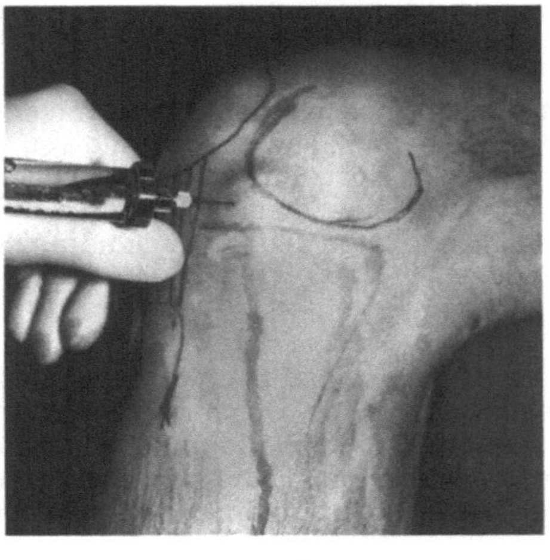

Figure 1. Schema for local infiltration with mepivacaine 1%

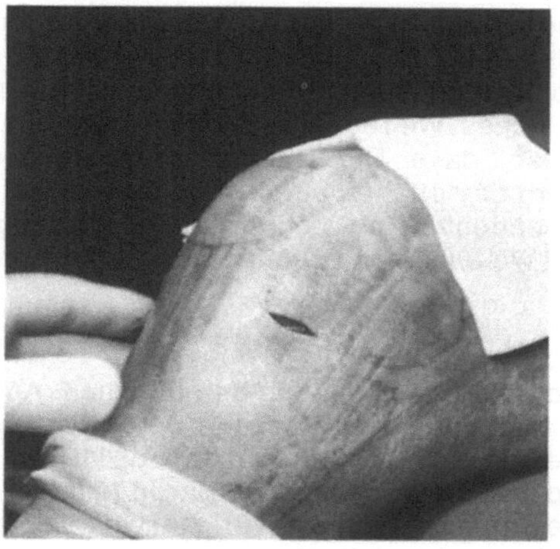

Figure 2. Horizontal skin incision over the anterior horn of the meniscus

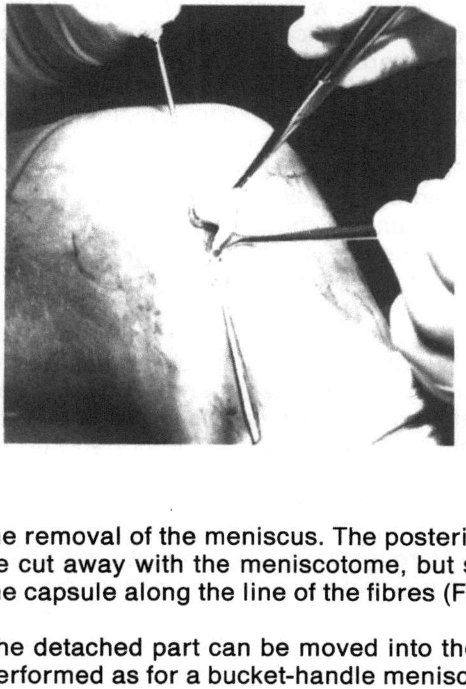

Figure 3. Removal of the meniscus through the mini-arthrotomy

the removal of the meniscus. The posterior horn of the meniscus should not be cut away with the meniscotome, but should be torn away in the area of the capsule along the line of the fibres (Figure 3).

The detached part can be moved into the intercondylar fossa. Resection is performed as for a bucket-handle meniscus. Remnants of the posterior horn can be removed with a small rongeur. The same procedure is applied for the lateral meniscus. The hiatus popliteus and the popliteus tendon should be treated carefully. When closing the wound care should be taken to have the incision of the capsule readapted with two resorbable sutures.

Aftertreatment

The aftertreatment is easy. Drains are not used. Active raising of the leg is already possible on the operation table. The musculus quadriceps can be activitated immediately since no tourniquet has been used. Anti-inflammatory drugs are then prescribed for the patient, who is told to tighten the quadriceps muscle with the knee stretched for 10 s, and this "1000 times a day". This will help to avoid the probability of effusion. The patient is usually able to walk immediatly and without crutches. We recommend full weight-bearing over the extended knee for the first 2 days. The best pain prophylaxis is to keep the leg elevated. From the 3rd day on the patient should try to walk as normally as possible. We give the patient an instruction sheet illustrating the best postoperative behaviour and we check each patient for the first time 2 days after the operation.

Results

A review of our patients operated on so far is soon to be published. Among 200 patients we had one case of infection. In three cases we had to repeat the meniscectomy (in two with the same method). About 94% of 118 patients who were re-examined confirmed that they would be prepared to undergo a similar operation again. It must be emphasized, however, that we try to make the operation as pleasant as possible for the patients, for example by playing music. A number of the dissatisfied patients were those who were frustrated because of problems with their health insurance (higher charges for the patients than when hospitalized). An aftertreatment with physiotherapy was necessary only in 20% of cases. To sum up, we have to point out that for this method the surgeon also needs wide experience in conventional meniscectomy. On the other hand, any kind of meniscal lesion can be treated in this way with an operating time of 7–20 min. The morbidity, at least as far as effusion and haemarthrosis are concerned, seems to be rather lower than with arthroscopic meniscectomy. One advantage that must certainly be pointed out is the excellent haemostasis during the operation and the possibility of immediate quadriceps activity.

Discussion

We think the meniscectomy by mini-arthrotomy and under local anaesthesia is certainly a good alternative to the arthroscopic operation. The outlay in terms of equipment is smaller, and no complicated organization is needed in advance, so that the intervention can easily be incorporated into even quite a busy programme. In a 60- to 70-kg patient acceptable blood levels can be maintained with the above-mentioned quantities of local anaesthetic agents, though it must be pointed out that Carbostesin by intraarticular injection will also be resorbed very well through the synovial membrane. This was measured by spectrometric evaluation. We have had no anaesthetic-related complications in over 200 operations. The so-called mini-meniscectomy allows rapid rehabilitation, which is especially important for athletes and self-employed patients.

References

1. Appel H (1970) Late results after meniscectomy in the knee joint. Acta Orthop Scand [Suppl] 133
2. Lysholm J, Gillquist J (1981) Endoscopic meniscectomy. Int Orthop 5:265–270
3. McGinty JB, Lawrence FG, Marwin R (1977) Partial or total meniscectomy. J Bone Joint Surg [Am] 59:736–766

Anterior Cruciate Ligaments

Clinical findings in acute anterior cruciate ligament ruptures: correlation with experimental data

P. Hertel

Abteilung Unfallchirurgie, Rudolf-Virchow-Krankenhaus
Augustenburger Platz 1, D-1000 Berlin 65
Federal Republic of Germany

Acute anterior cruciate ligament (ACL) ruptures most often occur during vigorous internal rotation near extension, accompanied by a forced quadriceps contraction. Other mechanisms for ACL ruptures are hyperextension and hyperflexion. External rotation always results in ACL rupture after rupture of the entire medial collateral ligament (superficial plus deep layer). The main symptoms of "isolated" ACL ruptures are somewhat similar to those of an acute patellar dislocation (Table 1).

Experimentally, ACL rupture has been investigated mainly by three different methods, using whole cadavers or cadaver knees: external stress indirectly producing different ruptures [10, 12], cuts made with instruments to cause definite ligament lesions and instabilities [5], and measurement of ligament length or tensions of intact knees [5, 9, 15].

Table 1. Symptoms of ACL ruptures and patellar luxations

	ACL ruptures	Patellar luxations
Collapse	+	+
Medial pain	+	+
Lateral pain	+	+
Haemarthrosis	+	+

Table 2. Theories of the function of the ACL

Tension of ACL bundles	Anteromedial bundle		Posterolateral bundle	
	Extension	Flexion	Extension	Flexion
Weber + Weber (1836) Fick (1911) Palmer (1938) Trillat (1959) Bousquet (1969)	Tense	Loose	Loose	Tense
Girgis (1975) Marshall (1975) Furman (1976) Abbott (1944) van Dijk (1983)	Loose	Tense	Tense	Loose
Hertel (1980)	Tense	(Loose)	Tense	Loose

The third method enables the areas of ACL tension sensitive to a ligament rupture to be found.

All cadaver experiments give only a certain approximation to the real situation, but they help us confirm or reject the sharply conflicting opinions [1, 4, 5, 7, 15] about function of the ACL (Table 2). We have recorded the relative tension of all major ligaments of the knee by a direct method [5]. The ligament laxity was measured perpendicularly to the direction of the ligament during flexion-extension, drawer and rotation movements (Figure 1). The main results are: 1. As found in previous investigations, there are two distinct parts of the ACL. Both parts are tense in hyperextension and hyperflexion. In flexion both parts are loose, but the anteromedial part is only about half as loose as the posterolateral part. External rotation lowers tension; internal rotation and anterior drawer movement raise tension of both parts of the ACL (Figures 2, 3).

2. Between about 0 ° and 30 ° flexion the ACL is the only tense ligament in internal rotation (Figure 4). The tension is pronounced during anterior

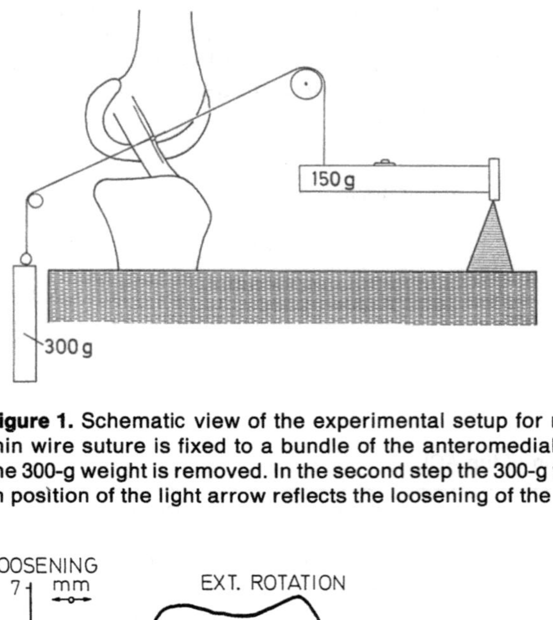

Figure 1. Schematic view of the experimental setup for measuring ligament loosening. A thin wire suture is fixed to a bundle of the anteromedial part of the ACL. In the first step the 300-g weight is removed. In the second step the 300-g weight is mounted. The difference in position of the light arrow reflects the loosening of the ACL

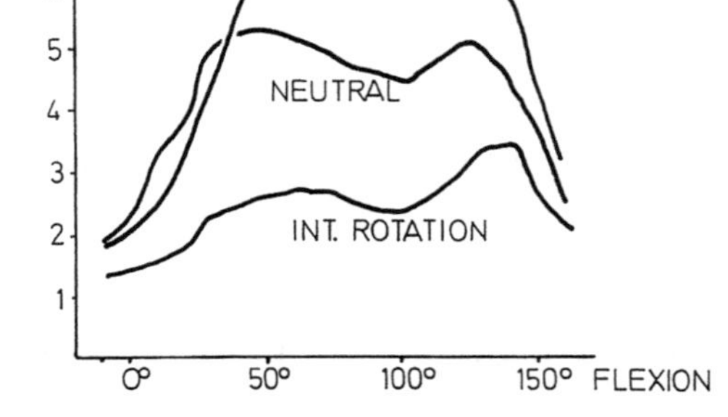

Figure 2. The anteromedial part of the ACL is tense in hyperextension, flexion and internal rotation. In external rotation more than in neutral rotation of the tibia there is a marked loosening of up to 7 mm between 40 ° and 130 ° flexion

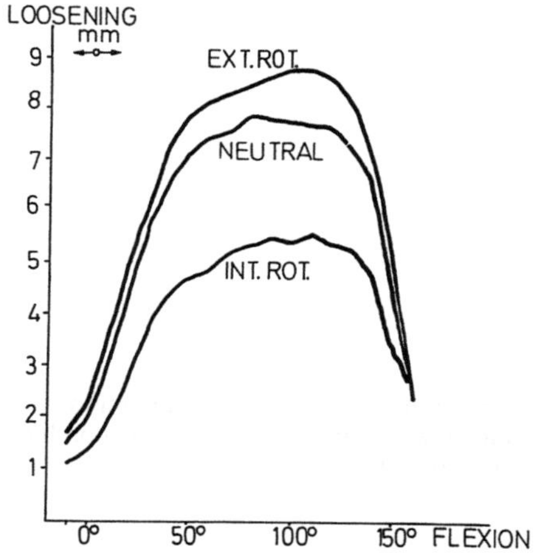

Figure 3. The posterolateral part of the ACL is generally looser than the anteromedial part, except in hyperextension and hyperflexion

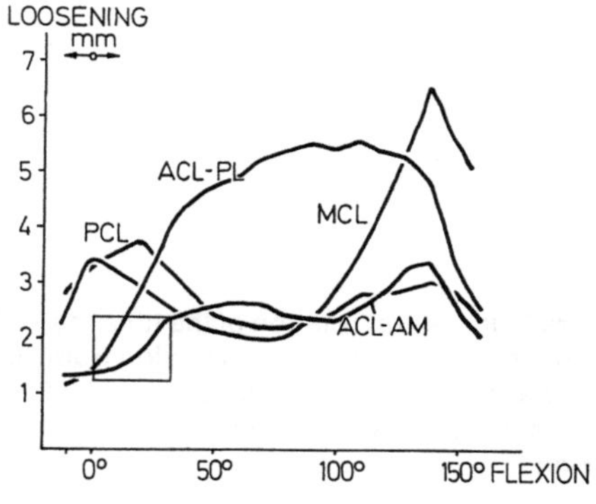

Figure 4. With internal rotation of the tibia and 0 ° to 30 ° flexion only the ACL (*ACL–PL+ ACL–AM*) is tense (*enclosed region*). The posterior cruciate ligament (*PCL*) and the medial collateral ligament (*MCL*) are loose. Flexing the knee between 50 ° and 100 ° the anteromedial part of the ACL, the PCL (anterolateral part) and the MCL become tense together. Internal rotation near extension combined with anterior drawer stress by quadriceps contraction is the reason for an isolated rupture of the ACL

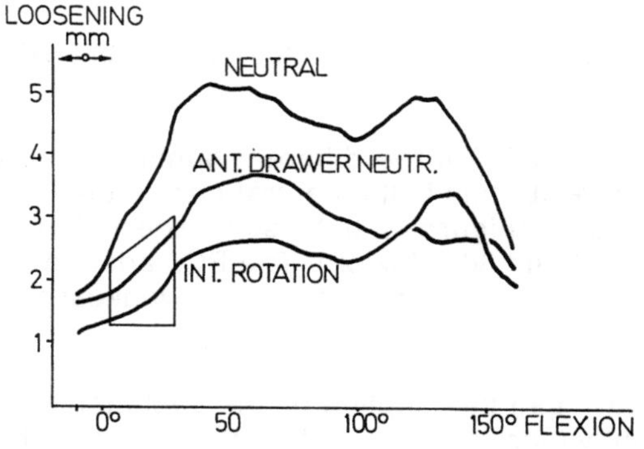

Figure 5. Anterior drawer and internal rotation act together causing tension in the ACL (*enclosed region*)

drawer stress (as caused by quadriceps contraction during a non-contact trauma; Figure 5). No other ligament exerts protection in this situation, in which most of the isolated ACL tears occur. The anterolateral capsule is too weak to withstand or is too lax to resist anterior-internal dislocation. Sometimes a small bony fragment at the capsular attachment is visible (sign of Se-

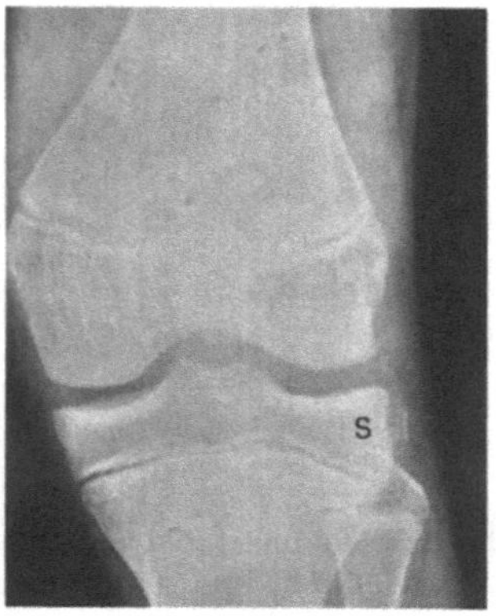

Figure 6. Sign of Segond (*S*): The bony detachment of the anterolateral capsular insertion at the tibia is combined with a rupture of the ACL

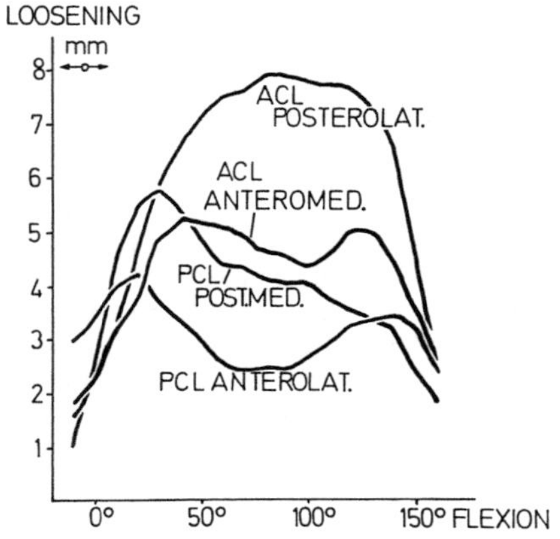

Figure 7. In neutral rotation of the tibia the PCL is tenser than the ACL during flexion from 30 ° on. The anterolateral (=central) part of the PCL is very tense between 50 ° and 100 ° flexion

gond), which is nearly always accompanied by a rupture of the ACL (Figure 6).

3. In the posterior cruciate ligament (PCL) three different bundles can be found. The anterolateral part of the PCL (this is the central part of the PCL) is tense not only in internal and neutral (Figure 7), but also in external, rotation of the knee (but not between 0 ° and 30 ° flexion). The PCL adds to the stability of the knee in all degrees of flexion and rotation. The weakest support is given near extension.

Proof of an acute rupture of the ACL can be supplied by the Lachmann test [14] near extension. This is a slightly more suitable test for the anteromedial than for the posterolateral part of the ACL (Figure 7). At 20 ° to 30 ° flexion the medial collateral ligament as an obstacle against anterior drawer movement is very loose in neutral rotation (Figure 8).

Real partial ruptures of the ACL are very rare. They cannot be detected by clinical means and should not be accepted by arthroscopic examination without examination of stability with the patient under anaesthesia. If the exam-

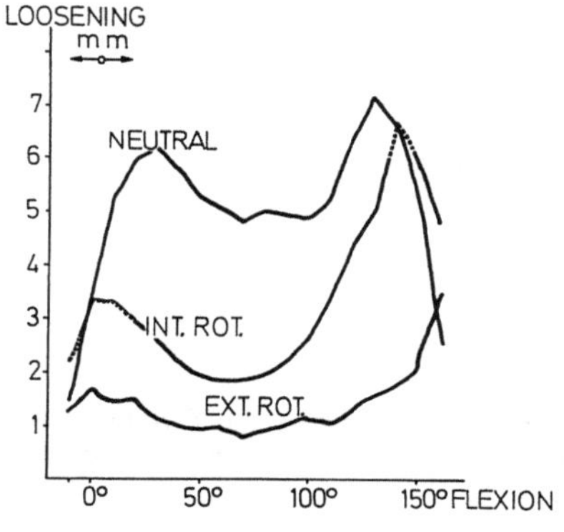

Figure 8. The medial collateral ligament is very tense and a restraint against anterior dislocation of the tibia in external rotation. In neutral rotation and 20 ° flexion (this position is held during the Lachmann test) the MCL is loose and allows the ACL to strike against the intercondylar notch

Table 3. History of pivot shift and jerk phenomenon

Jones (1906) Smith (1914) Hey Groves (1920) Palmer (1939)	Sudden anterolateral subluxation near extension	ACL rupture

ination with the patient under anaesthesia reveals a positive Lachmann test and pivot shift [3] or Jerk sign (Table 3), a complete rupture of the ACL is present, though some fibres may have shown apparent continuity during arthroscopy. The continuity can be divided on thorough investigation by the tip of a forceps.

The pivot shift or Jerk sign [6–8, 13] is positive in most acute ACL ruptures, but can only be examined with the patient under anaesthesia because testing is so painful. In some cases those tests are negative even if carried out with the patient under anaesthesia, due to strong muscular support. In such cases acute ACL rupture can be detected only by means of arthroscopy.

The pivot of a normal knee is at the medial tibial tubercle. After an ACL rupture the pivot shifts slightly to the medial side during pivot shift or jerk testing at 30 ° flexion. The pivot stays dislocated between extension and 30 ° flexion. At 90 ° flexion cutting the ACL produces no significant change in the pivot during rotation. Additional division of the posterolateral structures at 90 ° flexion markedly transfers the pivot to the anteromedial side of the knee. Unlike Nicholas [11] we found the pivots in complex instabilities to be generally on the opposite side of the lesion (Figures 9, 10).

Isolated ruptures of the ACL do occur rather frequently, but due to the rotational mechanism of most cases peripheral additional lesions are common. It is advisable to detect those lesions by arthroscopy immediately before surgery. Suitable lesions could then be treated by arthroscopic surgery if an additional approach were necessary.

Structure and function prove that the ACL is an important stabilizer of the knee. Suture, early augmentation or secondary reconstruction can restore a

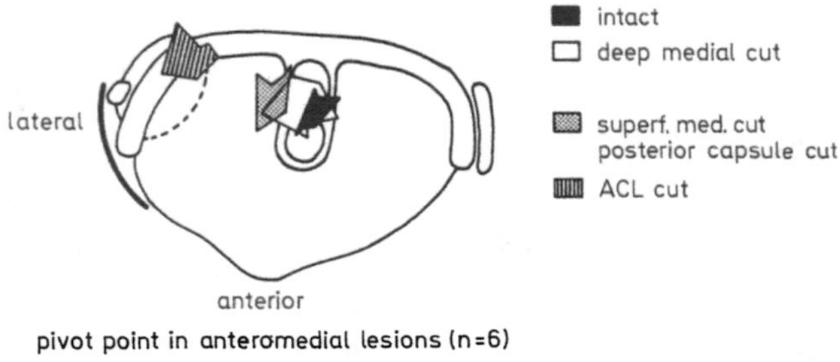

Figure 9. The pivot point of a normal knee is at the medial tibial tubercle. Cutting of the ACL alone does not change it. After sequential cutting of the medial structures the pivot changes position to the posterolateral corner of the knee

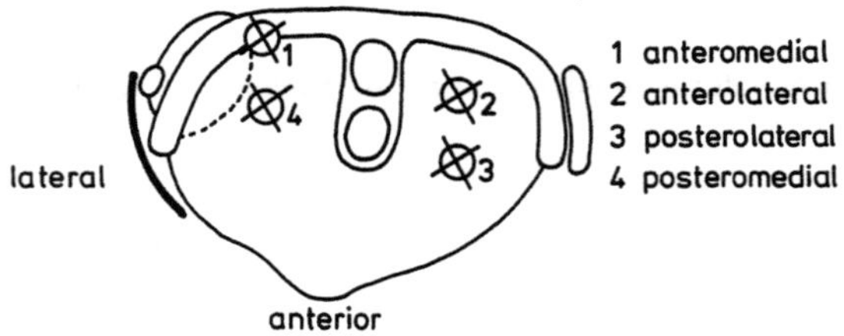

Figure 10. The pivot points of complex instabilities are generally located opposite the lesion

normal knee, though the clinical problem of the ACL has not yet been entirely solved [2]. But there is no question that it has been wrong to exclude this structure from therapeutic theory as Hughston has been done for some time [7].

References

1. Brantigan OC, Voshell AF (1941) The mechanics of the ligaments and menisci of the knee joint. J Bone Joint Surg [Am] 23:44–66
2. Feagin JA, Curl WW (1976) Isolated tear of the anterior cruciate ligament. 5-year study. Am J Sports Med 4:95–100
3. Galway RD, Beaupre A, MacIntosh DL (1972) Pivot shift: A clinical sign of symptomatic anterior cruciate ligament insufficiency. J Bone Joint Surg [Br] 54:763–764
4. Girgis FG, Marshall JL, Monajem A (1975) The cruciate ligaments of the knee joint. Anatomical, functional and experimental analysis. Clin Orthop 106:216–231
5. Hertel P (1980) Verletzung und Spannung von Kniebändern. Hefte Unfallheilkd 142:1–94
6. Hey Groves EW (1920) The crucial ligaments of the knee joint: Their function, rupture, and the operative treatment of the same. Br J Surg 7:505–515
7. Hughston JC, Andrews JR, Cross MJ, et al. (1976) Classification of knee ligament instabilities: Parts I, II. J Bone Joint Surg [Am] 58:159–172
8. Jones RS, Smith A (1913) On rupture of the crucial ligaments of the knee, and on fractures of the spine of the tibia. Br J Surg 1:70–89
9. Kennedy JC, Weinberg HW, Wilson AS (1974) The anatomy and function of the anterior cruciate ligament as determined by clinical and morphological studies. J Bone Joint Surg [Am] 56:223–235
10. Kennedy JC, Hawkins RJ, Willis RB, et al. (1976) Tension studies of human knee ligaments, yield point, ultimate failure, and disruption of the cruciate and tibial collateral ligaments. J Bone Joint Surg [Am] 58:350–355

11. Nicholas JA (1973) The five-one reconstruction for anteromedial instability of the knee, indications, technique, and results in fifty-two patients. J Bone Joint Surg [Am] 55:899–922
12. Noyes FR, Delucas JL, Torvick PJ (1974) Biomechanics of anterior cruciate ligament failure: An analysis of strain-rate sensitivity and mechanics of failure in primates. J Bone Joint Surg [Am] 56:236–253
13. Smith SA (1918) The diagnosis and treatment of injuries to the crucial ligaments. Br J Surg 6:176–189
14. Torg JS, Conrad W, Kalen V (1976) Clinical diagnosis of anterior cruciate ligament instability in the athlete. Am J Sports Med 4:84–93
15. Van Dijk R (1983) The behaviour of the cruciate ligaments in the human knee. Thesis, Catholic University, Nijmegen

Acute diagnosis and treatment in post-traumatic haemarthrosis

G. de Keizer

Department of Surgery, Maria Hospital
Tilburg
The Netherlands

Introduction

In the casualty department of a general hospital one is frequently confronted with patients with acute injuries of the knee joint. Traffic accidents and sports injuries are the major causes. Most patients with such an injury present with haemarthrosis. Apart from intra-articular fractures, it is often difficult to gain insight into the precise nature of the lesions in and around the haemarthrotic joint.

Until fairly recently it was common practice to treat these injuries by aspiration of the haemarthrosis, application of a compression bandage and some form of rest, followed by some form of physiotherapy and muscle exercises, if no gross pathology could be demonstrated at the first examination.

Some patients recover completely after such treatment. In other patients, however, complaints and functional disorders persist, the true nature of which will not become apparent until a late stage. Sometimes the chance of complete recovery appears to be lost at that moment.

The problem is that diagnostic facilities in the casualty department are rather limited.

To gain a good insight into joint stability, it is essential to eliminate pain and muscle spasms. For this reason it is desirable to perform stability tests under general anaesthesia or epidural anaesthesia.

Another point is to determine the origin of bleeding in a case of haemarthrosis. Mostly the causative intra-articular lesions remain hidden at physical examination, but these are easily detectable by means of arthroscopic examination. It is rather difficult, however, to perform this supplementary part of joint examination under the conditions of the casualty department.

For those reasons we decided some years ago to hospitalize patients with injuries of this kind, to analyse more precisely the status of the ligaments and the intra-articular structures.

Patients and method

All patients with post-traumatic haemarthrosis were included. Intra-articular fractures were excluded by plain X-rays.

Stability tests and arthroscopic inspection with the patient under general anaesthesia or epidural anaesthesia were carried out as soon as possible. The grade of instability was judged by clinical examination. In cases of apparent grade III instability operative repair of the ruptured structures was performed immediately. In these cases we omitted the arthroscopy. The joint was opened during operation to inspect the intra-articular structures directly.

In cases with no obvious instability and in cases with only a moderate degree of laxity, for which we felt conservative treatment was indicated, an arthroscopic examination was always added.

Arthroscopy was carried out with a pneumatic tourniquet after exsanguination of the limb. Before inspection the haemarthrosis was evacuated and the joint thoroughly irrigated with sterile saline until all fluid returned clear and colourless. After irrigation the intra-articular structures were inspected and the origin of bleeding determined. Depending on the nature of the observed lesions an operative intervention was subsequently carried out or not.

Although the approach with accurate diagnosis and final treatment in the acute stage seems to be a rational one, it is rather difficult to quantify the overall advantages and disadvantages of the acute policy as against a more moderate wait-and-see attitude.

To better assess the merits of the acute approach we studied retrospectively the records of all patients with knee injuries managed according to these guidelines during the years 1979 up to and including 1983.

Results

In those years 290 knee joints with post-traumatic haemarthrosis were clinically examined. Instability to such a degree that in our opinion immediate surgical repair of the ruptured ligaments was indicated was demonstrated in 57 joints. The interventions in these cases are listed in Table 1. The remaining 233 joints were inspected by means of arthroscopy. Despite careful inspection, in 17 joints we were not able to detect the origin of bleeding. In these cases the bleeding lesions were probably in the posterior compartment of the knee joint. In the remaining 216 joints we observed the lesions listed in Table 2. On account of the nature of the observed lesions an operative intervention was performed in 103 knee joints. These interventions are listed in Table 3. This clinical procedure was strictly adhered to, and the overall result is given in Table 4.

Table 1. Operative interventions in joints with grade III instability (57 joints)

Repair of ruptured ligaments	
Medial compartment	48
Lateral compartment	9
Anterior cruciate ligaments	18
Posterior cruciate ligaments	6
Related interventions	
(Partial) meniscectomy	10
Reinsertion of meniscus	6
Others	10

Table 2. Observed lesions by means of acute arthroscopy in 216 joints

Anterior cruciate ligament	
Complete ruptures	47
Incomplete ruptures	31
Ruptures of medial meniscus	46
Ruptures of lateral meniscus	18
Capsular tears and subsynovial haematomas	87
(Osteo)chondral fractures	60
Total lesions	289

Table 3. Operative interventions following acute arthroscopy (103 joints)

Reinsertion of anterior cruciate ligament	20
(Partial) meniscectomy	51
Reattachment of meniscus	7
Removal of loose bodies	19
Others	15
Total interventions	112

Table 4. Overall results of clinical examination of knee injuries with haemarthrosis (without fractures) ($N=290$ joints)

Grade III instability followed by operative repair of ruptured ligaments	57 joints
Operative intervention after arthroscopic inspection	103 joints
Non-operative treatment after arthroscopic inspection	130 joints

Discussion

Some authors, such as Noyes et al. [1], Gillquist et al. [2] and Eriksson [3], stress the importance of arthroscopy in the acute stage of injury. On the basis of our experience we are also convinced of the additional value of acute arthroscopy [4].

Thanks to the acute arthroscopy, in 93% of the joints examined it was possible to make an accurate inventory of the intra-articular lesions. It is important to know what is wrong in the joint, both in deciding whether to operate or not and in planning a good scheme for conservative treatment.

Based on the arthroscopic findings a final operative intervention was carried out in the acute stage in 44% of cases.

It is likely that most if not all of these injuries would have eventually come to operation after a useless period of conservative treatment, with persistent symptoms and subsequent damage to the joint.

Evacuation and irrigation of all intra-articular blood as a part of the procedure is probably also of prophylactic value to some extent; it has been shown by Puhl et al. [5] that even a single effusion of intra-articular blood can exert a destructive action on the superficial layer of joint cartilage. Irrigation prior to arthroscopy makes it possible to wash out all blood from the joint cavity.

Infections did not occur in our series either in the group of patients managed by arthroscopy alone or in those who underwent arthrotomy after arthroscopy.

Conclusion

The overall diagnostic usefulness of clinical examination under anaesthesia including stability tests and arthroscopy appears to be high. In our opinion the result of using the above-mentioned procedure justifies its application. It provides a sound basis for correct final treatment in the very early stage of these knee injuries.

References

1. Noyes FR, Basett RW, et al. (1980) Arthroscopy in acute traumatic haemarthrosis of the knee. J Bone Jt Surg [Am] 62:687
2. Gillquist J, Hagberg G, Oretorp N (1977) Arthroscopy in acute injuries of the knee joint. Acta Orthop Scand 48:190
3. Eriksson E (1983) The role of arthroscopy in examining the acute knee. Paper presented at the Symposium on Knee Ligament Injuries, Hilversum, 14 May 1983
4. De Keizer G (1983) Acute arthroscopy in post-traumatic haemarthrosis of the knee joint. Neth J Surg 35(3):94
5. Puhl W, Dustmann MO, Schulitz KR (1971) Knorpelveränderungen beim experimentellen Hämarthrosis. Z Orthop 109:475

The influence of haemarthrosis of the knee joint on the cruciate ligaments

W. Pförringer

Staatliche Orthopädische Klinik München
8000 München
Federal Republic of Germany

The hemarthrosis of the knee joint is known for its deterioration effects on the cartilage as well as on the synovial membrane of the joint. Influences on the cruciate ligaments were up till now unknown and have been studied by the following method.

Material and methods:
250 rabbits were used to study the influence of an hemarthrosis of the knee joint on the cruciate ligaments. The hemarthrosis was performed by infusion of autologous blood of the rabbit into the knee joint for different periods of time. The effect of immobilization of such a joint was studied as well. Examinations were performed biomechanically, histologically and electron-microscopically.

Results:
It was found that a hemarthrosis causes damage to the cruciate ligament in so far as the biomechanical stability deteriorates significantly for a period up to 4 months. The damage of the hemarthrosis is worse when a lesion of the synovial membrane covering the cruciate ligaments occurs at the same time as the hemarthrosis.
Histological and electron-microscopical studies show that the fibrous tissue of the ligaments gets into disorder and that soft tissue necrosis arises as well.
Immobilization definitely does not accelerate the healing process.

Discussion:
Hemarthrosis ot the knee joint always should be treated with the highest possible diligence. Arthroscopy is advisable to find the reason of the bleeding as well as to remove the hemarthrosis of the knee joint in the same procedure.
Since the deteriorating effects of the hemarthrosis seem to be based on biomechanical reactions it is even more advisable to remove the blood out of the joint. In athletes it must be considered that the strain bearing capacity of the cruciate ligament is considerably reduced for a period of 3 to 4 months and that athletic performance in this time should be discontinued.

Surgical or conservative treatment of the acutely torn anterior cruciate ligament; a randomized study with a short-term follow-up

M. Odensten, P. Hamberg, M. Nordin, J. Lysholm and J. Gillquist

Sports Trauma Research Group, Dept. of Orth. Surg., University Hospital Linköping Sweden

90 consecutive patients ranging in age between 13 and 49 years (mean 24.2) with an acute ACL rupture, underwent arthroscopy and clinical examination under anaesthesia within 5 days after injury. All patients showed a total midsubstance rupture of the ACL. The patients were randomized into two groups, surgical treatment and conservative treatment of the ACL. All associated injuries were sutured when necessary in both groups. Patients in group I, surgical treatment group had their ACL repaired with sutures and augmented with a strip from the iliotibial band. This group I underwent a control arthroscopy in mean 9.1 months after operation. 67 % of the patients had an excellent result with normal ACL, 27% were classified as good and 7% as poor. All patients were reviewed at the follow-up in mean 18.2 months after operation. The patients underwent clinical examination, a functional knee test isokinetic muscle strength (Cybex II) a standardized one leg jump, a figure of eight running and a functional knee score (Lysholm & Gillquist, 1982) was obtained.

95% of the patients in group I were stable at the follow-up review with a negative pivot-shift. In this group II patients was 85.0. 76% of the patients in group I achieved more than 84 points (good or excellent) while only 53% in group II were rated over 84 points ($p < 0.05$).

In the thigh muscle measurements the patients in group II (conservatively treated ACL rupture) had a significantly higher mean isokinetic quadriceps' strength than did group I patients, probably due to a longer rehabilitation time in this group. In running and jump tests we could not find any significant differences between the groups.

In earlier studies (Odensten, 1983) we have seen that unstable patients may overestimate their knee function in the early postoperative course and thereby achieve a high score. However, in the long run the unstable patients' score decreased as well as thigh muscle strength. The results in the one leg jump test and running tests depend on the thigh muscle strength. In a long-term perspective there will probably be separation between the groups in these tests.

The present study shows that early primary suture and additional augmentation seems to be the treatment of choice in patients with an acutely torn anterior cruciate ligament. However, before we can recommend this procedure we need at least another 2-3 years at which time we will present a long-term follow-up review of the same patients.

Isolated lesion of the anterior cruciate ligament

M. Weigert and C. Werhahn

Krankenhaus am Urban, Abteilung für Orthopädik und Traumatologie
D-1000 Berlin
Federal Republic of Germany

Among over 8000 arthroscopies performed in our special department for knee surgery in the course of the past 7 years, we found an isolated lesion of anterior cruciate ligament in 8 cases. Moreover, we detected 104 lesions of the anterior cruciate ligament, some of which were combined with minor defects such as lesions of the medial or lateral capsule.

Therefore in every case of suspected knee trauma we now perform acute arthroscopy as an ambulant procedure with local anaesthesia.

Suture or reinsertion is only possible within the first 4 weeks after the accident.

In cases in which primary reconstruction does not seem possible as well as in most chronic cases without signs of degenerative arthritis, we have performed our own double semitendinosus plasty for the past 1½ years.

Experiments with the double-running course of the semitendinosus tendon in cadaver specimens showed that movement and primary stability seemed better with the double-running tendon than with former methods of cruciate ligament plasty.

Operation technique
The patient is supine, with the leg exsanguinated by tourniquet. The medial Payr incision is made, preparing the semitendinosus tendon, which is cut proximally on the musculotendinosus transition. The muscle belly is sutured with the gracilis tendon. Two holes are prepared to the caput tibiae, one triangular hole in the fossa intercondylica as far back as possible. This hole has a blind ending; two small holes through the cortex of the femur for anchoring the suture begin on the end of the trigonum. The semitendinosus tendon is pulled into the dorsal hole of the caput tibiae, then fastened by a strong double suture in the femur and pulled out through the other hole in the tibia. Before tightening the sutures both tendons are covered by corpus adiposum genus according to Müller. During tightening of the sutures the position of the knee joint is 20 ° to 30 ° flexion and medial rotation. A Scotch cast is left on for 6 weeks; weight-bearing is usually allowed 10 weeks after the operation. Sports activities are not allowed until 16 weeks after the operation and competitive sports after 6 months.

In cases with signs of degenerative arthritis or recidive after cruciate ligament plasty, since last year we have inserted a prosthesis for replacement of the anterior cruciate ligament. We use two incisions and fasten a Gore-tex band by two screws on the femur and tibia. After this procedure only physiotherapy without weight-bearing is performed; no plaster at all is necessary. Weight-bearing is allowed after 6 weeks. Our own histological investigation on sheep and humans showed perfect incorporation of the Gore-tex by connective tissue.

Results

We use the grading scale of Müller, with three degrees of instability and four categories of results. The results after reconstruction of the anterior cruciate ligament by suture or reinsertion in 77 cases are:

Very good	18%
Good	65%
Moderate	14%
Bad	3%

Results after double-running semitendinosus plasty for 48 cases are:

Very good	28%
Good	52%
Moderate	16%
Bad	4%

Results after Gore-tex plasty, 12 cases so far, are:

Very good	25%
Good	50%
Moderate	25%

All these 12 cases had previously had at least one tendon plasty and signs of degenerative arthritis.

Conclusion

For detection of isolated ruptures of the anterior cruciate ligament the Lachmann test is significant and acute arthroscopy is mandatory.

In cases in which reconstruction of the anterior cruciate ligament is not possible, results after double-running semitendinosus plasty seem superior to former methods.

In recidive cases and cases with severe cartilage degeneration, cruciate ligament plasty prosthesis seems to be very promising.

Fresh injuries of the anterior cruciate ligament treated by suture in combination with augmentation plasty

R. Meyrat and B. Noesberger

Department of Orthopaedics and Traumatology, Regionalspital CH-3800 Interlaken Switzerland

The recommendations of how fresh lesions of the anterior cruciate ligament (ACL) should be treated are various. Repair of the ligament alone leads to a good functional result only in 30% of cases. As the suture of the ACL alone often does not guarantee stability, there is the problem of how it could be reinforced. With intra- or extra-articular augmentation plasty the result in relation to stability should be improved.

As early as 1936, Bosworth and Bosworth described an extra-articular repair. Later other authors described various techniques. All of them used the tractus iliotibialis for this plasty in one way or another. Other authors, as documented by Kennedy et al. (1978), have had disappointing results with this type of procedure and therefore prefer intra-articular graft augmentation.

Augmentation plasties have been performed at the Regionalspital Interlaken since 1978. Isolated avulsions of the ligament with a convincing morphological structure are sutured only. Of course, the external capsular and ligamentar apparatus is – when damaged – reconstructed exactly. In all other cases where a suture is still possible an additional augmentation plasty is performed.

From 1978 to 1982, 131 fresh injuries of the ACL were operated on at the Regionalspital Interlaken. In 50 patients only suture of the ACL was performed; in 67 cases an additional augmentation plasty was carried out. As many of our patients are foreign tourists or seasonal workers, only 26 of these 67 patients could be clinically controlled by the authors personally. It was decided to send a questionnaire about possible problems to all the patients, as suggested by the AOSSM study group. Of 57 questionnaires dispatched, 51 (89%) were returned. Eight patients are abroad with unknown addresses, one died of an unrelated cause and one patient had a new ACL lesion after another trauma. Of 67 injuries, 45 (67%) were the result of skiing accidents; 23 patients had other sports accidents, 4 domestic accidents, 2 car accidents and only 1 an accident at work. The age of the patients operated on was 33 years on average. The youngest patients were aged 17 years at the time of surgery, and the oldest was 79 years.

The following lesions of the ACL were found: 42 femoral avulsions, 13 intermediate ruptures and 12 combined lesions.

The femoral avulsions were mostly repaired by a suture over the top. For the augmentation plasty the following techniques were used: 35 Hughston, 21 Ellison, 2 Andrews, 2 Lemaire and 7 intra-articular augmentation plasties.

The aftertreatment consisted of a closed cast in 30 ° flexion of the knee for 6 weeks. All patients were sent for physiotherapy, which varied widely from case to case. The period of therapy varied from 0 to 40 weeks, giving an average of 9.5 weeks.

At the time of follow-up 33 patients never suffered pain, while 12 patients sometimes had slight pain. Five patients complained about moderate and one patient about severe pain. A slight sensitivity to change in the weather was indicated by about 50% of the patients, while only 17 were never influenced by the weather.

Thirty-three patients never had symptoms of giving way in the operated knee. An unstable knee joint was complained of by seven patients only during sports activities, by nine occasionally and by two patients with normal daily activities.

The actual sports activity documents the results attained with the operation quite well: 25 patients perform the same sports as prior to injury and nine patients do the same sports but at a lower performance level. This group includes three ski racers. Six patients have changed their favourite sport, some of them not because of the accident. Four patients feel significantly limited in their sports activities and two patients no longer participate in sports at all.

It is surprising that 45 (80%) of the patients judge the attained result as good, 4 classify the result as moderate and 2 consider it poor.

The following results were obtained during the follow-up control of 26 patients:

The anterior drawer test produced a distance of 5 mm in 4 cases and 10 mm in 2 cases.

Seven patients showed a positive Lachmann test (shifting of more than 2 mm, distinct stop). These patients were X-rayed in the anterior-posterior direction to check on the instability. Naturally these examinations were performed without anaesthesia. It is interesting that there was no correlation between the X-rays and the anterior drawer test result found during follow-up controls. This phenomenon was probably caused by muscular tension during X-rays. A pivot shift could be provoked in three patients. We think that the measurement of the circumference of the thigh is still a good method to determine atrophy of the quadriceps muscle, even though nowadays muscular strength can be measured mechanically, e.g. by Cybex. Fifteen patients showed atrophy of the treated leg; five showed no difference. In six patients a larger circumference was found on the treated leg.

Considering the results of the follow-up, symptoms and sports activities we divided the patients into four groups according to W. Müller (1978);

1. Very good — Instability up to 2 mm
No problems
Same sports activities as before the accident

2. Good	Instability up to 5 mm Slight problems Sports activities slightly reduced Usually no giving way
3. Moderate	Instability up to 10 mm Moderate problems Occasional giving way Sports activities significantly reduced
4. Bad	Instability over 10 mm Severe problems Frequent giving way No sports possible

Very good and good results were found in 42 of the 51 cases (82%) in the follow-up:

Very good	18	35.3%
Good	24	47.1%
Moderate	7	13.7%
Poor	2	3.9%

The age of the patients seems to have a definite influence on the results obtained.

With regard to the physiotherapy it is noticed that the patients with poor results needed more therapy. The results of the thigh measurements mentioned before distinctly show that the training performed was inadequate. After rehabilitation, proper muscle training is lacking.

Comparing the results of the various operation methods, no significant difference can be found:

Table 1. Results and operation methods (51 patients)

	Very good	Good	Moderate	Poor
Hughston	12	9	3	2
Ellison	3	9	2	–
Andrews	1	–	1	–
Lemaire	–	2	–	–
Intra-articular augmentation plasty	2	4	–	–

It is noticed that the Ellison procedure shows only few very good results. This could have several reasons:

1. This operation method seems to provide more stability than, for example, the Hughston procedure. Therefore it was chosen for severe lesions or in combination with difficult sutures.
2. The method is technically more demanding.
3. Dislocation of the Gerdy tubercle or screw fixation may cause persistent pain.

On the basis of the results presented here, we conclude that suture of the injured ACL combined with augmentation plasty has a good chance of success and can be recommended.

It cannot be determined which method of reinforcement should be chosen. Possibly this is not significant. It is of much more importance that an additional repair is performed at all.

References

1. Bosworth DM, Bosworth BM (1936) Use of fascia lata to stabilize the knee in case of ruptured crucial ligaments. J Bone Joint Surg [Am] 18:178
2. Ellison AE (1979) Distal iliotibial band transfer for anterolateral rotatory instability of the knee. J Bone Joint Surg [Am] 6:330
3. Johnson LL (1979) Lateral capsular ligament complex: Anatomical and surgical considerations. Am J Sports Med 7:156
4. Losee RE, Johnson ETR, Southwick WO (1978) Anterior subluxation of the lateral tibial plateau. J Bone Joint Surg [Am] 60:10
5. Galway RD, Beaupre A, McIntosh DL (1972) Pivot shift: A clinical sign of symptomatic anterior cruciate insufficience. J Bone Joint Surg [Br] 54:763
6. Hughston JC, Andrews JR, Cross MJ, Moschi A (1976) Classification of knee ligament instabilities: II. The lateral compartment. J Bone Joint Surg [Am] 58:173
7. Kennedy JC, Steward R, Weber DM (1978) Anterolateral rotatory instability of the knee joint. An early analysis of the Ellison procedure. J Bone Joint Surg [Am] 60:1031
8. Andrews JR, Sanders R (1983) A "mini-reconstruction" technique in treating anterolateral rotatory instability. Clin Orthop 172:93
9. Feagin JA, Blake WP (1983) Postoperative evaluation and result recording in the anterior cruciate ligament reconstructed knee. Clin Orthop 172:143
10. Müller W (1978) Rotational stability of the knee. Prog Orthop Surg 3:59
11. Frösch P, Noesberger B (1982) Die anteromediale Instabilität des Kniegelenks. Dissertation, University of Berne

The treatment of recent ruptures of the anterior cruciate ligament with early augmentation

A. Mitsou, N. Piscopakis and J. Parker

Department of Sport Injuries, University of Athens
Kifisia – Athens
Greece

The treatment of recent ruptures of the anterior cruciate ligament (ACL) is controversial. The poor results of end to end suturing of the ACL in recent ruptures of the mid portion of it, led the authors to attempt augmentation of the suturing by the use of a transplant.

Material and methods

Our report refers to 37 knees with recent injury of the mid-portion of the ACL to which primary suturing of the ligament and augmentation of it, was carried out. The surgical technique consisted of use of reversed pull-out sutures for the ACL and then reinforcement of it with a part of the fascia lata (over the top). Evaluation was based on the subjective and functional problems of the patients and with the objective evaluation of the clinical test for the ACL.

Results

The final evaluation was completed from 32 patients with a follow up of 10 to 40 months. The average age of the patients was 22 years old and all were athletes of various sports. Our results were excellent in 62,5%, good in 31% and poor in 6,2%.

Discussion

From our study we believe that the method of choice in recent ruptures of the mid portion of the ACL is the primary suturing of the ligament and augmentation of it. This conclusion was drawn because the greatest percentage of our results was excellent in that 93% of the patients returned, to a great extent to their former standard of athletic activity and 33% of them took part again in professional football.

Summary

Primary suturing of recent ruptures of the mid portion of the ACL with augmentation of it was carried out in 37 knees. Our results from 32 patients were excellent in 62,5%, good in 31% and poor in 6,2%. All of our patients were athletes of various sports.

Factors of importance for cruciate repair and reconstruction

J. Gillquist

Department of Orthopaedic Surgery, University Hospital
S-581 85 Linköping
Sweden

Since the time of Hey Groves and Ivar Palmer operative treatment has been the rule for a torn anterior cruciate. In acute cases we use the simple repair originally described by Palmer: several U sutures are used to reattach the torn ligament. The results reported in the literature with this repair are not consistent, but many Scandinavian authors have suggested good results in short-term follow-ups. One problem with acute knees used to be correct early diagnosis. Diagnosis on the basis of clinical examination alone led to a very high frequency of isolated anterior cruciate lesions. With the advent of arthroscopy the acute diagnosis became more detailed and the whole spectrum of lesions in acute knees could be demonstrated and treated. However, if diagnosis was delayed primary suture was not feasible. The ligament had to be reconstructed. Of the several techniques for reconstruction it seems that use of part of the patellar tendon is the most common today. Again, results in follow-ups have varied and hardly any prospective controlled studies on the technique are available. This presentation will discuss some factors influencing the outcome of treatment of the torn anterior cruciate ligament.

Anatomy

Several studies are available on anterior cruciate anatomy, but there seems to be none where anatomical data are used to influence current surgical treatment. The normal ligament is 25–35 mm long, with a mean of 31 mm. It makes an angle of 28° with the long axis of the femur when the knee is flexed to 90°. Both attachments are about 2 cm long in a sagittal plane. The distance from the anterior border of the tibia to the centre of the tibial attachment is 24 mm. The femur attachment is within the posterior 25% of Blumensaat's line. When the ligament is sectioned longitudinally and horizontally no anatomical separations into different bundles can be found within the ligament. The effect of different attachments was examined in several knee specimens by pulling a thread through different drill holes. The central points of both attachments were found to be isometric. No motion of the thread occurred over the whole range of motion. Attachments anterior or posterior to these points were non-isometric and led to shortening or elongation of the ligament in flexion and extension. This accounts for the popular belief that the ligament has different bundles. Being non-isometric the anterior and posterior parts of the ligament are subjected to varying tension during flexion-extension. Thus different parts of the ligaments are tensed in different positions, as was already pointed out by Palmer. We found that the over-the-top position was very unfavourable, with more than 30% change in length during motion. If an over-the-top reconstruction is tightened in flexion the patient will end up with an extension block or a ruptured ligament. If it is tightened in extension the ligament will allow a 1-cm drawer in flexion. There is no way to attain both a full range of motion and stability throughout unless the ligament substitute is placed in the isometric point. This also means that for there to be any chance of success the substitute has to be at least 31 mm long in its intra-articular portion. What are the conditions in acute rupture? We measured the length of the remaining ligament in all acute cases during the course of 1 year. All patients were operated on within 5 days of the accident. The useful length of the stump was measured. The mean was found to be 20 mm and none was longer than 25 mm. This means that primary simple suture cannot bring the stump into contact with the femur at the normal attachment. If one reaches the femur it is always too far forward in a non-isometric position. This may explain the rather unsatisfactory results of our controlled long-term follow-up of simple acute suture. At 2 years the results looked good, with a majority of patients having good function and stability, but at 4 years more than 50% had instability and less than adequate function. In contrast, patients with a partial rupture had unchanged normal function after 6 years. Thus, healing had a greater chance if at least one part of the ligament was intact and still attached to the proper insertion point. This is the philosophy behind repair with reinforcement or augmentation. The gap between the stump and the femur is bridged by a substitute, usually a strip from the iliotibial tract. In a prospective randomized study we were able to demonstrate a better result 2 years after the accident with this method than with conservative treatment. However, this study also demonstrates that many patients have a good result with conservative treatment only. About 80% of the conservatively treated patients had no major problems with the knee over the first 2 years. An important goal for future research will be to define patients who have a reasonable chance of success with conservative treatment as well as the ones who need an acute operation.

The anatomical measurements are important also in reconstructing the anterior cruciate. An important part of the reconstruction of an old injury to the anterior cruciate is recreation of the normal tunnel width. In young specimens the normal mean width is 21 mm. In a series of old unstable knees the mean was 15 mm. Some were even as narrow as 10 mm. There is no chance that a cruciate substitute could survive in that space. All osteophytes on the lateral femur condyle and on the roof of the tunnel should be removed. The tunnel should be measured to make sure it is restored to 21 mm. This will create a good space for the new ligament. Adequate graft length is also important. From a series of measurements of patellar tendon length it was quite obvious that it generally was about 30% too short to reach the anatomical insertion site if left attached to the tuberosity. This means that a free graft or some kind of pedicled graft has to be used to get the substitute in the isometric position.

If a free graft is used there is the problem of revascularization and survival of the graft. It was shown in the early 1970s by Alm that the tendon was revascularized to survive both in the human and in the dog. These studies were repeated by Clancy, who verified Alm's results. However, with the free graft there is a period when the graft is devoid of all blood supply. In order to speed up vascularization, a so-called vascularized graft with a stalk from the medial retinaculum or the fat pad has been suggested by Noyes and Clancy. In terms of blood vessels this is obviously a good method. Whether it makes any difference in the clinical situation is not known, since no controlled studies are available. To obtain and maintain proper stability the correct tension of the substitute must be achieved. What the tension should be is not known at present. We have been using a simple tensiometer in order to get at least the same tension every time. Perhaps the tension should take up something like half of the elasticity of the substitute. If the substitute is too tight close to maximum elongation, a sudden impact load may break it. Orientation of the collagen in the substitute is probably dependent on load. Therefore, load on a transplanted tendon must increase over a period of time. Whether early range of motion exercises will speed up recovery of strength in the graft and result in a more stable knee is not known. Immediate fixation of the substitute should be achieved with the device that allows stability testing. It should be possible to perform a Lachmann test as well as a pivot shift test to make sure the knee is stable. Stability of the joint has to be achieved at operation with any type of graft. There will be no increase in joint stability afterwards: only a decrease can be expected. The stability achieved can be measured with a stability-measuring device, which can be sterilized.

In order for the transplant to survive the correct position is very important. A non-isometric position will ultimately lead to graft failure and instability. This calls for a reproducible and accurate operative technique. It is preferable if the motion between the graft and the attachment channel is as small as possible, to diminish wear at the inner ends of the channels. This is accomplished by drilling the two channels through the femur and tibia in a straight line. A good compromise is to drill the two channels in a straight line with the knee in 90° flexion, which is an easily defined position of the knee.

Using a recently designed patented drill guide we drill both channels simultaneously in the proper position. The length of the intra-articular portion automatically becomes the desired 31 mm, and if the guide is aligned correctly with the long axis of the femur the angle of 28° is achieved. The channel through the bone has to fit as tightly as possible to the transplant in order to speed up bone healing. The inner ends of the channels should be rounded off with a special router to avoid wear of the transplant against any sharp edges. With this placement technique any substitute can be used as well as an artificial ligament. Compared with free-hand drilling the drill guide system improves the accuracy threefold. It is also important that the position of the channels is checked with a test ligament. This should not move at all in the channels when the joint is taken through a full range of motion.

Evaluation

If different techniques are to be compared in terms of end-result, accurate and reproducible evaluation systems have to be used. It is also vital that different operative techniques are compared in prospective, randomized trials where as many factors are controlled as possible. Otherwise there will never be any progress in knee ligament surgery. The evaluation system has to be aimed at stability and function. There are various stability-measuring machines available today, which are more or less elaborate. If the error of measurement is controlled, these machines represent an improvement over the estimation of instability in +, + + or + + +. However, the change from instability to stability is often very small – it may be a matter of a few millimetres. Therefore a high level of accuracy is a necessary feature of the machine, and the measuring technique must be reproducible. Knee function can be evaluated with scores and different tests. Elsewhere in this volume we present an evaluation system using the Lysholm score and a standardized functional test. These tests are very important in order to decide whether rehabilitation is complete or if one operation gives a superior functional result to another.

Normal values can be established for different groups of athletes and this information can be used to set the goal for rehabilitation after knee ligament surgery.

Hopefully better operative techniques, better evaluation systems and better scientific designs will ultimately provide us with the preferred treatment of the ruptured anterior cruciate.

Postoperative comparison of 155 acute and 211 old anteromedial knee instabilities grade III

M. Kolb, C. J. Wirth and M. Jäger

Orthopaedic University Hospital
8000 München
Federal Republic of Germany

155 acute anteromedial knee instabilities grade III were reevaluated between 1 and 10 years postoperatively. Acute knee instabilities were treated by suture of the medial collateral ligament, refixation of the anterior cruciate ligament, occasionally by primary anterior cruciate plasty and by suture or removal of the medial meniscus.

Old knee instabilities were treated by the method described by Nicolas, modified Nicholas procedure with additional replacement of the anterior cruciate ligament, and modified O'Donoghue procedure with replacement of the anterior cruciate ligament. Always a medial meniscectomy was performed. The follow-up examination was performed after the criteria and point system as described by Marshall (1977).

Generally speaking, results after immediate treatment were better by 20% when compared to late repairs. Good to excellent results were obtained already after one year in acute anteromedial knee instabilities in 70%. These results do not change much up to the tenth year postoperatively. In old knee instabilities good to excellent results were obtained in 55% not before the 5th postoperative year. There was no further improvement up to the seventh year. The operation modified after Nicolas with replacement of the anterior cruciate proved to be the best operative method. Due to the medial meniscectomy there was almost always a medial osteoarthritis of varying degree which influenced the subjective result and the overall results.

We conclude from this study that follow-up examinations after acute anteromedial knee instabilities are relevant at the earliest after one year, after old repairs at the earliest after 3 years.

Our experience with treatment of injured knee ligaments

V. Pokorny

Research Institute of Traumatology
Brno
Czechoslovakia

Material and Methods

More than 1,700 knee injuries were operated in our Research Institute of Traumatology in the period from 1964 to 1982. These were mostly injuries of meniscus (1,186 patients), ligaments were treated with 558 patients. The majority of patients in the latter group were operated on for chronic instability (488 operations), number of acute operations was 70. The ratio between primary and reconstruction operations of ligaments is 7:1 and this relation is considered unfavourable. The reason is that serious knee injuries are sent late for special examination and treatment or that primary treatment, both conservative and operative, is not sufficient or complete in some cases.

Results

Operation results with 117 patients were checked after 5 – 8 years. 32 patients were operated on within 4 days after the injury and 85 patients because of chronic instability. We tried to evaluate the functional capacity of the operated knee objectively with the help of our own system of points. We evaluated the atrophy of muscles, mobility extent, passive instability, functional capacity, pains, exsudates and changes of life regime. When comparing both groups of patients, the advantages of primary operation treatment are indisputable.

Discussion

When examining the acute injury medically it is necessary to consider the complex anatomical structure of the knees. When examining it thoroughly we find there are much less patients with the injury of only one joint structure and more frequently there occurs a simultaneous injury of more anatomical structures even when in various extent and with various clinical manifestation.

Summary

It should be stressed that emergency treatment of injured ligaments is always more advantageous than the reconstruction due to chronical instability. Restitution of knee stability is the best cure for arthrosis after injury.

One thousand operations for ligamentous lesion of the knee joint 1971–1983

K. Franke

Dept. Surgery, Municipal Hospital Berlin-Pankow
DDR-1100 Berlin
German Dem. Rep.

During twelve years from 1971 until 1982 in our hospital were operated on 2 595 knee joints after an injury. Among them were 878 patients with different ligamentous injuries. This number will have increased to about 1000 at the end of 1983, which will be the background of the conference paper.

Our procedure to repairing ligamentous lesions is standardized:
ACL: since 1968 free graft from the patellar tendon, since 1980 occasionally gracilis tendon transfer;
PCL: gracilis tendon transfer (Lindemann);
LCL- distension: capitulum-fibulae-transfer to lateral tibial plate (Trillat);
MCL-distension: insertion transfer downward the tibial plate;
MCL + LCL insufficiency: free graft from patellar tendon (Brückner) or plastic repair with lyophilized tissue;
capsule instability: dorsal insertion's attachment (Trillat) or reinforcement of collateral ligament and anterior capsule by lyophilized tissue (our method).

Analysis of 878 patients hints at the following facts:

- male: female ratio = 2,8 : 1
- 71,4% had already a chondromalacia
- primary operation within 3 days: 1971..1980=5%; 1981/82:12,4%
- cause of injury: sports 63,3%; traffic 14,3%; work 12,4%; at home 10%
- 95,9% of all collateral ligament injuries were medial ones
- isolated ACL-ruptures were found in 7,3% of all ligament lesions, whose pattern is shown below:

51,1% (n=449) combined plastic repair of collateral ligament and fibrous capsule or primary suture;
18,9% (n=166) collateral ligament alone;
47,4% (n=416) cruciate ligament's replacement or suture;
7,3% (n= 64) intercondylar eminence transposition;
3,4% (n= 30) intercondylar eminence avulsion.

New ideas about knee joint biomechanics have influenced also our indications and methods of repairing ligamentous injuries. As far as 1975 the majority of operations was an isolated ACL or MCL repair. Since 1976 combined methods are dominating:

kind of lesion	1971–75	1976–80	1981/82	1971–1982
cruciate ligament(s)	139	61	34	234
collateral lig.	48	176	84	308
ligaments combined	65	147	112	336
				878 patients

Functional results of knee joint surgery are determined by
- interval between accident and sufficient operation,
- thereby influenced extent of cartilage destruction, and
- efficiency of rehabilitation, starting as early as possible.

An analysis of 390 ligamentous lesions operated on between 1971 and 1977 confirmed these relations. Patients with only one operation obtained a good physical load capacity in 80%. Among those with two ore more operations this optimum was only reached by 66%.

The active pivot shift test – the role of the popliteus muscle

L. Peterson and M. I. Pitman

Dept. of Orthopaedic Surgery, Östra Hospital
Gothenburg
Sweden

This study was stimulated by the ability of one of us (L.P.) to actively perform a pivot shift test upon his anterior cruciate deficient knee. Subsequently this phenomenon has been observed in other patients. The purpose was to define and analyze the active motor involved in this abnormal active motion in the knee with Antero-Lateral Rotatory Instability.

Quigley has noted the role of the Popliteus muscle in internal rotation of the tibia and has discussed its possible effects upon rotatory instability. Basmajian analyzed the function of the Popliteus muscle electro myographically and defined its role as an internal tibial rotator especially in the first 20° of flexion to unlock the screw home mechanism.

Three subjects with proven ACL deficient knees who were actively able to perform the pivot shift phenomenon were studied. The test is reproducible with the subject sitting, the knee flexed to 90° and the foot on the floor. The subjects then can actively sublux the lateral tibial plateau anteriorly. Needle electrodes were to record the activity of the popliteus muscle on active performance of this test, and to attempt to reproduce the test by electrical stimulation of the popliteus.

In all 3 patients, the role of the popliteus as the active motor was demonstrated electromyographically. No other muscle could be implicated in the movement.

The popliteus has a role as an active motor in producing ALRI in the ACL deficient knee. Active internal tibial rotation at the start of flexion may dynamically increase the instability. Advancement of the arcuate complex in cases of lateral corner instability associated with ALRI may actually strengthen the role of the Popliteus in producing the ALRI rather than preventing it.

This study reinforces Quigley's thesis that advancement of the Popliteus may be used in the treatment of AMRI by increasing its internal rotatory strength. If the popliteus is used as a substitute for the PCL, the knee may be deprived of its active synergistic force in prevention of PLRI-which it performs by rotating the lateral tibial plateau anteriorly. Transfer of the popliteus to replace the PCL may be biomechanically incorrect.

The use of electric stimulation may provide an objective clinical method to demonstrate rotatory instability.

Intra-articular reconstruction of the anterior cruciate ligament. An experimental comparison of length changes of different positions of the reconstructed ligament

T. Hoogland and B. Hillen

Ignatius Hospital
Breda
The Netherlands

Purpose of the study

The study was designed in order to evaluate the most favourable positions of the tunnels and fixation points for the intra-articular reconstruction of the anterior cruciate ligament. In particular the "over the top" repair was compared to tunneling the plasty through the lateral femoral condyle.

Material and methods

An anatomical model was developed to test different positions of intra-articular ACL-reconstructions. Four cadaver knees were tested in an identical fashion. In each knee 12 different positions were tested. All ligaments of those knees were preserved, except the ACL was excised.

The drill-holes were made in the tibial plateau: one at the anterior site of the ACL-insertion: one in the middle of the ACL-insertion and one psoterior at the ACL-insertion. Two tunnels were drilled in the lateral femoral condyle: one origination anterior at the femoral insertion of the ACL and one posterior at the ACL-insertion. More over a hole was made in the posterior capsule "over the top" of the lateral condyle.

A 5 mm wide plastified steel cord was fixed just beneath the insertion of the medial 1/3 of the patella tendon and subsequently routed over the tibial plateau into the femoral tunnels, "over the top" and through the separate tibial tunnels. That way 12 different positions of ACL reconstructions could be tested: Fig I. (positions 1A, 1B, 1C, 2A, 2B, 2C, 3A, 3B, 3C, 4A, 4B and 4C) The rope was freely mobile and kept under a constant tension of 45 Newton force. The knees were then slowly put through a full range of motion and all length changes of the artificial reconstructed ligament were measured at the exit.

Table I
Average maximum length changes in millimeters of the 12 different positions of the reconstructed ACL in 4 cadaver knees.

		Femoral positions		
		A.	B.	C. (over the top)
Tibial positions	1.	8,1	2,6	4,0
	2.	8,2	2,7	5,7
	3.	9,2	3,3	8,5
	4.	8,4	3,9	9,9

Results

The results of all three knees were rather identical. The average maxium length change over a full range motion (0°-130°) are recorded in Table I.

The greatest stretch free range of motion was found in the graft positions where it was guided through the tunnel posteriorly through the lateral femoral condyle.

Discussion and summary

The results indicate that the "over the top" repair is an unfavourable position of the anterior cruciate ligament reconstruction from a mechanical standpoint.
It is likely that this type of repair in human knees will lead to excessive stretching and insufficiency of the recontructed tissue. The same thing seems true when the graft is led through a tunnel anteriorly to the anatomical origin of the ACL at the femoral condyle. Leading the plasty through a tunnel posteriorly through the lateral femoral condyle appears a much more desirable route. The position of the tibial tunnel is less crucial but the more anterior tunnel seems most favourable.

The technique of intra-articular cruciate reconstruction

W. Müller

Leitender Arzt der Orthopädischen Abteilung Kantonsspital Bruderholz
CH-4101 Bruderholz
Schweiz

Introduction
More and more, we are finding that operations which strive to replace the lost function of the cruciate ligaments but fail to duplicate the anatomy of the cruciate ligaments are rarely successful in restoring full performance to the knee joint in the long term.

Even the results of intra-articular cruciate reconstructions have proved somewhat disappointing. We have learned, however, that a detailed knowledge of the anatomy and function of the cruciate ligaments is fundamental to the improvement of operating technique and thus of the operative result.

Clinical manifestations of cruciate ligament insufficiency
The well-known anterior and posterior drawer have long been the most obvious signs of cruciate deficiency, but they are not helpful in understanding the fine functional problems that result from this condition. The patient is the first to recognize that the knee is not as steady as before and has lost its "closure" internally, even though the examiner may be unable to demonstrate objective change.

The principal causes of this unsteadiness are the destruction of the delicate guidance system of the knee and the disintegration of the rolling-gliding mechanism. A secondary cause is the failure of rotational control. Without sound cruciate ligaments, the longitudinal axis of rotation wanders, and even the automatic terminal rotation of the knee which limits extension and prevents hyperextension is impaired. One expression of this is instability of the knee *near the terminal phase of extension* as described by Lachman and Trillat. A very clear manifestation of deficient rotational control is the presence of rotatory instabilities in all four quadrants of the knee, especially when the instabilities involve entire compartments.

The isolated vs. combined ligamentous injury
It is questionable whether a true isolated cruciate ligament rupture can occur. As a rule, there will be an occult associated injury involving the connection between the medial meniscus and the posterior oblique ligament, the Kaplan attachment of the anterolateral femorotibial structures (where a traumatic elongation of only a few millimeters can produce anterolateral rotary instability), or the popliteus corner.

The occurrence of an isolated PCL rupture caused by a blow to the upper tibia with the knee flexed is a more likely entity than the "isolated ACL rupture".

Interim conclusion: In every operation where repair or reconstruction of the cruciate ligaments is proposed, it is essential that these secondary or co-stabilizers of the knee be carefully evaluated and restored to their normal anatomic position and length. This is the only way in which a cruciate ligament that is undergoing healing can be adequately protected from harmful stresses. This applies equally to the ligament substitute, which is susceptible both to interstitial damage and to avulsion from its sites of attachment.

Isolated ruptures of the peripheral ligaments are also rare, for even a linear instability with, say, a 2+ medial opening of the joint space will produce a concomitant lesion or at least a distention of the central pillar.

The intra-articular cruciate reconstruction
Anatomic imitation is the guiding principle for intra-articular reconstructions. The free lengths of the cruciate ligaments are so short that a positioning error of 2 or 3 mm will mean an error of plus or minus 10%–20% in the length of the substitute.

Also, care must be taken that there are no osteophytes present that could elongate or damage the ligament substitute.

Both cruciate ligaments are usually composed of two or more main fascicles. Several authors have already developed techniques with which at least two main bundles can be reconstructed.

The posterior cruciate ligament
Injuries of this ligament are becoming increasingly frequent as a consequence of motorcycle accidents, dashboard injuries, and injuries sustained in hard contact sports.

In many instances the outcome in the conservatively treated or untreated knee is so poor that reconstructive surgery becomes the only option for restoring the patient to an acceptable level of occupational or recreational activity. It is in reconstructions of the posterior cruciate ligament (PCL) that we have made the most satisfying progress in the past three years compared with the results of previous years.

Tightening an existing scarred and lax PCL
Often there will be a very good but scarred collagenous band that has the proper strength and thickness, but is too long. Only 5 mm of excess length can produce a 2+ or 3+ posterior drawer.

A laxity of this type can be adequately managed by proximal advancement of the femoral insertion of the PCL through a channel prepared with a drill and curette. The amount of advancement corresponds to the length excess of the ligament (e.g., 5 mm in the example above). The tightness is maintained with a suture tied around a "mooring screw" (e.g., a Jakob type screw) on the lateral aspect of the medial femoral metaphysis (Figure 1 a, b, c).

As with all posterior instabilities, it is necessary to follow the repair with the insertion of a transpatellar Steinmann pin according to Grammont's tech-

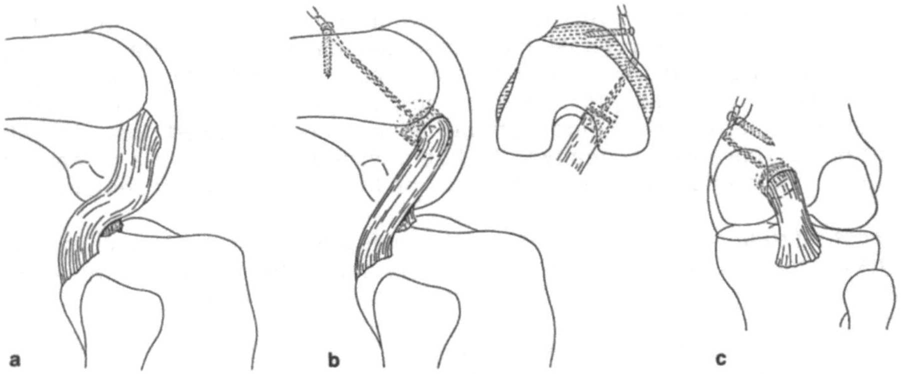

Figure 1 a–c. Tension is restored to the lax but qualitatively good PCL by pulling it into the femur after undermining its insertion (**b** and **c**)

nique to serve as a postoperative splint (Figures 2a, b, c). The quadriceps apparatus is temporarily fixed with Backhaus clamps to ensure that the patella is correctly positioned when the tibia is centered.

This type of therapy requires immediate postoperative mobilization on a Kinetec machine (CPM machine) to protect the atypically loaded cartilage. With this program the pin splint may be left in place for 6–8 weeks and even up to 12 weeks (!) in selected cases, allowing a range of flexion/extension of 85-5-0 degrees (Figure 2c). Following removal of the pin, the knee will

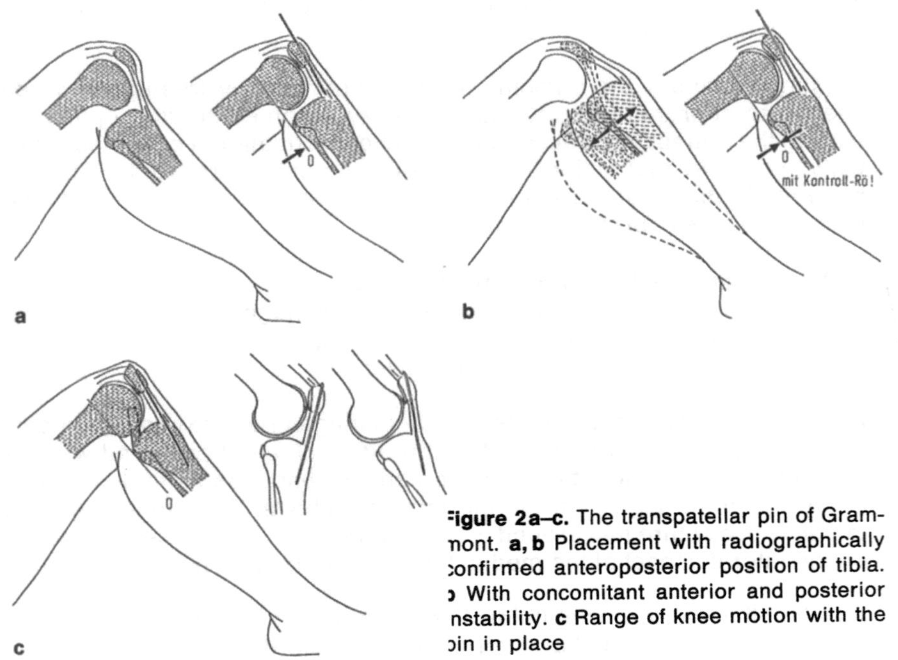

Figure 2a–c. The transpatellar pin of Grammont. **a, b** Placement with radiographically confirmed anteroposterior position of tibia. **b** With concomitant anterior and posterior instability. **c** Range of knee motion with the pin in place

quickly gain additional motion (e.g., 120-0 degrees by the 14th to 16th week) without loss of stability.

Reconstruction and partial reconstruction of the PCL
In cases where there is no serviceable posterior band that would make a tightening operation feasible, it is necessary to make use of substitute tissue. In many cases the surgeon will find a good residual band of collagen and scar tissue that can be used to reconstruct at least one main bundle of the PCL – usually the posterior, more longitudinally oriented bundle that is close to the joint capsule. It can be tightened proximally by the method described above or, if the situation warrants, it may be tightened transtibially as described below.

The second bundle – usually the anterior, obliquely oriented one – is replaced by a graft: *partial posterior cruciate reconstruction*.

In the absence of a useful residual collagen band, a *complete posterior cruciate reconstruction* is indicated. This involves the use of a larger graft to replace primarily the obliquely oriented part of the ligament. The part of the patellar tendon graft belonging to the galea aponeurotica patellae is placed posteriorly and has more of a longitudinal orientation, mimicking the posterior longitudinal bundle of the ligament.

Technique of cruciate reconstruction using a strip of patellar tendon with a vascularized fat pad pedicle
We have practiced this technique in several hundred patients over a four-year period. It is an extension of our previous technique, which we adapted from the ideas of Noyes and Clancy.

T. Drobny tested this technique experimentally in sheep and confirmed by microangiography that the transplanted central third of the patellar tendon had a blood supply and that its vascular attachments with the infrapatellar fat pad were preserved. After one year the two pedicled grafts in the sheep had only about half the tensile strength of a normal ovine cruciate ligament, although when harvested the grafts had approximately the same tensile strength as the normal ovine ACL. The two free patellar tendon grafts without vascular pedicles that were transplanted as controls had somewhat lower tensile strengths at one year, although they had been quickly vascularized by the fat pad (which is more closely apposed to the graft in the ovine knee than in the human knee). The pattern of vascularity in the free grafts appeared to be somewhat less regular than in the pedicled grafts.

Reconstruction of the PCL
Our technique for reconstructing the PCL differs from that of Clancy in that we prepare a square cavity in the femur into which the corresponding bone block on the graft is fitted. A graft inserted into a round tunnel must hang over an edge, is not very anatomic, and is subject to shear during motion of the femur. With our inlaid-block technique the tendon fibers are transferred together with their "blue line," and they maintain their broad, firm, and anatomically correct attachment to bone. Figure 3 a and b illustrate the technique of harvesting the pedicled graft and show its final position after insertion of

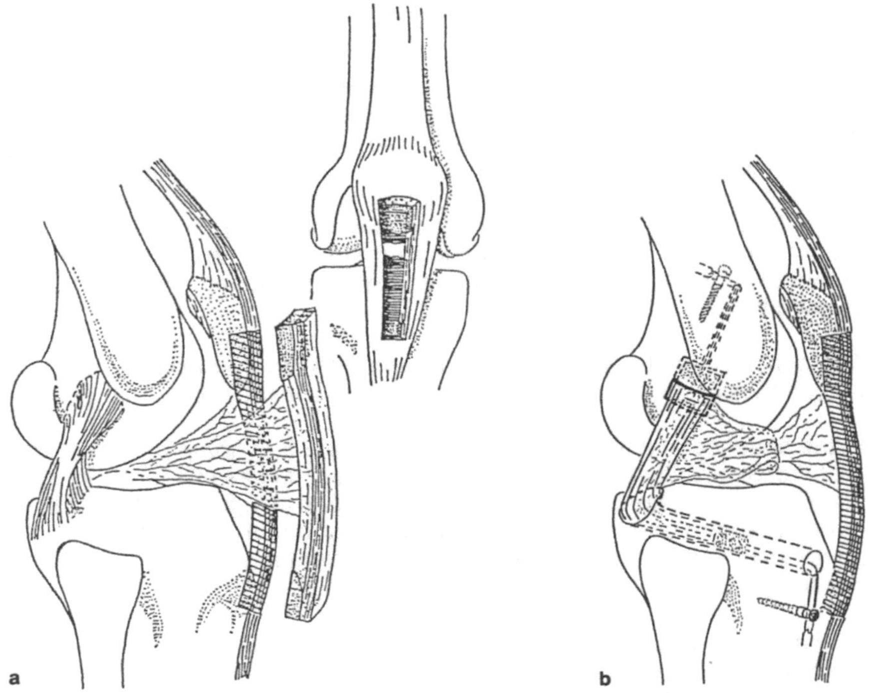

Figure 3 a, b. Reconstruction of the PCL with the vascularized patellar tendon graft

the block into the femur. Care must be taken beforehand to develop an adequate length of vascular pedicle, and problems may be encountered when attempting to pass the distal bone plug into the tibial channel. We have found it helpful to insert the graft within a urethral catheter. The position of the tibial drill hole is critical to the success of the transfer. We first drill a 4.5-mm pilot hole from the anterior side of the tibia between the tuberosity and Gerdy's tubercle. The bit is directed toward the most distal and lateral point of the tibial insertion of the PCL, while an index finger is placed posteriorly to keep vulnerable neurovascular structures away from the drill. We then enlarge the pilot hole posteriorly with curettes of increasing size, extending the bony opening medially and superiorly as required and rounding it at the edges (important!).

With the drill hole thus prepared, the distal end of the graft is pulled into the channel with the help of suture passers, catheters, or other guiding instruments until it is taut.

To be safe, each bone block is secured with two No. 3 Polydec sutures tied over a mooring screw.

As in all procedures on the PCL, it is necessary to tighten the fibers of the posterior oblique ligament, repair the popliteus corner and, at the appropriate time, insert a transpatellar Steinmann pin to serve as a protective splint (see above).

Reconstruction of the ACL
A few cases of anterior cruciate insufficiency can be managed by distal advancement of the ligament insertion, analogous to the PCL, but this is very unusual.

With the markedly improved results of our current reconstruction technique, we are far less inclined than we were two or three years ago to preserve an old, avulsed, and well-vascularized ACL, free its adhesions with the PCL, and reinsert it into the femur.

The problem of the site of femoral attachment is of central concern. During flexion/extension to 135°, the femoral attachment of the ACL rotates "in place" more than 90°. It is at that site on the femur that the bipartite to tripartite structure of the ACL has its greatest significance. A circular attachment at the opening of a drill hole leads to stress concentration at the edge of the hole and a 90° torsion of the (new) ligament, whereas a broad, fanlike insertion (duplicating normal anatomy) allows for more favorable loading and stress distribution. The danger of a second avulsion at the femoral end, as can occur in contact sports, is reduced. Our technique for the bipartite ACL reconstruction is described below.

Technique of ACL reconstruction using a vascularized strip of patellar tendon
As in reconstructions of the PCL, primary attention is given to the femoral attachment of the graft.

The object is to attach the patellar bone block with its "blue line" to the medial aspect of the femoral condyle. The blue line should be placed at the anatomically correct site, as in the normal femoral insertion of the ACL.

Also, the ligament substitute should have at least two sites of attachment to the femur.

This goal is made difficult by the *normal structure of the patellar tendon*. The patellar tendon consists of two parts, each having its own fiber orientation and its own vascular network with few interanastomoses. The *anterior part of the patellar tendon*, making up $^1/_3$ to $^1/_4$ of its thickness, consists of quadriceps tendon fibers which converge on the anterior patellar surface to form a galea aponeurotica and then pass as a discrete anterior layer to the tuberosity. The nutrient vessels enter the tendon from its anterior side, from the tuberosity, and from the patellar side.

The *deep, main part of the patellar tendon* extends from the bone of the tuberosity to the bone of the patella and thus makes an ideal bone-to-bone substitute for the main component of the ACL. It is supplied with important blood vessels by the attached infrapatellar fat pad.

Our two-part graft (Figures 4a, b) consists first of a bone-to-bone component extending from the anchoring hole in the femur to the tunnel in the upper tibia (posterolateral bundle).

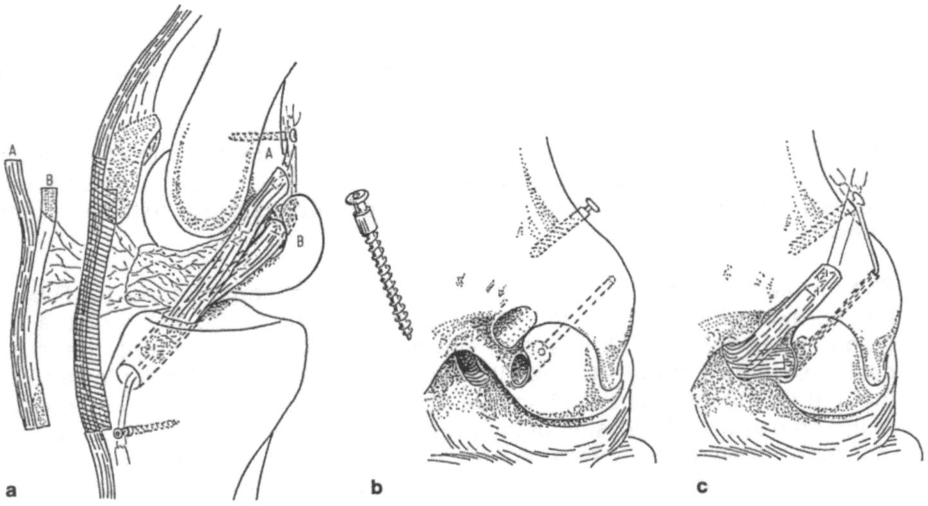

Figure 4 a–c. a Reconstruction of the ACL with the vascularized patellar tendon graft. **b** Preparation of the femur. **c** Posterior view of the femur after attachment of the graft

The anterior, proximal part of the galea is sharply released from the patella, grasped and pulled "over the top" in a shallow groove to substitute for the anteromedial bundle of the ACL. The vascularized fat pad pedicle remains attached to the central portion of the graft between the bone blocks. It provides an anastomotic supply to the thinner, anterior tendinous strip, which also will be quickly vascularized by the cancellous bone in the over-the-top position.

As with the PCL, each end of the graft is secured with two Polydec sutures passed through the bone block and tied over a screw. The tibial screw is placed about 15 mm distal to the tunnel outlet. The femoral screw is placed in the lateral metaphysis proximal to the isometric point of Kaplan's attachment of the iliotibial tract. After the threads have been tied over the screws, the free ends of the threads may be utilized to fix the deep layers of the tract and the sunken strip.

Graft tension is tested by hand when the threads are tied. Too much tension can exhaust the "reserves" of material flow too rapidly and impair the capillary circulation. We consider it more important that the graft is positioned anatomically and can function isometrically. Under *protection*, the new ligament will be able to adjust its tension spontaneously to physiologic values in the first weeks and months after surgery. Any artificially created excess of tension would fall to unknown values within minutes as a consequence of material flow.

Reconstruction of peripheral co- or secondary stabilizers
On the medial side
The medial collateral ligament itself, being dynamically stabilized by the vastus medialis, is seldom elongated to a point that would justify special reconstructive measures.

On the other hand, it is crucial to the protection and rotational control of the knee that a lax posterior oblique ligament ("posterior medial collateral ligament") be tightened proximally in its meniscofemoral portion or distally in its meniscotibial portion, or else reattached to the bone. The simple technique of Hughston and Eilers has proved very effective for proximal as well as distal repairs.

On the lateral side

a) With a coexisting anterolateral instability (without a significant posterolateral component), it is sufficient to refix Kaplan's iliotibial tract attachment to the femoral metaphysis. This is most effectively done by attaching a sunken strip of the iliotibial tract to the femur.
b) With coexistence of a chronic 2+ to 3+ posterolateral instability, we additionally perform a "popliteus bypass" using a pedicle graft from the iliotibial tract. The objective is to restore the pattern of interaction among the ligamentous systems of the central pivot and the medial and lateral periphery as primary and secondary stabilizers of the knee.

The accuracy of clinical examination of injury of the knee joint

J. Lauritzen, J. Jensen and O. Simonsen

Department of Orthopaedic Surgery, County Hospital
Åarhus
Denmark

Acute knee injury involving lesions of the ligaments often but not always results in haemarthrosis. Conversely, some patients with acute traumatic haemarthrosis in the absence of fractures will have ruptures elsewhere in the capsule with no ruptures in the ligaments. The bleeding into the joint can be so slight that it does not produce a clinically significant swelling.

Many patients with acute ligamentous lesions have obvious instability, but a large proportion will be so anxious and in so much pain from muscle spasm that it is not possible or easy to investigate for instability in the first days after the injury.

The distortion of the knee is a dynamic process, during which the kinetic energy will be absorbed in the different parts of the tissues while these are stretched or ruptured partly or totally. At the same time, the distortion can produce other lesions, especially in the menisci and the cartilage. Such simultaneous lesions are nearly impossible to diagnose clinically in the acute phase.

Nonetheless, haemarthrosis and instability are still the best criteria for the clinical diagnosis of an acute torn knee ligament, and we find it important to examine knee ligament injuries in the acute phase.

The catchment area of the department of orthopaedic surgery in the County Hospital in Aarhus, Denmark, has a population of 160000. The casualty ward is open day and night, its 30000 consultations per year being conducted by junior doctors in training. All patients with acute knee injuries involving haemarthrosis or instability are admitted. The day after admission the patient is normally investigated clinically by a senior orthopaedic surgeon before operation. The instability tests are normally repeated under anaesthesia and reevaluated, and then all patients are examined by arthroscopy before operation. Arthroscopy and operations are carried out by experienced senior orthopaedic surgeons.

This procedure was followed during the period 1.1.1981 to 1.9.1983, and retrospectively we have evaluated the accuracy of our clinical and arthroscopical diagnoses, taking the findings during surgery as the final diagnosis for the cases operated on and the arthroscopical findings as the final diagnosis for other patients.

This series consists of 218 patients. The majority were male and the mean age was 29 years, very few being more than 45 years of age.

Clinically, 168 were found to have an effusion with blood in the joint, while 50 were included only because of suspected clinical instability. In half of these the arthroscopic investigation demonstrated blood in the joint, but the rest had only instability and no blood.

The instability tests were unfortunately not all repeated under anaesthesia before arthroscopy in 69 cases, but all patients underwent arthroscopy in a bloodless field using a probe; at arthroscopy we overlooked only two partial and two total ruptures of the medial collateral ligament.

In the 27 patients who had no blood in the joint but in whom a clinical examination had suggested instability we found the following lesions: 4 partial ruptures MCL and 11 totally isolated MCL ruptures, 1 MCL rupture with an old ACL rupture, and 2 more old ACL ruptures, 1 of them with a concomitant medial meniscal tear. In 9 cases we found no lesions on arthroscopy.

Among the 23 cases where blood was first recognized during arthroscopy we found a variety of different lesions, and in 8 cases combined ligamentous lesions were found. There were 12 patients with ruptures in the ACL and altogether 12 with lesions in both ligaments and menisci, which gives the same frequency as in the material as a whole.

If blood can be detected in the joint by aspiration or lavage the patient should be examined by arthroscopy.

If the presence of blood in the joint after a knee distortion can be definitely excluded acute arthroscopy and surgery are unnecessary, because either would reveal only isolated tears in the medial collateral ligament, which might cause slight instability.

In the total of 218 cases we found 15 with no lesions according to arthroscopy, 26 with only capsular sprains, mostly caused by patellar dislocation or subluxation, 3 with isolated meniscal lesions, 81 with isolated lesions of only one ligament, one third with only partial rupture, 24 with rupture of one ligament plus a meniscal lesion, and 69 with combined ligament lesions.

To evaluate the reliability of the clinical findings as diagnostic indicators for each single lesion with and without anaesthesia we have used a formula for calculating diagnostic specificity, diagnostic sensitivity and total agreement rate (Table 1).

The predictive value for a positive test (Table 2) is the number of lesions of the specific structure divided by all with positive clinical findings.

Table 1. Formula used in evaluation

Clinical test	Lesion present	Lesion absent	Total
Positive	a	c	a+c
Negative	b	d	b+d

Table 2. Predictive value of test results

Predictive value for positive test (PV pos.):	$\frac{a}{a+c}$
Predictive value for negative test (PV neg.):	$\frac{d}{b+d}$
Total agreement rate (TAR):	$\frac{a+d}{a+b+c+d}$

The predictive value for a negative test is the number of cases with no lesions of the specific structure divided by the number of all those with negative clinical findings.

The total agreement rate is the number of cases with plus the number of cases without findings divided by the total number of all findings.

We have calculated these values for each single structure, i.e., collateral ligaments, cruciate ligaments and menisci. For the ligaments the calculations were worked with the findings both with and without anaesthesia. For the meniscal lesions the calculations were naturally only worked for findings before anaesthesia.

Figure 1 illustrates the calculations. It is clear that generally the reliability with which a ligament lesion can be diagnosed by stability tests is lower than the reliability with which a lesion can be excluded, and that it is nearly impos-

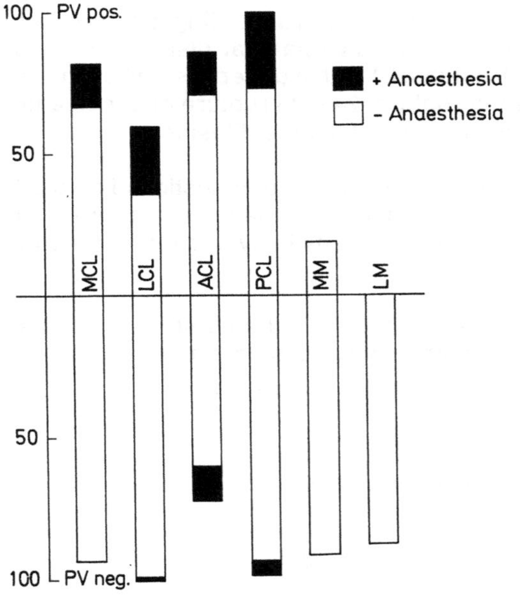

Figure 1. Reliability of stability tests with and without anaesthesia for diagnosis of ligamentous lesions

sible to diagnose lesions in the menisci by clinical tests when combined lesions are present. The exclusion of lesions in the menisci is more accidental. The reliability of a diagnosis or exclusion of a lesion is greater in PCL than in ACL lesions. This is in accordance with the findings of Butler (1980), who in cadaver knees proved that there were more secondary stabilizing structures for the anterior drawer than for the posterior drawer test.

It is also clearly seen that the reliability of diagnosis of lesions in the ligaments is higher when the stability tests are carried out with the patient under anaesthesia than when the patient is conscious, but even then the number of both false-positive and false-negative findings is much too high in the case of anterior cruciate ligament lesions.

Arthroscopy revealed more lesions in all structures than it had been possible to diagnose by stability tests even during anaesthesia, and we discovered many simultaneous lesions in the menisci. Arthroscopy also revealed lesions especially in the anterior cruciate ligament when these were not suspected after the stability tests.

The total agreement rate for the clinical findings of a total of 296 ligamentous and meniscal lesions was only 83%. The total agreement rate for the clinical findings in the 248 ligamentous lesions alone was only 82%. The total agreement rate for the findings of ligament lesions when stability was evaluated with the patient under anaesthesia was higher, it but still contained 10% of failures.

From a practical point of view with reference to treatment planning, we have put the following question to ourselves: Which treatment, and in the case of an operation which incision, would we have decided on had we evaluated the patients on the basis of our clinical findings alone? This was compared with the treatment selected on the basis of our arthroscopical investigation. To answer this question we have reviewed the 148 patients who were tested both before and during anaesthesia and then underwent arthroscopy. There were 53 for whom we should have selected conservative treatment, but 13 of these needed a surgical operation (Figure 2a); and there were 95 for

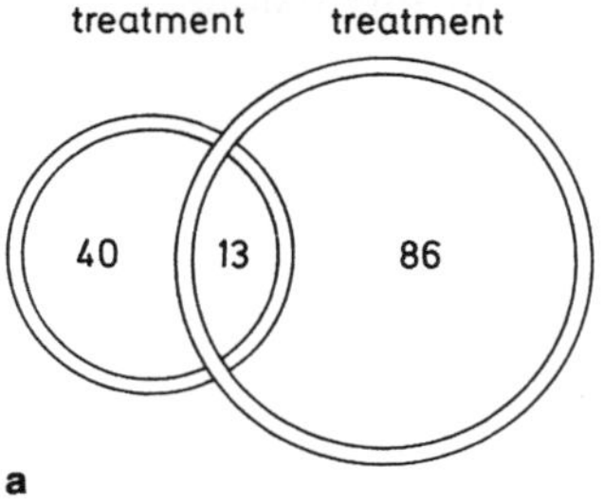

a

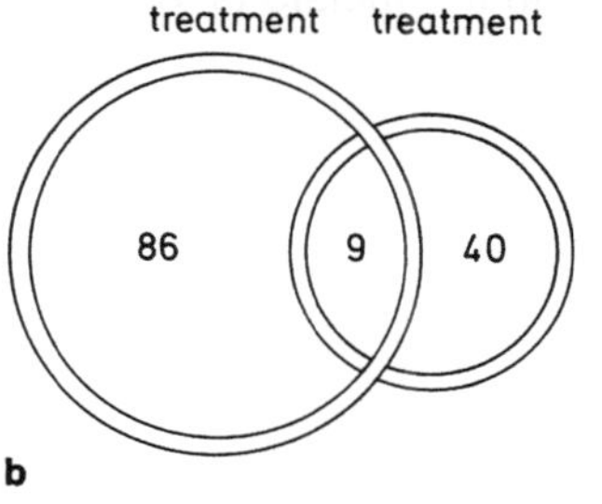

b

Figure 2a, b. Revision of treatment planned: Artrhoscopy revealed the necessity of surgical treatment in 13 patients previously thought to require only conservative measures (**a**) and the superfluity of surgery in 9 patients for whom it had initially been planned (**b**)

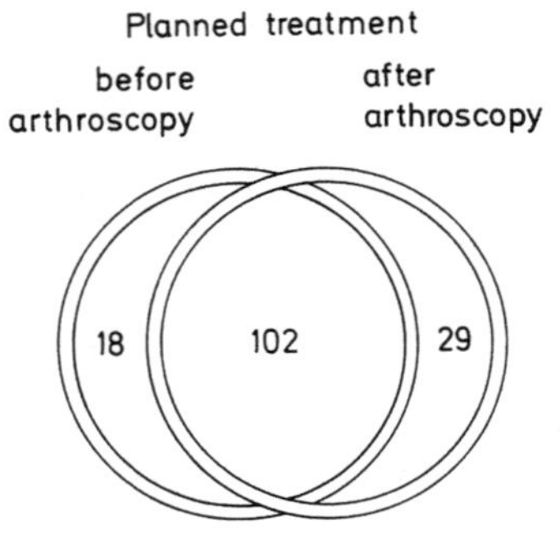

Figure 3. Overall changes in treatment planned following arthroscopy

whom we should have selected operative treatment, though 9 of these needed only conservative treatment (Figure 2b). Even the incisions selected for the operations were different after the arthroscopical investigation from those we would have made had the operations been planned on the basis of the stability tests alone.

In all, the treatment planned was changed in 47 of the 149 patients after the arthroscopical investigation (Figure 3).

Believing as we do in the value of primary repair of knee ligament lesions, on the basis of this investigation we have reached the following conclusions.

1. Traumatic distortion of the knee joint with blood in the joint very often means rupture of one or more structures which need to be corrected surgically, whereas patients without blood in the joint can be treated by conservative methods even if instability is clinically suspected.

2. A clinical investigation for instability, even when done with the patient anaesthetized is insufficient for diagnosis of the different, often combined, ligamentous lesions. Arthroscopy is superior and is necessary if all lesions are to be found, especially in the menisci and the anterior cruciate ligament.

3. Arthroscopy is the best investigation for use in planning the treatment and selecting the incisions to be used for repair of the different lesions.

The clinically stable knee with haemarthrosis

H. Hempfling

Second Surgical Clinic
Nuremberg Medical Centre
Federal Republic of Germany

Clinically and radiographically apparent injuries of the knee, with or without haemarthrosis, normally do not present a problem of surgical diagnosis, in contradistinction to post-traumatic haemarthrosis occurring in the clinically stable knee without osseous injury. Bleeding into the knee joint may be secondary to a capsular injury requiring nonoperative treatment, a cartilage fracture requiring operative treatment, or an isolated rupture of the anterior cruciate ligament (ACL). It is important to recognize that the prognosis of an injury requiring operative treatment depends critically on the timing of surgical intervention. To avoid missing the most favourable time for intervention, arthroscopy should be performed promptly so that a definitive diagnosis can be made.

The clinical examination of the acutely injured knee generally is limited to a few select manoeuvers because of pain. Radiographic evaluation should be routinely done in four planes. If the diagnosis still is not established by that time, arthroscopy may be performed under local anaesthesia, following the same aseptic rules observed for knee operations. The choice of anaesthetic technique should be discussed with the patient. If the sole intent is to establish a diagnosis, the examination may be done under local anaesthesia. If surgery is to follow the arthroscopy, a general or peridural anaesthetic is indicated.

We have reviewed 2000 arthroscopies performed in recent years at our centre. In 196 of these cases, or about 10%, arthroscopy was advised for clinically stable knees with haemarthrosis that showed no evidence of osseous injury.

The following disorders were diagnosed by arthroscopy of the acutely traumatized knees:

Stable knees with haemarthrosis (n = 196)

ACL injuries	59	30.1%
Chondral & osteochondral injuries	46	23.5%
Patellar dislocations	31	15.8%
Fractures	18	9.2%
Capsular & synovial membrane injuries	18	9.2%
Meniscal tears	16	8.2%
PCL injuries	2	1.0%
Other injuries	6	3.1%

Most frequent were injuries involving the ACL, articular cartilage, and injuries accompanying patellar dislocation.

The examination of fractures with the arthroscope – especially radiographically undisplaced fractures of the upper tibia and longitudinal undisplaced fractures of the patella – allows the extent of cartilaginous injuries to be assessed and also provides an opportunity to irrigate the joint and clear it of blood.

Tears involving the retinacula and synovial membrane occurred predominantly in the area of the femoropatellar articulation, showing an overall incidence of 9%. Fresh meniscal tears were relatively uncommon, and we saw only two cases of isolated posterior cruciate injury in the present series.

The category of "other injuries" included two isolated, intra-articular ruptures of the popliteus tendon and two tears of the infrapatellar synovial fold. In two patients the source of the haemarthrosis was not apparent.

Our review of arthroscopic examinations of stable knees with haemarthrosis during 1982 showed that the femoropatellar articulation was involved in almost 62% of cases overall. The percentage involvement of the ACL appears to be of major significance in the occurrence of haemarthrosis.

Haemarthrosis in the stable knee
Incidence of isolated ACL ruptures (literature survey)

Beaufils	n= 53	ACL=39	74%
Scheuer	n= 96	ACL=66	68%
Gillquist	n= 69	ACL=31	45%
Hertel	n= 67	ACL=21	32%
Benedetto	n= 74	ACL=40	54%
Benedetto	n= 41	ACL=20	49%
Hohlbach	n= 26	ACL= 5	19%
Dehaven	n= 88	ACL=52	59%
Glinz	n= 48	ACL=18	38%
Hertel	n= 62	ACL=11	18%
Noyes	n= 85	ACL=62	72%
2nd Clinic Nuremberg (1984)	n=196	ACL=59	30%

Reports in the literature place the incidence of isolated ACL ruptures between 18% and 74%. In our series of 196 patients, ACL injuries were responsible for intra-articular haemorrhage in 30% of cases. Besides the complete, usually femoral avulsion injury (Figure 1) we also saw intrasynovial femoral avulsions in which arthroscopy (after irrigation of the joint) showed that the torn ACL had retracted into an intact synovial sheath.

The spectrum of chondral and osteochondral injuries, primarily in the area of the femoropatellar articulation, ranges from cartilaginous haematomas and contusions (Figure 2) to extensive cartilaginous fractures with the presence of cracks and fissures (Figure 3). In rare cases we noted the avulsion of large

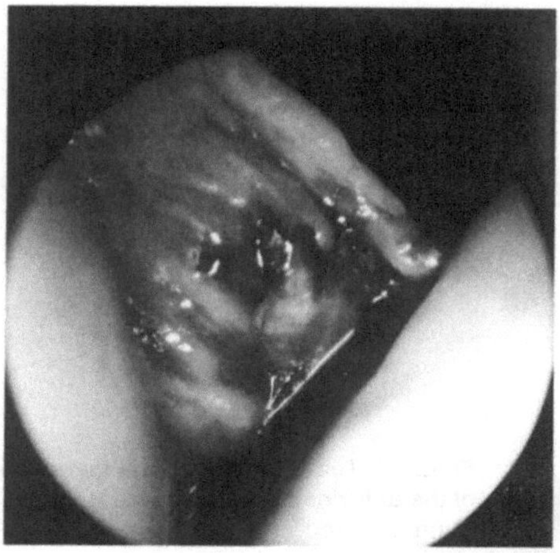

Figure 1. Femoral rupture of the anterior cruciate ligament

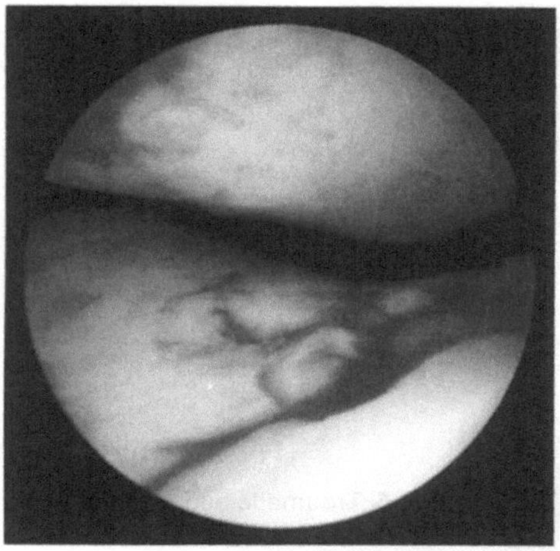

Figure 2. Contused cartilage in the femoropatellar articulation

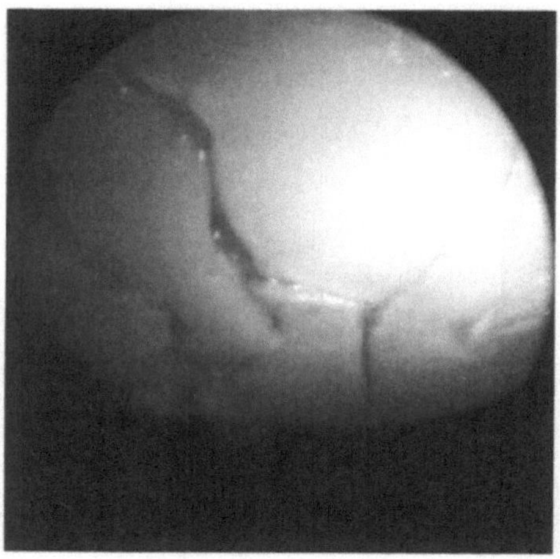

Figure 3. Cartilage fracture of the patella

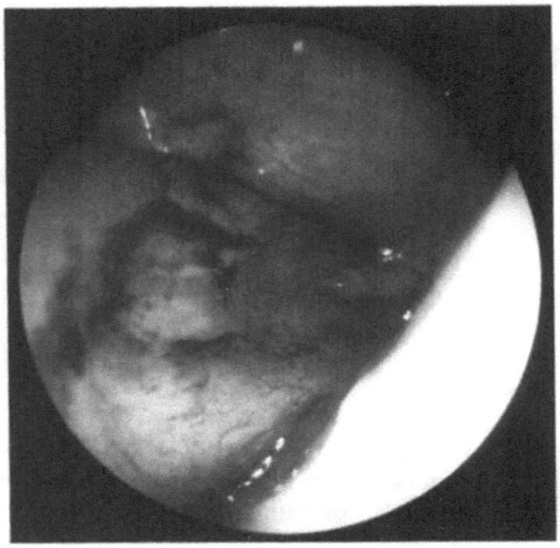

Figure 4. Tear of the synovial investment of the anterior cruciate ligament. Stability is unimpaired

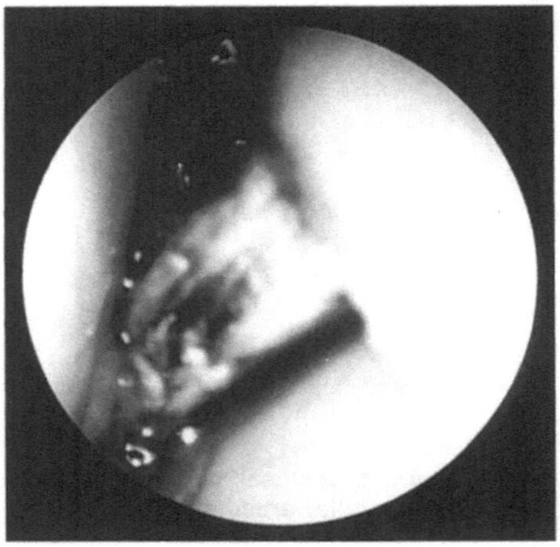

Figure 5. Traumatic bucket-handle tear of the medial meniscus

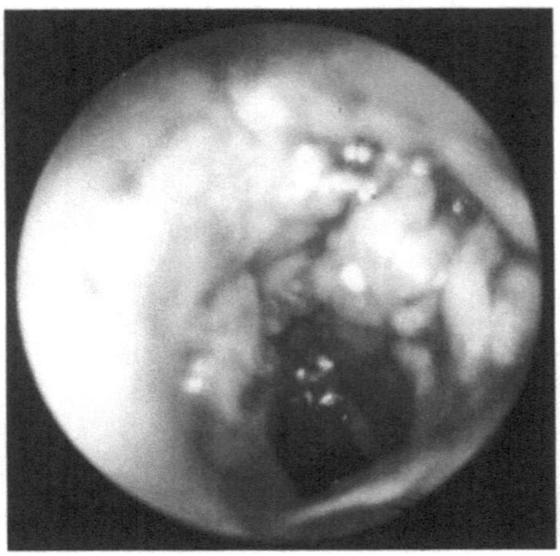

Figure 6. Femoral avulsion of the popliteus tendon

cartilage fragments that required early reduction and fixation. With all cartilaginous injuries of the femoropatellar articulation, one should carefully consider the question of patellar dislocation, which leaves behind characteristic lesions at sites of predilection in the femoropatellar articulation.

Most tears of the synovial membrane and retinacula occurred in the region of the medial retinaculum. The possibility of a previous patellar dislocation should always be considered when such lesions are found, and isolated tears (e.g., of the synovial sheath of the ACL, Figure 4) may occur without loss of stability. Acute meniscal tears (Figure 5) rarely occur in isolation; nevertheless they show an incidence of 8% in our series and are important in view of current thinking on the value of operative meniscal reattachment, especially in acute injuries.

Other injuries leading to haemarthrosis included tears of the plicae (e.g., the infrapatellar synovial fold) and two cases of isolated femoral avulsion of the popliteus tendon, causing the tendon to retract through the popliteal hiatus and present as a tendinous stump deep in the hiatus with concomitant injury to the synovial sheath of the tendon (Figure 6).

In summary, acute arthroscopy may be regarded as a necessary study in the clinically stable knee without osseous injury in cases where an accurate diagnosis is desired.

The reliability of the lateral pivot-shift as a clinical sign of anterior cruciate insufficiency

C. Kieser and C. Junker

Chirurgische Klinik Stadtspital Zürich
CH-8000 Zürich
Switzerland

McIntosh and Galway considered the lateral pivot-shift as a clinical sign of anterior cruciate insufficiency though later it was classified as anterolateral rotatory instability. Its sensitivity and specificity is studied.

Material and methods

The reports of 869 arthroscopies combined with an examination of ligamentous stability done in general anaesthesia were retrospectively analysed. Reports lacking a sufficient description of the ligament or of stability were excluded as well as reports of knees with previous surgery of the anterior cruciate.

Results

A positive subluxation test was observed in 207 of 277 cases with a tear of the anterior cruciate (74,7%). The rate of positive tests depended on the experience of the examiner and of the completeness of the rupture. A high rate was observed in knees with bilateral meniscal ruptures (88%), but a lower rate in isolated tears (62,5%). The specificity of the pivot-shift phenomenon was 98,6%; of 592 knees with an intact anterior cruciate only 8 had a false positive subluxation test. Two of them had a lesion of the posterior cruciate ligament, two a bucket-handle tear, one a patellar osteoarthritis and three no visible lesion.

Discussion

A negative McIntosh test, even done in general anaesthesia, does not exclude a tear of the anterior cruciate ligament. A positive test is highly specific of a rupture of the anterior cruciate and cannot be produced by any other ligamentous lesion unless a rupture of this ligament is present.

Summary

About 75% of the knees with a tear of the anterior cruciate ligament had a positive McIntosh test, proved by examination in general anaesthesia. 98,6% of all knees with a positive lateral pivot-shift had a tear of the anterior cruciate. Anterior subluxation of the lateral tibial plateau is not a very sensitive, but a very specific sign of anterior cruciate ligament laxity.

The anterior cruciate ligament deficiency syndrome

M. Wagner, W. Scharf and R. Schabus

I. Universitätsklinik für Unfallchirurgie
A-1097 Wien
Austria

In the athlete with a neglected anterior cruciate deficiency, the recurrent episodes of pivot shift may cause a characteristic sequence of pathological events in the knee. The consequences of anterior cruciate deficiency and lateral pivot shift are several; with time, an unresolved deficiency causes an increase in instability with all associated problems.

Material and methods

This paper reports on a series of 100 patients with anterior cruciate ligament deficiency seen from January 1981 to December 1982; these patients represent a consecutive group.
History, clinical and operative findings are studied.

Results

In our series of 100 patients with anterior cruciate ligament deficiency 82 patients were male and the average age was about 26 years.
More than 60 patients were injured while practising athletics.
Most of the patients had already suffered one or more operations prior to diagnosis of the anterior cruciate deficiency (the most frequently performed procedure was medial meniscectomy).
At operation, the authors found an incidence of a medial meniscal tear in more than 70 percent, of a lateral meniscal tear in 50 percent and of chondral erosions in about 60 percent of the cases.

Discussion

The loss of anterior cruciate ligament function produces overloading of other knee ligaments increasing their changes of potential deficiency; failure to repair the anterior cruciate deficiency causes progressive deterioration and dysfunction:
- meniscal tears
- giving way episodes
- reinjury
- pivot shift phenomenon.

Summary

The "anterior cruciate ligament deficiency syndrome" is a series of predictable pathological events which may occur in the patients (mostly athletes) whose anterior cruciate ligament deficiency is ignored. Recurrent pivot shift episodes produce stretching of supporting capsular structures and increase instability. If meniscal or articular cartilage damage has not already occurred as part of the initial trauma, this may occur with the trauma of repeated subluxation. The final outcome may be a knee which is completely destroyed and unable to be salvaged by soft tissue reconstruction.

Anterior cruciate ligament reconstruction by two-armed quadriceps tendon transplant: technique, biomechanics and first results

J. Hassenpflug

Department of Orthopaedic Surgery, University Kiel
D-2300 Kiel
Federal Republic of Germany

For the replacement of the anterior cruciate ligament a double-layered strip ot the quadriceps tendon is used which remains distally fixed to a trapezoid piece of bone from the patella. This piece of bone is inserted into the tibia head. One of the two arms of the transplant is guided through a canal in the condyle. The other arm is fixed "over-the-top". It has been demonstrated by biomechanical investigations in autopsy knees that the "over-the-top" arm is able to protect the transcondylar arm against early distension. Extraarticularly an ELLISON-procedure is performed.

50 knee joints were operated on in this manner. All of them were controlled more than 1 year after surgery. At that time the stability of the knee joint was tested and the patient's personal assessment was recorded. The results appear to be very promising so far.

A modified Andrews technique in antero-lateral rotatory instability of the knee

G. Fonda and G. L. Canata

Il Divisione Ortopedica, Centro Traumatologico Ortop
Torino
Italy

The lateral tibial subluxation in anterior cruciate ligament (A.C.L.) deficient knee is an important factor of instability. Some surgical techniques utilize the ilio-tibial band to prevent the typical "giving way" of these knees. Recently Andrews proposed a simple technique of lateral stabilization utilizing this band. In this paper we propose a modified Andrews technique. Since 1980 twenty patients with combined antero-medial and anterolateral instabilities have been treated with a modified Andrews technique in association with other stabilizing techniques.

Surgical technique

After a lateral hockey-stick skin incision, the ilio-tibial band is divided longitudinally 4 cm anterior to its posterior margin. The posterior part of the band is then fixed to the femur slightly distal and anterior to the insertion of the lateral intermuscular septum on the linea aspera. This is done with a bicortical screw and a washer keeping the knee flexed approximately at 30°. Then the anterior part of the ilio-tibial band is sutured on the posterior. After surgery the knee is placed in a cast with 40° of flexion. At 40 days the cast is removed.

Results

Every patient has been evaluated 10 months or more after surgery, considering symptoms, stability and kind of sports activities possible after surgery. 90% of them were able to take part in sports activities and showed good results. No patient complained of giving way symptoms.

Discussion

In the short term follow-up the results of this modified Andrews technique are promising and give support to the concept that a strong extra-articular reconstruction is effective in stabilizing an A.C.L. deficient knee even without closely approximating the biomechanical function fo the A.C.L.

Summary

20 patients with combined anteromedial and anterolateral instability of the knee have been treated since 1980 with a modified Andrews technique in association with other stabilizing techniques. After a short term follow-up 90% of the patients showed good results and were able to resume their sports activities.
These results indicate that a strong extraarticular reconstruction is effective in stabilizing A.C.L. deficient knees.

A new method of replacing the anterior cruciate ligament

R. Passl

Casualty Deparment, Hospital of St. John of God
A-7000 Eisenstadt
Austria

Introduction

The anterior cruciate ligament is a slightly twisted band consisting of three bundles: the anterior medial, the intermediary and the posterior lateral. The specific points of attachment of each fasciculus to the tibia and the femur produce the rotation, which occurs to a greater or lesser extent, depending on the degree of flexion of the knee. This rotatory motion is an important part of the functioning of the anterior cruciate ligament.

The anterior medial bundle travels from the medial side of the anterior tuberosity to the intercondyloid notch. When the leg is extended it is taut, and widest at the top; it is relaxed and widest at the bottom when the leg is bent (Figure 1 A). The posterior lateral bundle extends from the lateral dorsal aspect of the tuberosity backwards and outwards into the intercondyloid notch, and so lies relaxed and under the anterior medial section when the leg is extended (Figure 1 A). When the knee is flexed, the femoral attachment of the posterior lateral bundle is widest at the top, and is stretched taut in front of the other two bundles (Figure 1 B).

The intermediary bundle, which lies between the two other parts of the anterior crucial ligament described above, resembles the anterior medial bundle in its behaviour. That is, in extension and inward rotation, both the anterior

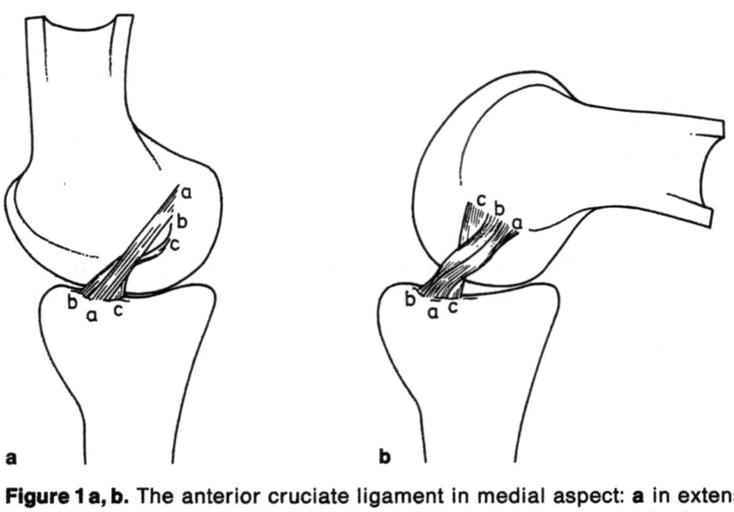

Figure 1 a, b. The anterior cruciate ligament in medial aspect: **a** in extension; **b** in flexion. *aa*, anterior medial bundle; *bb*, intermediary bundle; *cc*, posterior lateral bundle

medial and intermediary bundles are taut, and pressed against the intercondyloid boundary. Bearing these anatomical facts in mind, the Casualty Department of the Hospital of St. John of God in Eisenstadt has, since the beginning of 1982, replaced defective anterior crucial ligaments by the plantaris tendon.

Operating procedure

The plantaris tendon in the same leg is located and removed. After exposing the knee joint, three channels are bored with a 3.2-mm drill beside the tibial tuberosity to the anterior medial part of the intercondyloid spine in the form of a triangle. Then the lateral femoral condyle is exposed. Somewhat above the Kaplan fibres two channels are drilled in the intercondyloid notch in line with the original attachment of the cruciate ligament. The plantaris tendon is now threaded through the tibia and stretched outwards over the top with the leg extended. Then it is led back from the side through two channels, following the direction of the posterior lateral bundle. This part of the tendon is stretched and attached with the joint at a 90° angle. At this point of the operation it can be checked if the replacement ligament is correctly sited by bending and stretching the knee joint. In flexion, the posterior lateral bundle should become taut, while the anterior medial one should relax and vice versa. In other words an anterior drawing movement should not be possible either in flexion or in extension of the limb.

Finally, the remaining portion of the plantaris tendon is drawn through the two remaining channels, following the direction of the intermediary bundle. With the knee half bent, the plantaris is sutured under moderate tension to the prepared loop of tendon on the outside of the lateral femoral condyle (Figure 2).

Following a suggestion of Müller [1], after completion of the reconstruction, we now suture a pedunculated part of the infrapatellar fat pad over the plantaris tendon.

Results

Since the beginning of 1982, 23 replacements of the anterior cruciate ligament by the plantaris tendon have been carried out. We have been able to follow 21 of these clinically for periods ranging from 6 to 24 months, and some

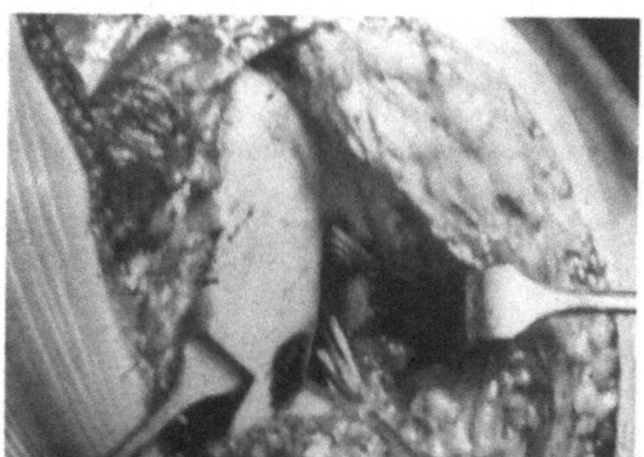

Figure 2. Operating procedure. All three bundles have been replaced

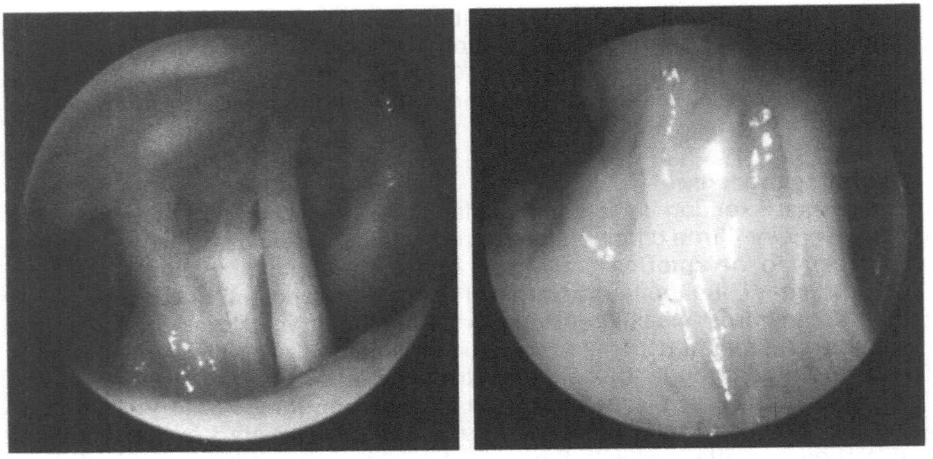

a b

Figure 3 a, b. Arthroscopic examination: **a** A well-integrated cruciate ligament after 1 year of full participation in sport. The structure of the fasciculi is clearly distinguishable. **b** Plantaris tendon with pedunculated fat pad after 1 year

of them have also been examined arthroscopically (Figure 3). (Two patients underwent operations less than 6 months ago.) Of the 21 patients investigated, 15 had been distinctly unstable prior to their operation, with frequent episodes of giving way. Although the remaining six also evidenced anterior drawing signs, they could bring them under good muscular control.

Subjective results. Table 1. Of the 21 patients, 15 resumed their sporting activities, 8 of them competitively. The remaining six do not now engage in any sport – but two of these never did, even before their injury.

Objective postoperative findings. Table 2. There are four cases of limited knee flexion. One patient can only bend her knee up to 125 °, the three others up to 135 °. Postoperative giving-way episodes have occurred solely in the case of the patient with the greatest degree of limitation in knee flexion. Her quadriceps has atrophied 2 cm, although 1 year has passed since her operation. We consider this operation to be a failure; the patient herself, however, is subjectively satisfied: preoperatively she had had up to ten giving-way episodes per day, but in the year since her operation has had a total of only two.

Table 1. Subjective results of 21 replacements of the anterior cruciate ligament by the plantaris tendon 1–2 years after operation

Ability to walk	Full	Limited	Change of occupation
Ability to work	21	–	–
Ability to engage in sport	Unlimited	As hobby	No sport
	8	7	6
Pain	Never	Sometimes	Frequent
	15	6	–

Table 2. Objective results of 21 replacements of the anterior cruciate ligament by the plantaris tendon 1–2 years after operation

Movement	Full	Limited flexion (20°)	Limited extension (5°)
	16	4	3
Giving way	Never	Sometimes	Often
	20	1	–
Anterior drawing sign in flexion or extension	None	Some indication +	Marked + +
	14	7	–
Atrophy of quadriceps	None	1–2 cm	2 cm
	15	5	1

Discussion

Up to now, no intra-articular plastic replacement of the anterior cruciate ligament has been able to reproduce the characteristic structure of this ligament. The torsion – of prime importance in guiding the rolling-gliding motion of the knee joint – is effected by the three constituent bundles having separate points of attachment to the tibia and the femur. Because of this, each of the three bundles is tensed differently in the course of knee movement. The anterior medial part of the anterior cruciate ligament is in the state of greatest tension when the knee is extended, the posterior lateral when the knee is bent; the intermediary bundle is tensed above all during extension and inward rotation. (An intact posterior cruciate ligament is of course presupposed in all these deliberations.) The importance of reconstructing the anterior medial and the posterior lateral bundles has been pointed out in recent years, in particular by Müller. His modified Brückner-Erikson method cannot, however, reproduce the differing states of tension of the different bundles. Our sample is too small as yet to demonstrate that this is as significant as we believe it to be. We must await the results of future such operations.

Reference

1. Müller W (1982) The knee. Springer, Berlin Heidelberg New York

Extra-articular stabilization a.m. Losee in chronic anterolateral rotatory instability in the knee

A. O. Mølster, T. Strand, A. Skredderstuen, L. Engesaeter, T. S. Raugstad and A. Alho

Haukeland Hospital and Hagavik Orthopaedic Hospital
Bergen
Norway

In the period 1979-81, 34 patients with symptomatic anterior cruciate ligament insufficiency and a positive Slocum test were operated on. Twenty-nine patients, 6 females and 23 males aged 16-63 years (median 29) were available for follow-up examination, and were included in our study. A knee function score was obtained at follow-up, and was reconstructed for the preoperative status (Lysholm & Gillquist 1982). The maximum score possible was 100 points. The preoperative median value was 56 points (rang 22-77). At follow up (median time 23 months, range 15-49 months), median knee score was 90 (range 14-100). According to the knee score, 21 pat. had a good/excellent result (< 77 p) Subjective evaluation by the patients gave excellent or good results in 21 patients, fair in 3 and poor in 5 patients. Nine patients (1/3) had a positive Slocum test at follow-up, the rest (2/3) were classified as stable concerning ALRI. The excellent and good results were significantly related to the absence of anterolateral instability.

Anterior cruciate ligament reconstruction

J. A. Feagin, Jr.

Post Office Box 2770
Jackson, WY 83001
USA

Introduction
The anterior cruciate ligament (ACL) is not so named to reflect a preoccupation with an anatomic structure. It is the *crucial* ligament. Crucial, not because the knee cannot function without it, but because it stands as a challenge to the soft tissue surgeon. When the repair or reconstruction of this ligament is solved, then the soft tissue surgeon can approach his task with the same confidence, same aggressiveness, and the same certainty as we now approach hard tissues – thanks to the contributions of Charnley, Wagner, Weber, and the AO school.

Our problem with the ACL is the result of a classic misadventure in medicine. We tried to go too far too soon without the basic scientific knowledge.

Initially we tried to ignore the complex rotationally unstable knee because the cruciate ligament proved to be difficult or unreliable to repair. This attitude has not been tenable because the world has become a sporting culture with more leisure time, more emphasis on competition, and a more efficient shoe-turf relationship.

Consequently, a very real epidemic of functionally unstable knees daily challenges our reconstructive skills.

Subsequently, we tried to share our knowledge and concern but without a commonality of terms. This led to 10 years of misunderstanding and misadventure – of which we as North Americans perhaps contributed the most to the confusion.

Finally, we have appropriately returned to the proper place – the anatomic and kinematic laboratory – in an attempt to gain some understanding of the problem. That is where we are today and that is where we will remain until we better understand the biology of soft tissue healing.

My experience is consistent with the literature, and the literature supports the following three points:

1. Primary repair of the ACL is untenable.
2. Augmentation is essential.
3. Extra-articular substitution is suspect.

The case against primary repair
My initial clinical experience with primary repair was gratifying for 2 years. There was then, however, gradual failure with return to competition in a

sporting population. We now know both from the laboratory and from follow-up of these patients that the blood supply is so impaired by the initial injury that there is not sufficient tensile strength or quality of tissue for the ligament to sustain itself. Thus, I no longer do primary repairs, although an interesting article in the literature documents the efficacy of repairing the ACL to the posterior cruciate ligament, and I sometimes use this procedure in children with open epiphyses.

The case for augmentation
Though still crude in nature, intra-articular augmentation surgery has held up over 5 years. The results of many investigators worldwide, using a variety of tissues, is such that this surgery can be approached with confidence if it is done with care and precision.

Fixation at either end of the graft and isometricity are critical to the success of these procedures.

The case against extra-articular substitution
Although the final chapter on extra-articular substitution surgery has yet to be written, it of necessity interrupts the harmonious relationship between the primary and secondary stabilizers and thus, with rare exceptions, the idea of extra-articular substitution for the ACL is anathema to me.

What of prosthetics?
We have done prosthetic research for 10 years. The quest has and will continue to be for a biodegradable substance. Nevertheless, our current results with autogenous intra-articular augmentation are such that it would be difficult to justify a transition to prosthetic materials at this time. To attempt the transition to prosthetic materials at this time would risk repeating the already disastrous wasting of the past 10 years, for we lack the basic science as it relates to prosthetics.

Recommendations
1. Do not do primary repairs. They fail too often.
2. If you believe the knee needs stability, then augment the ACL either primarily or secondarily with patella ligament; this is the best substitute.
3. Be patient – prosthetics are coming, but perhaps too soon and without sufficient testing, so that there is the capacity for great harm.

We can be optimistic with what we have today if we apply conventional intra-articular augmentation surgery hand in hand with our best surgical techniques.

Repair of the anterior cruciate ligament with meniscal tissue – a recommendable procedure?

D. Hager and H. Seiler

Chirurgische Universitätsklinik, Abtlg. Unfallchirurgie
Homburg/Saar
Federal Republic of Germany

The repair of the anterior cruciate ligament (ACL) with meniscal tissue has been recommended long ago and seems to be generally abandoned. Modern trends in arthroscopic surgery use menisci again for the substitution of this ligament in the ACL-deficient knee and made us review patients, who underwent this procedure in the past with open surgery.

Material and methods

Out of 20 patients with 20 knees, treated over a five year period, 12 were followed-up after mean time of 24 months. In 5 cases, there was a fresh mopend-tear of the ACL, in 12 meniscal graft was used as substitution in chronic instabilities. In recent tears meniscal tissue served as reinforcement of the ruptured ligament. Usually bucket-handles of lateral meniscus, never normal menisci, were used for the procedure. The usual pattern of lesions in fresh cases was rupture of the ACL combined with tear of the medial collateral ligament, lateral meniscus and sometimes additionally medial meniscus, the type of chronic instabilities was mostly antero-lateral and antero-medial.

Results

In no patient the operated knee was subjectively fully restored. In recent tears (meniscal reinforcement) only 2 knees were fully stable. An arthroscopic control in one patient of this group revealed a totally absorbed graft. In late cases (meniscal substitution) the range of instability was at least 2+. The subjective rating of the patients even in the presence of gross subluxation nevertheless was not always bad.

Discussion

Especially pathological and meniscal tissue shows little vascularity and resistance against tension forces. This presumes the clinical results after meniscal reinforcement or substitution of the ACL. They are not satisfying because only in 2 fresh cases of the restored knees complete stability was gained. The procedure therefore should not be revived.

Summary

12 out of 20 patients were followed up 2 years after reinforcement with meniscus in mop-end-tears of ACL or substitution with meniscus in chronic ACL ruptures. Only 2 knees were fully stable, the usual result especially after meniscal substitution of the ligament was a grade 2 or 3 instability.

The behaviour of fascia lata transplants as a substitute for the anterior cruciate ligaments in dogs

T. J. G. van Rens, A. van den Berg, W. Kuyper, and R. Huiskes

Dept. of Orthopaedics, University of Nijmegen
Nijmegen
The Netherlands

Substitution of the cruciate ligaments by fascia lata strips is still controversial. Both the material used for this cruciate substitution and the method of fixation of the transplant to bone are subjects of continuing discussion.

Material and methods

We studied the macroscopic, the histologic and the mechanical behaviour of standard size pedicled fascia lata transplants fixed to the femur and tibia with the so-called bone peg fixation technique (Van Rens, 1977) in 23 adult Labrador dogs (46 knees).

The post-transplantation period varied from 0 days to 3 years. The dogs were not immobilised nor splinted.

Results

Macroscopy: 3 transplants failed. These knees became arthritic to some extent. Microscopic examination: the transplant becomes necrotic in a few days. However, on the fourth day a reactive and simultaneous process of cellular infiltration, followed by new bone formation at the site of transplant fixation and ingrowth of young connective tissue, is seen. Synovial lining of the free part of the transplant starting in the ligament surrounding intra-articular blood clots is seen within 2 weeks post-operatively.

In 8 – 10 weeks the fascia lata transplant is substituted by newly formed dense fibrous tissue with collagen fibres at the bone ligament junction, strongly resembling Sharpey fibres. As from then, the transplant closely resembles the normal A.C.L., but it has coarser fibre bundles showing a more undulent course, and a hypertrophic synovial lining. 14 Knees were used for mechanical testing in an Instron Testing machine one year postoperatively. The tests were performed with a force scale of 200 kg/20 cm and a speed of 5 mm/min.

The mechanical data were compared with six normal contralateral knees. The data demonstrate that the transplants are less stiff than normal ACL's with a factor of 50% and that the yield point is 1/3 of the normal ACL. Normal ACL's rupture at the tibial insertion, whereas the reconstructed ACL's rupture interligamentarily.

Conclusion:

Although cruciate substitution with bone peg fixation demonstrates an excellent ingrowth of the transplant into bone and the histologic appearance strongly resembles the normal ACL, its mechanical properties are inferior to those of a normal ACL with a factor of 50% for stiffness and 1/3 for the yield point.

Lit.: Van Rens, Th., "Fixation of ligamentous structures in the knee". In: Injuries of ligaments and their repair, Chapchal, Georg Thieme, Stuttgart, 1977, p. 90-94.

Patellar tendon graft with a fat pad pedicle for anterior cruciate ligament reconstruction

T. K. Drobny[1], W. Müller[1], A. Wentzensen[2] and S. M. Perren[3]

[1] **Department of Orthopedic Surgery, Kantonsspital Bruderholz, CH-4101 Bruderholz/BL, Switzerland**
[2] **Berufsgenossenschaftliche Unfallklinik D-7400 Tübingen, Federal Republic of Germany**
[3] **Schweizerisches Forschungsinstitut, Labor für experimentelle Chirurgie CH-7260 Davos-Platz/GR, Switzerland**

Surgical technique, experimental viability testing, and long-term study of healing processes in the sheep compared with a free graft (microangiography, tensile testing).

Introduction

The method of cruciate ligament reconstruction using a strip of patellar tendon attached to the infrapatellar fat pad is briefly described. Two key questions are addressed: (1) Does the attached fat pad indeed represent a vascular pedicle and, if so, (2) is there a marked difference in the healing of the pedicled patellar tendon graft as a cruciate substitute compared with the free graft?

The first question was investigated using disulphine blue vital staining and microangiography in the knee joint of the sheep. Based on the positive results of these tests, a long-term study was instituted in the sheep to compare the healing of the pedicled graft with that of the free autogenous graft as cruciate substitutes on the basis of microangiography and tensile testing.

Since the fall of 1978, 706 reconstructive procedures on the knee ligaments have been performed at our district hospital in Bruderholz. Of these operations, 637 were cruciate ligament reconstructions. Since August of 1981, a strip of patellar tendon with an attached portion of the infrapatellar fat pad has been our standard substitute for the anterior cruciate ligament (ACL). By late February of 1984 we had performed 213 ligament reconstructions using this method.

Surgical technique

The knee joint is approached through an extended lateral parapatellar incision about 25 cm long. The tibial channel is drilled from the anteromedial aspect of the upper tibia. To avoid unnecessary kinking of the graft at the edge of the tibial drill hole, the drill bit is directed toward the femoral insertion site of the ACL. We use a 4.5-mm ASIF drill bit and enlarge the tunnel with sharp curettes to the necessary calibre of 8–10 mm.

Next the knee is flexed about 120° for drilling of the femoral hole. In this position the drill hole can be correctly placed and directed without an aiming device, the hole being drilled in a medial-to-lateral direction. Again we use the 4.5-mm ASIF drill bit for this purpose, and we curette a notch in the lateral

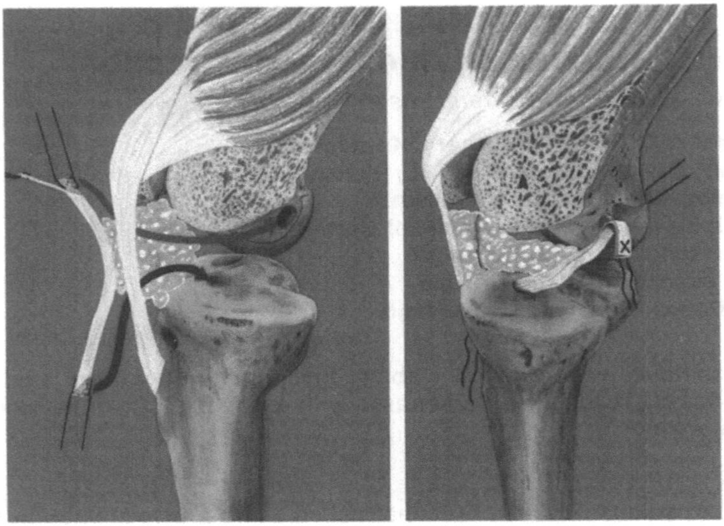

a b

Figure 1.

femoral condyle to receive the bone block on the proximal end of the graft. The accuracy of the placement and size of the drill holes are crucial to the success of the operation.

The graft is harvested from the central one-third of the patellar tendon. Its proximal and distal bony insertions are freed to provide a bone block at each end of the graft. We divide the proximal end of the graft into two strips. One strip is pulled "over the top" of the femoral condyle and replaces the anteromedial bundle of the ACL. The part of the graft attached to the bone block is pulled through the femoral condyle and replaces the posterolateral bundle of the ACL. The attachment of the infrapatellar fat pad to the undersurface of the graft is preserved as a pedicle (Figures 1a, b).

An L-shaped incision is made in the fat pad so that the graft with its vascular pedicle can be turned 180° for insertion into the joint. As mentioned, passage of the proximal end of the graft is partly transcondylar and partly over the top.

After the graft has been attached to the femur, it is pulled taut distally and anchored to the tibia (Figure 2).

The fat pad attachment to the patellar tendon graft is maintained to facilitate revascularization of the graft and promote its consolidation. The fixation technique for the proximal end of the graft offers three additional advantages:

1) Bone-to-bone union is better than the healing of ligament to bone.
2) The normal insertion sites of ligaments and tendons exhibit a peculiar microarchitecture, called the blue line, which compensates for differences in the elastic moduli of the collagen and bone. In this procedure the actual insertion site is transferred together with the graft.

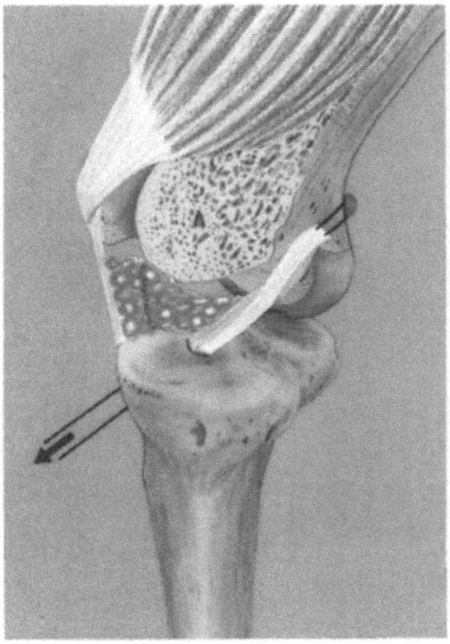

Figure 2.

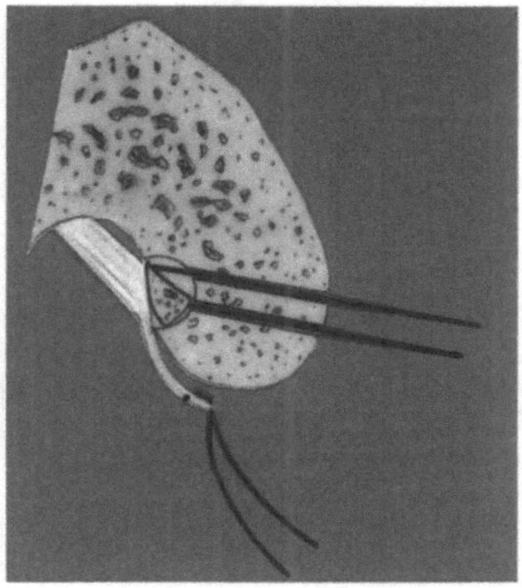

Figure 3.

3) Division of the proximal end of the graft into two strips duplicates the bipartite architecture (anteromedial and posterolateral bundles) of the normal ACL (Figure 3).

The vascularity of the pedicled graft was demonstrated in the knee joint of the sheep by vital staining with disulphine blue. Figure 4a shows the prepared graft with its fad pad pedicle, and Figure 4b shows the same graft 5 minutes after vital staining with disulphine blue. The stain clearly demonstrates blood flow in the graft via the vascularized fat pad pedicle.

Subsequent microangiography confirmed the results of the disulphine blue tests (Figure 5a). It also demonstrated some vascularity in the patellar tendon graft based distally on the tibial tuberosity (Figure 5b), but to a lesser degree than in the graft attached to the fat pad.

As the microangiograms of a normal knee joint indicate, these vessels are derived from the periosteal capillary plexus of the patella and the tibial tuberosity. Also, solitary vessels may occur that bridge an otherwise avascular zone of the insertion site.

With regard to its collagen architecture and the number and distribution of its cellular elements, the patellar tendon is very similar histologically to the normal ACL, as our study in the sheep has demonstrated.

The mechanical properties of the patellar tendon graft, such as stiffness and tensile strength, also have proved to be very similar to those of the normal ACL.

On the basis of these investigations, we were able to conclude that the patellar tendon graft with a fat pad pedicle indeed possesses a blood supply. It

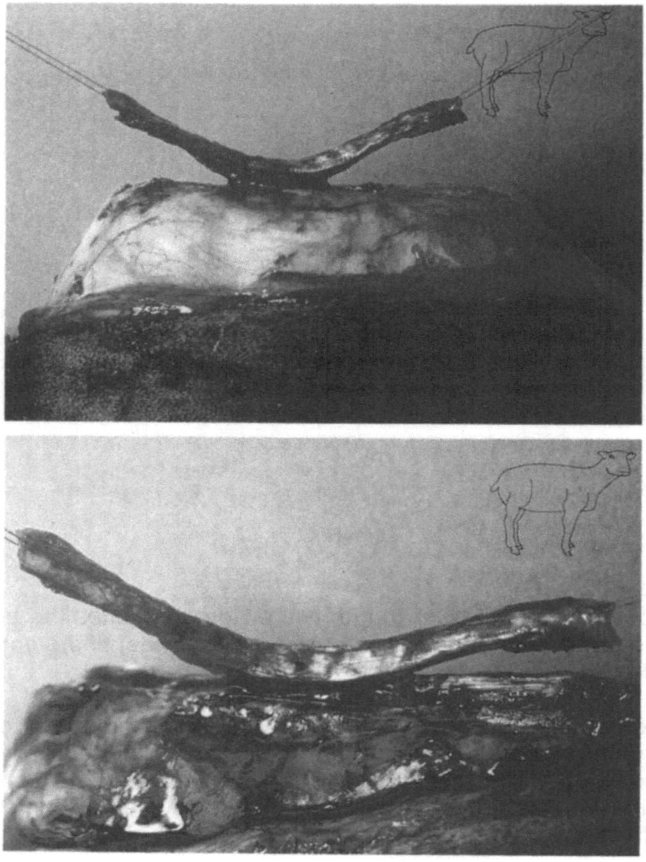

a

b

Figure 4.

remained to determine whether the healing of the graft is significantly influenced by the presence of the vascular pedicle.

To answer this question, we conducted a long-term study in a total of 18 sheep, which were divided into 2 groups. In one group the ACL was replaced by an autogenous patellar tendon graft with a fat pad pedicle. In the second group, the same surgical technique was used to replace the ACL with a free autogenous patellar tendon graft. The healing of these grafts was compared by microangiography. Microangiograms were obtained by injecting 500 ml of barium sulphate contrast medium into the femoral artery at the time the animal was sacrificed. The timing of sacrifice was as follows: The first sheep was killed immediately after the reconstructive surgery, and the other animals were sacrificed at 2, 4, 6, 8, 26, and 52 weeks postoperatively. This gave us the opportunity to study revascularization processes over a period of 1 year after the surgery. Two grafts from each group were subjected to tensile testing at 1 year postoperatively.

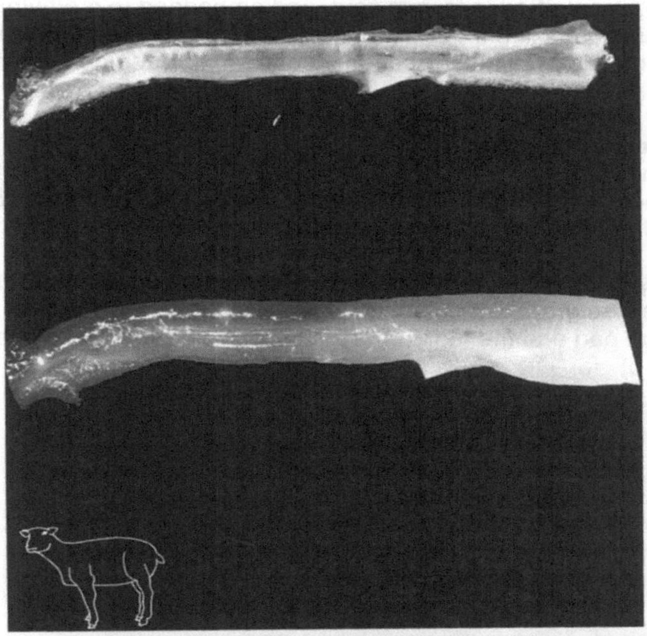

Figure 5 a.

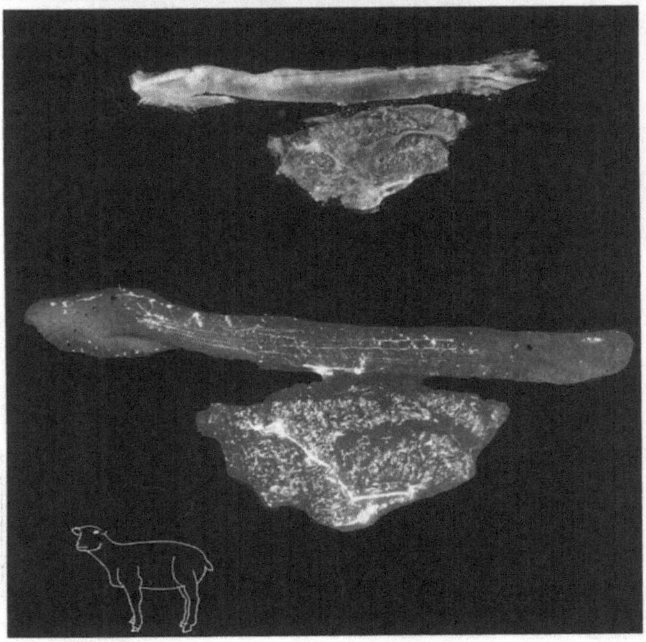

Figure 5 b.

For the microangiograms, the knee joints of the euthanized sheep were fixed in formalin in toto, decalcified in formic acid, and embedded in methylmethacrylate. Sagittal sections 1 mm thick were cut from the centre of the methacrylate blocks, and it is from these sections that the microangiograms were prepared.

Group A: free patellar tendon graft
(Microangiography)
As one would expect with a free graft, the immediate postoperative microangiograms showed nothing but an avascular strip of tissue (Figures 6a, b).

At only 2 weeks postoperatively we observe longitudinally oriented blood vessels within the free graft. Note also the close association of the graft with the infrapatellar fat pad and the ingrowth of vessels from the fat pad into the graft (Figures 7a, b).

a 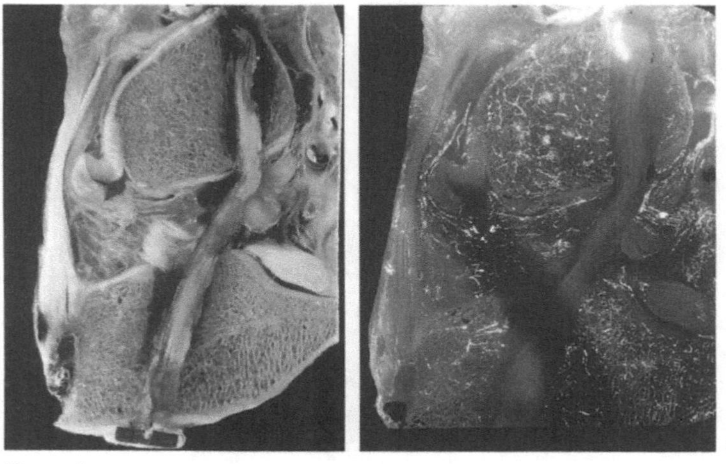 b

Figure 6.

a 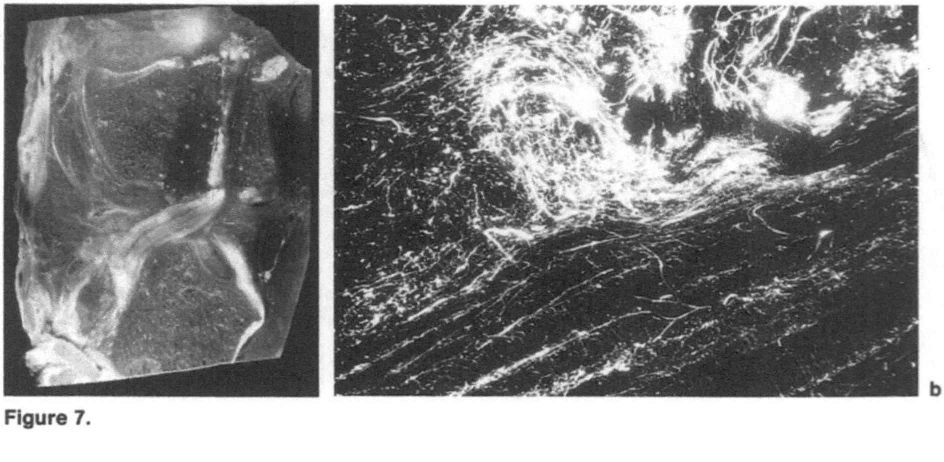 b

Figure 7.

a 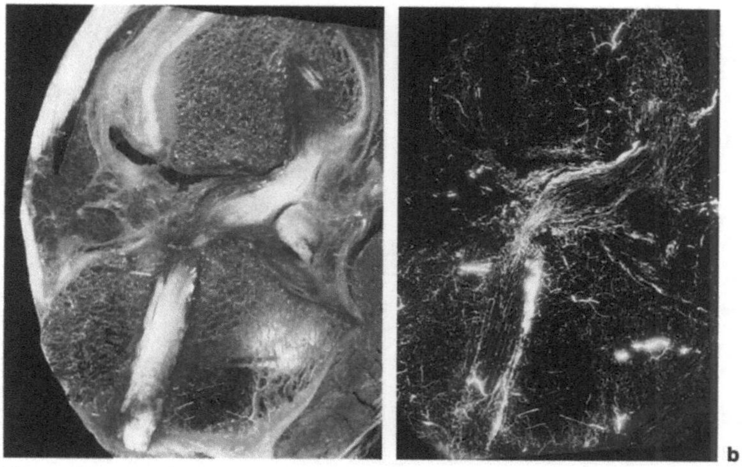 b

Figure 8.

a 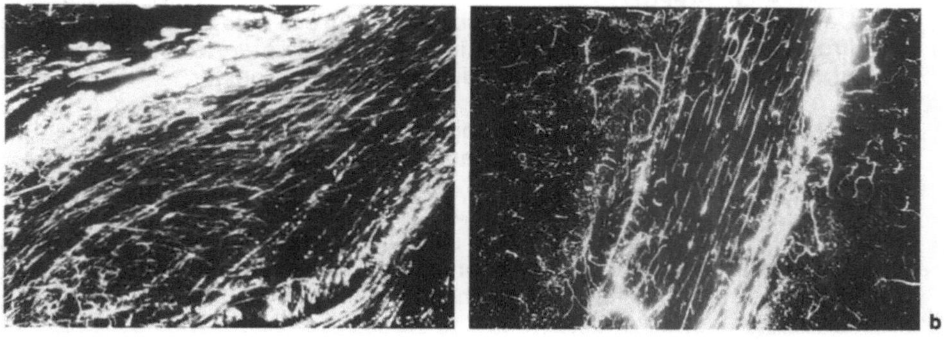 b

Figure 9.

This basic pattern of vascularization is evident throughout the period of the study, as the microangiograms at 6 weeks (Figures 8a, b) illustrate. The high-power views of the intermediate portion of the graft show that it derives its major blood supply from the adherent fat pad. Some vascularization of the graft through the drilled bone channels is also apparent (Figures 9a, b).

The one-year result in the group with the free grafts is rated as excellent both grossly and microangiographically.

In the 2 sheep in which the graft was exposed at 1 year postoperatively, the graft was found to be completely adherent to the infrapatellar fat pad. The fat pad had to be cut away to gain access to the graft.

The tensile strengths of these 2 grafts are far below the desired value, however (Figure 10). The shaded area in the graph represents the range of tensile strength of the normal ACL. Both of the graft curves are far outside and below this range. Both the stiffness and the rupture strength of the ligament substitutes are relatively low.

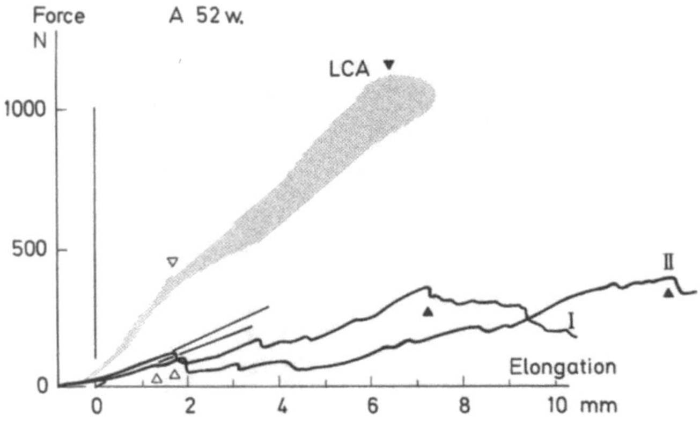

Figure 10.

Figure 10.

Group B: patellar tendon graft with fat pad pedicle
(Microangiography)
Despite our standardized technique, the failure to obtain contrast filling in the first animal of this group makes it impossible to state whether the pedicled graft still has a blood flow immediately after the transfer.

But as in the first group, microangiography showed obvious vascular filling with attachment of the graft and fat pad at 2 weeks postoperatively (Figures 11 a, b).

Further microangiograms in this series show the same pattern of graft perfusion with obvious vascular connections across the fat pad-graft interface. Figures 12 a, b and 13 a, b show the situation at 6 and at 52 weeks postoperatively.

Like the free grafts, the gross appearance of the pedicled grafts was very good. But again, the grafts showed substantially lower tensile strengths than the normal ACL at 1 year after surgery (Figure 14).

a 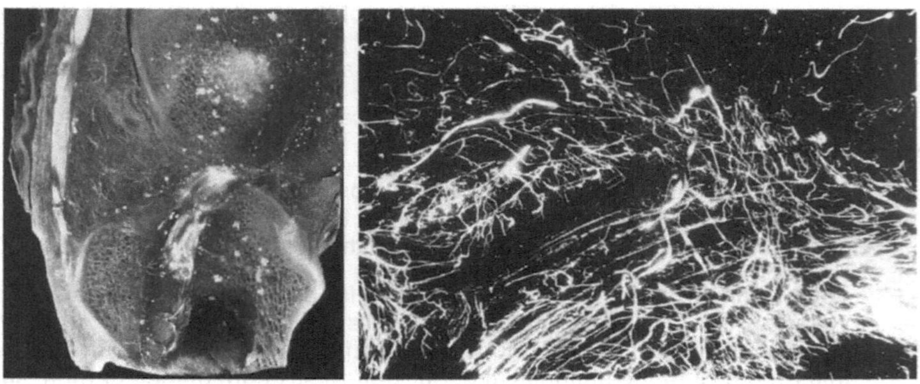 b

Figure 11.

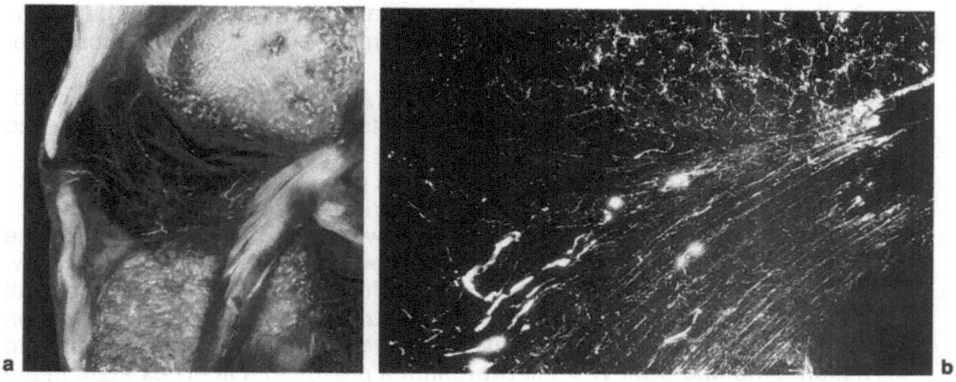

Figure 12.

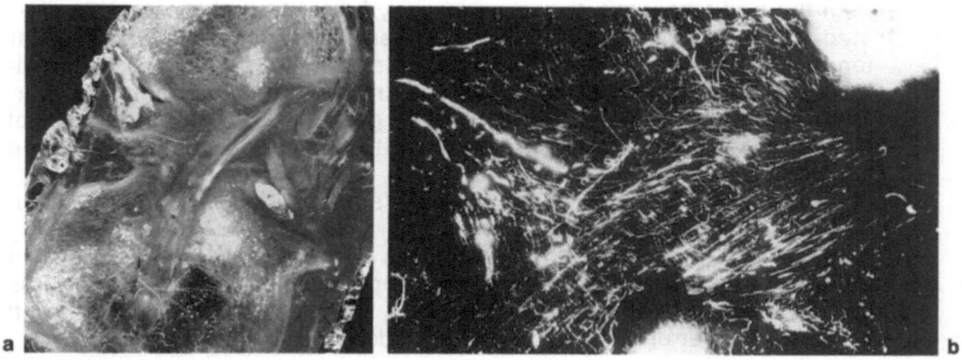

Figure 13.

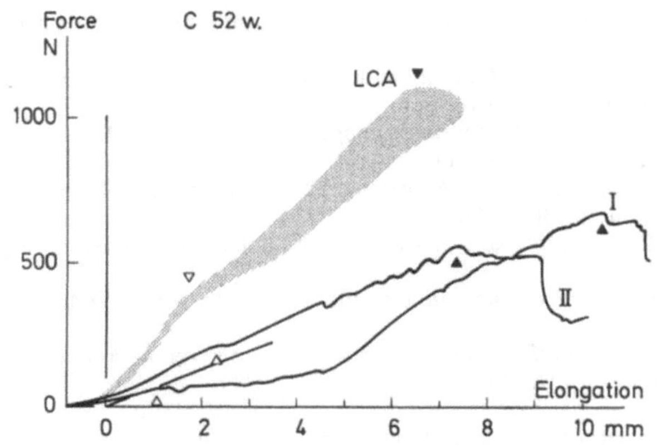

Figure 14.

Summary

1. On the basis of our experience and these investigations, the proposed surgical procedure is in every respect commensurate with biological, mechanical, and kinematic requirements.
2. The patellar tendon, as an autogenous graft material, is a very good potential substitute for the ACL by virtue of its histologic characteristics and mechanical properties.
3. The patellar tendon graft with attached fat pad is vascularized, and so the fat pad pedicle may be regarded as a nutrient pedicle.
4. Because of a methodologic error, we were unable to prove that the pedicled graft retains its blood flow immediately after the transfer. However, we were able to show that both the free graft and the pedicled graft had a blood supply just 2 weeks after surgery. Thus, revascularization took place within the first 14 days after the operation. It is reasonable to assume that the graft vessels represent a plexus that is preexistent in the tendon at the time of the transfer, and that the plexus subsequently gains attachment to vessels invading from the fat pad and the drilled channels. With the pedicled graft, this process may be facilitated or even accelerated by preserving the original attachment of the fat pad to the patellar tendon. However, the fat pad pedicle, at least in the sheep, has no significant influence on further healing of the graft or on the result at one year.
5. The initial biomechanical quality of both grafts, free and pedicled, is not reattained at 1 year after surgery despite the good appearance of the grafts.
6. The infrapatellar fat pad of the sheep is so large that, in contrast to humans, it completely fills the joint cavity after closure and immediately covers all intra-articular structures. This facilitates revascularization of the free patellar tendon graft in the sheep. In the human knee joint, it is likely that the fat pad pedicle will have a more noticeable effect on graft survival. Further clinical studies are needed to resolve this question.

References

1. Alm A, Stroemberg B. Transposed medial third of patellar ligament in reconstruction of the anterior cruciate ligament
2. Alm A, Gillquist J (1973) Reconstruction of the anterior cruciate ligament by using the medial third of the patellar ligament. Acta Chir Scand
3. Alm A (1973) Survival of part of the patellar tendon transposed for reconstruction of anterior cruciate ligament. Acta Chir Scand, p 139
4. Arnoczky SP, Tarwin GB, Marshall JL (1982) Anterior cruciate ligament replacement using patellar tendon. J Bone Joint Surg [Am] 46
5. Brückner H, Brückner H (1972) Bandplastiken im Kniebereich nach dem Baukastenprinzip. Zentralbl Chir 97:65–77
6. Chiroff RT (1975) The experimental replacement of the anterior cruciate ligament. J Bone Joint Surg [Am] 57
7. Clancy WG, et al. (1981) Anterior and posterior cruciate ligament reconstruction in rhesus monkeys. J Bone Joint Surg [Am] 63
8. Clancy WG, unpublished
9. Cooper RR, Misol S (1970) Tendon and ligament insertion. J Bone Joint Surg [Am] 52
10. Davies DV, Edwards DAW (1948) The blood supply of the synovial membrane and intra-articular structures. Ann R Coll Surg Engl
11. Dolgo-Saburoff B (1929) Über Ursprung und Insertion der Skelettmuskeln. Anat Anz, 68

12. Jones GK (1963) Reconstruction of the anterior cruciate ligament. A technique using the central one third of the patellar tendon. J Bone Joint Surg [Am] 45
13. Müller We (1982) Das Knie. Springer, Berlin Heidelberg New York
14. Rubin P (1964) Microangiography: facts and artifacts. Radiol Clin North Am 2:499
15. Scapinelli R (1968) Studies on the vasculature of the human knee joint. Acta Anat 70
16. Tillmann B, Thomas W (1982) Anatomie typischer Sehnenansätze, -ursprünge und Engpässe. Orthop Praxis 12:910–917
17. Whiston TB, Walmsley R (1960) Some observations on the reaction of bone and tendon after tunneling of bone and insertion of tendon. J Bone Joint Surg [Am] 42/2
18. Clancy WG (1983) Anterior cruciate ligament functional instability. A static intra-articular and dynamic extra-articular procedure. Clin Orthop Rel Res, No. 172
19. Paulos LE, Butler DL, Noyes FR, Grood ES (1983) Intra-articular cruciate reconstruction. II. Replacement with vascularised patellar tendon. Clin Orthop Rel Res, No. 172
20. Lambert KL (1983) Vascularised patellar tendon graft with rigid internal fixation for anterior cruciate ligament insufficiency. Clin Orthop Rel Res, No. 172

Arthroscopy and electron microscopy following anterior cruciate reconstruction

W. Hackenbruch[1], *H. Schmiebusch*[1], *W. Müller*[2] *and J. Staubesand*[2]

[1] **Department of Orthopedics, Kantonsspital Bruderholz**
[2] **Institute of Anatomy, Division I, University of Freiburg**

Continuity-disrupting injuries of the cruciate ligaments are unable to heal spontaneously because of the anatomy of the structures involved. Surgical reconstruction is an essential preliminary to ligamentous healing in such cases, and this accounts for the increasing frequency with which these operations are advocated and performed [3, 5, 7, 9, 10, 13]. A variety of techniques have been described in the literature [1, 3, 7, 9, 10, 14]. All are costly and require prolonged postoperative care. The results of the operations are not entirely satisfactory, due largely to the complex anatomic arrangement of the cruciate ligaments [5, 9] and their precarious blood supply [15, 17].

Despite the logical demand for surgical reconstruction, the therapeutic cost must be weighed against the anticipated functional gain. Subjective complaints may be mild owing to the compensatory effect of secondary stabilizers (peripheral capsuloligamentous structures) and sound muscular function.

It has been difficult in the past to conduct meaningful follow-ups of surgical results. Previous publications have dealt mostly with clinical examinations, which are of limited value in evaluating the condition of the cruciate ligament. Complaints and subjective performance ability (sports) depend largely on muscular function. Coexisting injuries (e.g., of the cartilage) also have a major bearing on subjective complaints (pain). The clinical examination can provide objective criteria for mobility, swelling, effusion, and muscular function. However, the most important parameter is stability, which can be evaluated with differentiated clinical tests. But the results of these studies are difficult to interpret with accuracy, because the secondary stabilizers can greatly influence the apparent degree of cruciate stability.

The following methods of objective investigation are available:

1. *Tensile testing:* Tensile tests are possible only in animal studies and have been conducted by Salamon, O'Donoghue, Drobny, and Oakes.
2. *Histologic investigations:* Most previous studies of this type have been done in laboratory animals, and only isolated observations are available in human patients following reoperations (Alm).
3. *Arthroscopic examinations:* Arthroscopy is an invasive study that provides information on the gross appearance of the anterior cruciate ligament (ACL) but not on its mechanical strength or structure. Isolated observations have been reported in man, most involving follow-up examinations after anterior cruciate reconstructions [6, 8].

Table 1.

Electron microscopic biopsies taken at operation:	17
Electron microscopic biopsies taken at follow-up arthroscopy:	25

Table 2.

Electron microscopic studies, biopsy from:		
Anterior cruciate ligament	After replacement with free graft from central third of patellar tendon	17
	After replacement with patellar tendon graft with fat pad pedicle	7
	After pull-through suture	3
	After distal bony avulsion	1
	After replacement with iliotibial tract	1
	After unspecified reconstruction	2
Control specimens:	Anterior cruciate ligament	6
	Posterior cruciate ligament	1
	Patellar tendon	2
	Laboratory animals	2
		42

The three investigations listed above give qualitatively different answers to the question of the mechanical load capacity of the reconstructed ACL. Tensile testing is the most accurate method of investigation in theory, but it is inappropriate for human medicine. Histology is of only limited usefulness, because the excision of a large biopsy specimen would weaken the reconstructed ligament and jeopardize the surgical result. Certain criteria for mechanical load capacity can nevertheless be derived from the histologic picture. Arthroscopy, which is the most rational investigation in man, can give information on the caliber of the ACL, its synovial investment, and its degree of tension.

In our search for objective follow-up investigations, we have made use of electron microscopy as well as a combination of arthroscopy and electron microscopy (Table 1). With electron microscopy it is possible to perform a morphologic examination on a very small volume of resected tissue that will not compromise the stability of the knee or cause other problems for the patient. The examination requires a specimen only about 1 mm × 1 mm in size, which is immediately fixed in a buffered gluteraldehyde solution after its removal. The specimen is stored and transported at a constant temperature (about 4 °C), and subsequent processing follows the standard rules of electron microscopy.

Some of the biopsies were taken at reoperation, but most were obtained during the course of a follow-up arthroscopic examination. Additional control specimens were taken from the ACL, posterior cruciate ligament (PCL), and patellar tendon, and two were taken from laboratory animals (Table 2).

The specimens taken at operation were either from joints in which an anterior cruciate reconstruction had previously been performed and a reoper-

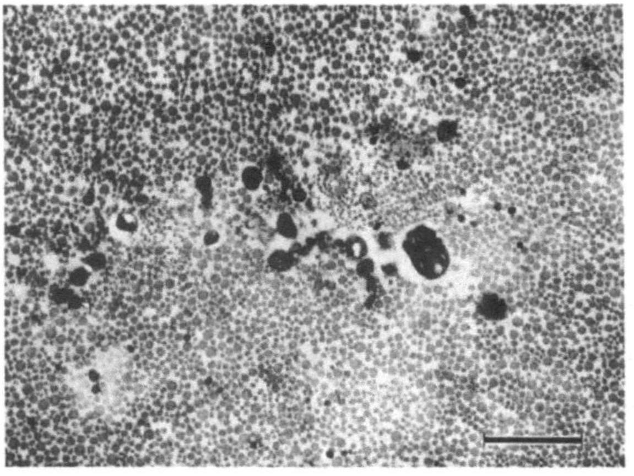

Figure 1 a. Electron micrograph of a PCL with a normal ultrastructure and minimal cellular ingrowth. We see a fairly homogeneous pattern with a symmetric arrangement of fibrils.

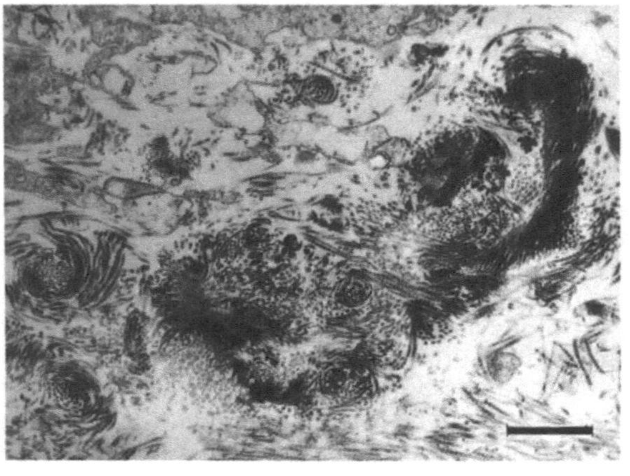

Figure 1 b. ACL, biopsy taken from the same patient during the implantation of a total knee prosthesis. Gross inspection shows extensive destruction and partial absorption of the ligament in the setting of chronic rheumatoid arthritis. Electron microscopy shows an irregular arrangement of collagen fibrils with scarring and cellular ingrowths

ation was required for significant residual instability, or they were control specimens taken for purposes of comparison.

We biopsied both the ACL and PCL during a total knee arthroplasty in a 72-year-old woman with chronic rheumatoid arthritis. At operation we found the typical presentation of advanced degenerative disease of rheumatic origin. THe ACL showed extensive destruction and was largely resorbed; the PCL was fairly well preserved. This is consistent with the electron microscopic picture, in which the PCL shows a normal ultrastructure, while the ACL shows an irregular fibrillary pattern with cellular ingrowth and scarring (Figure 1). Another control specimen was taken from a grossly healthy ACL during a meniscus operation in a 63-year-old man (Figure 2). The specimen shows a regular arrangement of collagen fibrils.

One biopsy was taken during an anterior cruciate reconstruction using the central one-third of the patellar tendon. Electron microscopy of the patellar tendon shows a completely homogeneous pattern with a symmetric arrangement of fibrils (Figure 3).

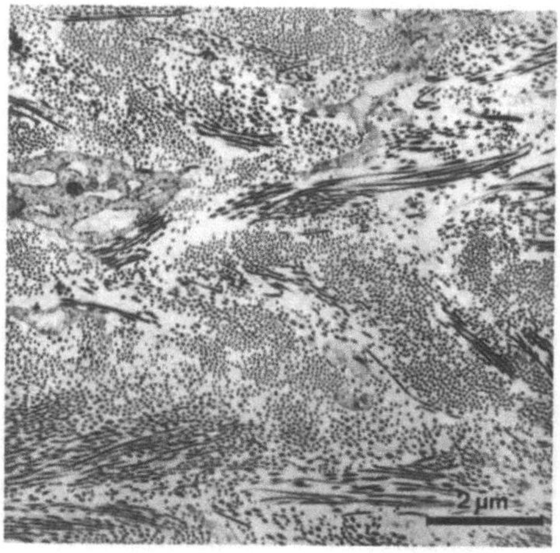

Figure 2. Electron micrograph of a grossly healthy ACL. Note the regular fibrillary pattern and homogeneous ultrastructure (specimen from a 63-year-old man)

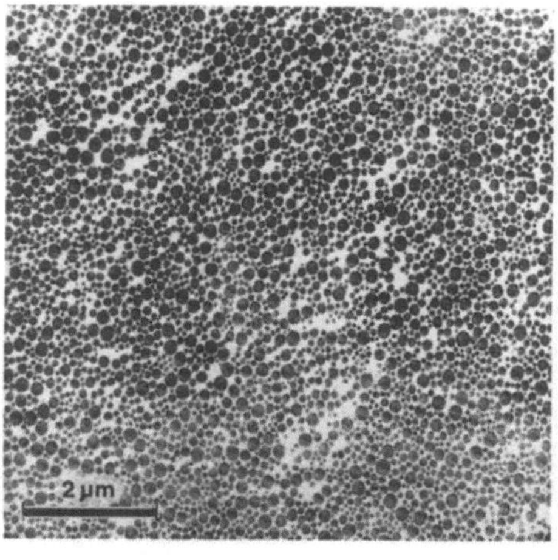

Figure 3. Electron microscopy of the patellar tendon in this young patient shows a completely homogeneous and symmetric fibrillary pattern

Several reoperations for significant residual instability or other complaints afforded the opportunity to biopsy a reconstructed cruciate ligament. One 28-year-old man had to be reoperated on 2 years after an ACL reconstruction performed elsewhere. The main cause of residual instability in that patient was a faulty femoral insertion of the cruciate substitute. On gross examination the graft appeared viable and had good synovial coverage, but it was markedly lax in extension because its direction was too vertical (Figure 4).

Three cases in this series were reoperated on following an unsuccessful repair of the ACL. In all cases electron microscopy showed cellular ingrowth into the scarred ligament, a finding consistent with the functionally deficient status of the ligament remnant (Figure 5).

To date we have performed combined arthroscopic and electron microscopic examinations in 25 patients. All involved follow-up arthroscopies after ante-

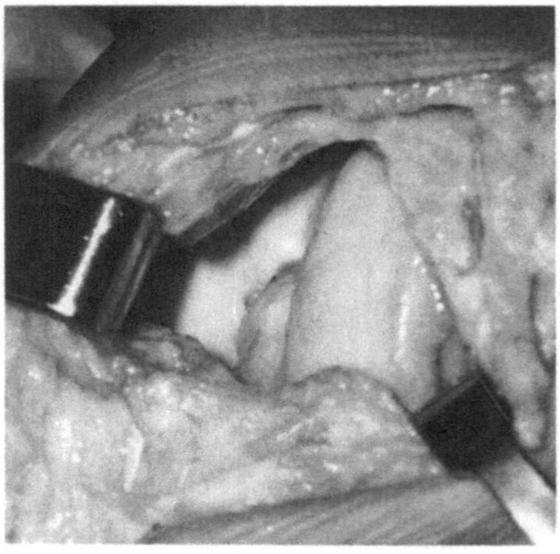

Figure 4. Photo taken at reoperation after a prior anterior cruciate reconstruction. The graft is viable, but its direction is too vertical

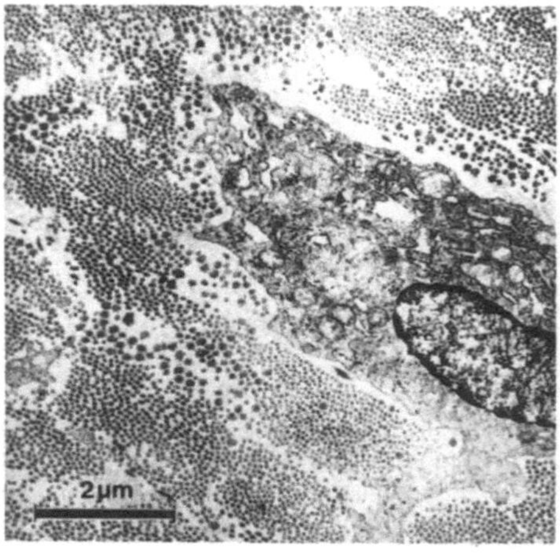

Figure 5. Electron micrograph of a scarred, insufficient ACL 5 years after a primary repair in a 32-year-old woman. The ultrastructure shows cellular ingrowth, scarring, and irregular collagen fribrils

rior cruciate reconstructions. In most cases the ACL had been replaced with a free graft taken from the patellar tendon (Figure 6). In the past 3 years we have routinely left a portion of the infrapatellar fat pad adherent to the patellar tendon graft to provide a vascular pedicle; a smaller number of follow-ups are available for this technique (Figure 7).

All arthroscopic follow-up examinations were performed under local anesthesia as outpatient procedures. The majority were done in patients with mild residual complaints (chondropathy, meniscal tab tear, etc.). Arthroscopy of the previously operated knee can pose technical difficulties, because adhesions may limit opening of the joint space and synovial scarring can obstruct vision. The gross appearance of the ACL provides useful information on its condition. An hourglass constriction (Figure 8) and a nonphysiologic direction of the ligament are pathognomonic for insufficiency.

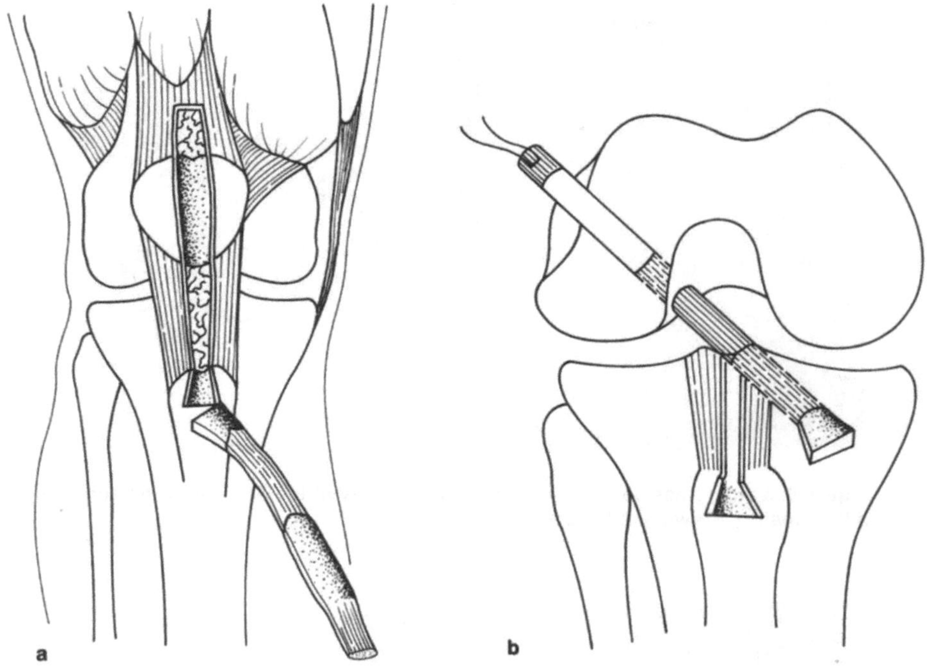

Figure 6. a Schematic drawing of the removal of a free graft from the central one-third of the patellar tendon; **b** Drawing showing the replacement of the ACL by the free graft

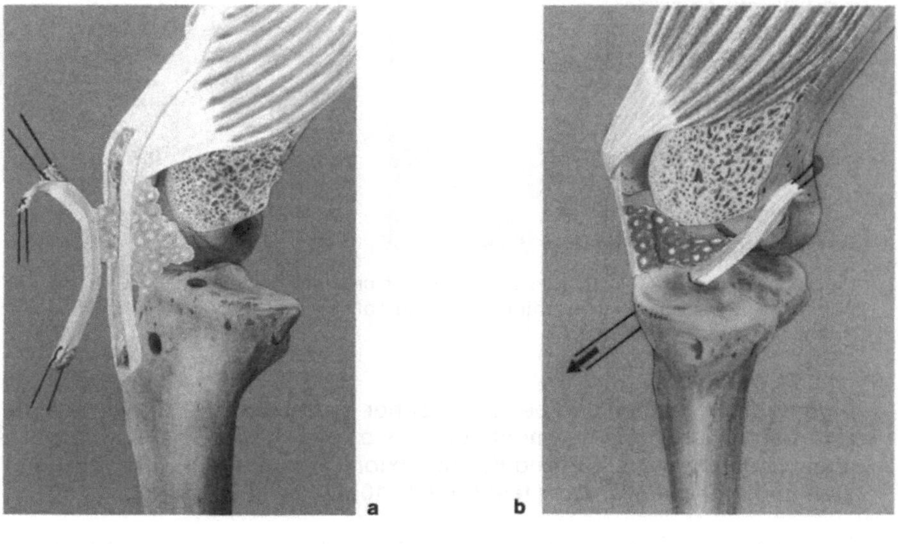

Figure 7. a Drawing showing the preparation of the patellar tendon graft with a fat pad pedicle for reconstruction of the ACL; **b** Drawing showing the pedicled patellar tendon graft in place

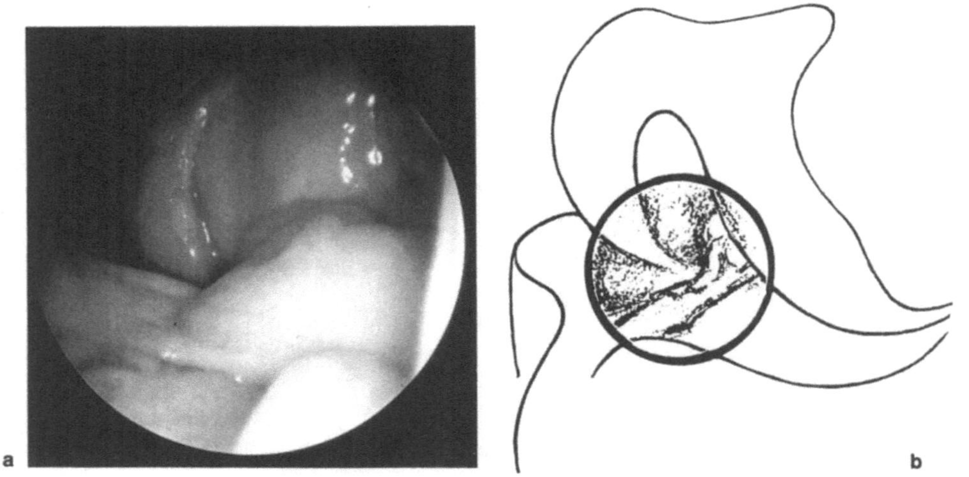

Figure 8. a Hourglass constriction and marked laxity of the ACL following surgical repair; b Explanatory drawing of the arthroscopic view

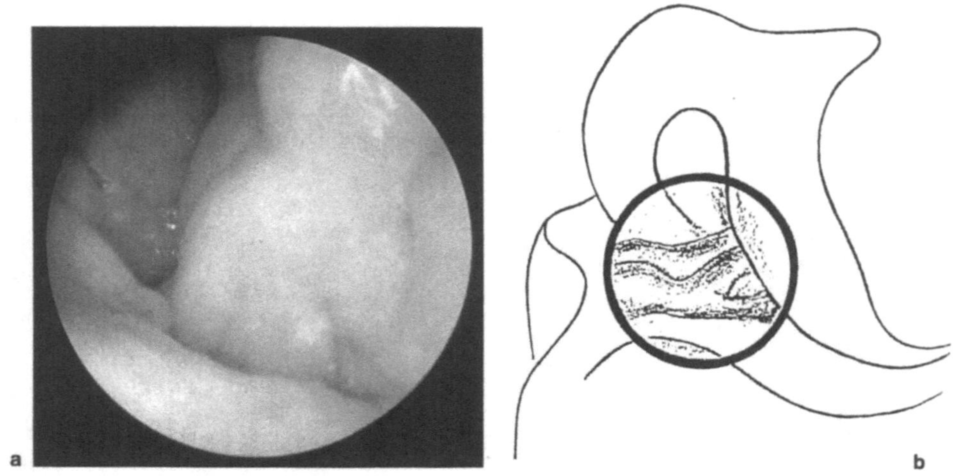

Figure 9. a Arthroscopic picture after anterior cruciate reconstruction with the pedicled patellar tendon graft, showing mild laxity in 50 ° of flexion; b Explanatory drawing of the arthroscopic view

Ligamentous tension can be tested either by the anterior drawer test during arthroscopy or with a ligament hook. As a rule, the ACL substitute will show slight laxity between 40° and 60° of flexion (Figure 9) but will show good tension in the anterior drawer test (Figure 10).

In 25 cases a tissue specimen about 1 mm × 1 mm in size was retrieved through the arthroscope with fine biopsy forceps for electronic microscopic evaluation. In agreement with clinical and arthroscopic findings, the patellar tendon graft shows a uniform cross section with a regular fibrillary pattern

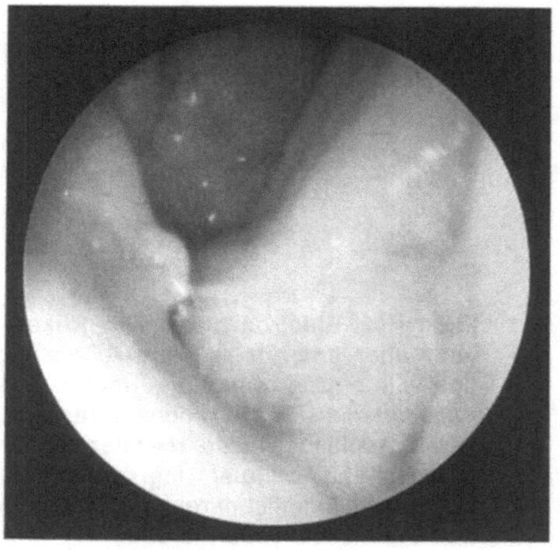

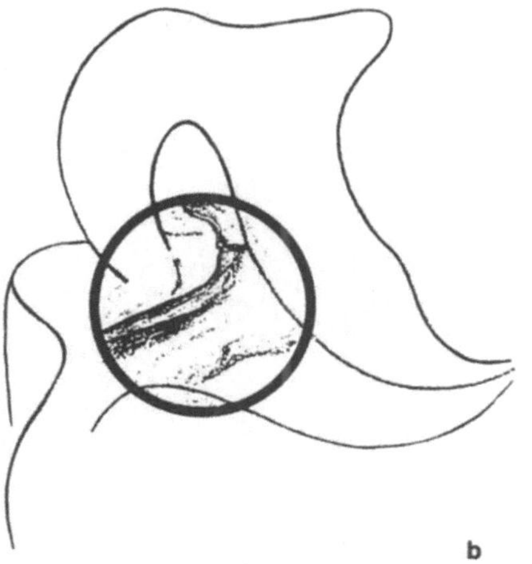

Figure 10. a The same graft shows good tension in the anterior drawer test and a firm, sufficient, viable structure; b Explanatory drawing of the arthroscopic view

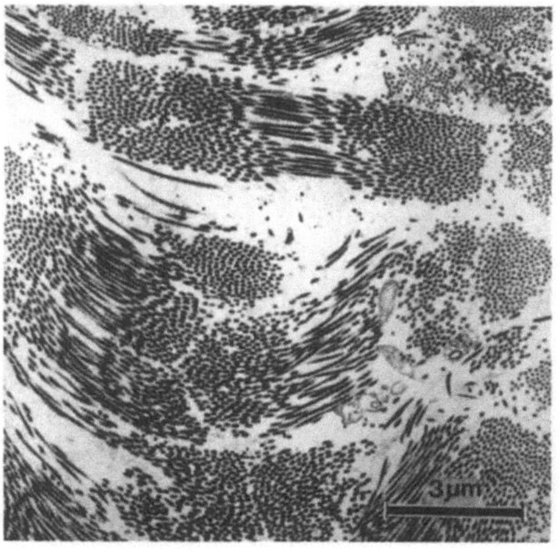

Figure 11. Electron micrograph taken 1 year after anterior cruciate reconstruction with a free patellar tendon graft in a 36-year-old man. We see a relatively uniform arrangement of fibrils with symmetric calibers; the clinical and arthroscopic results are good

(Figure 11). On the other hand, the repaired ACL (Figure 5) or an ACL reconstructed from the iliotibial tract (Figure 12) shows dysplastic collagen with irregularly arranged fibrils of varying diameters.

The nonhomogeneous material of our investigations and the small case numbers do not permit statistically valid conclusions to be drawn. Further experience is needed in order to make a more meaningful assessment of functional capacity based on the morphologic picture. Nevertheless, a definite trend is apparent which provides useful, though not yet definitive, guidelines for therapeutic decision-making.

The average length of electron microscopic follow-up after anterior cruciate reconstruction has been 26 months (3–68 months). It is still too early to char-

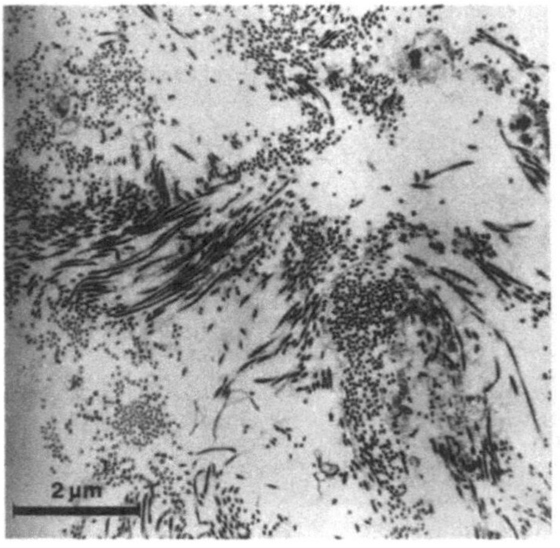

Figure 12. Electron micrograph taken 1 year after anterior cruciate reconstruction with a strip of iliotibial tract in a 19-year-old male. There is considerable collagen dysplasia with an irregular fibrillary pattern and cellular ingrowths. This patient has significant residual instability, and the clinical result is poor

acterize the collageneous structure of the substitute (remodeling) as a function of time after surgery, and further investigations are needed to resolve this question.

Posterior Cruciate Ligament

Replacement of the two cruciate ligaments with a single transplant derived from the extensor apparatus (crossed quadriceps ligamentoplasty)

J. L. Lerat, L. Dupré Latour, C. Tarquini and P. Dumont

Department of Orthopedic Surgery and Traumatology, Centre hospitalier Lyon Sud
France

Introduction

The technique of crossed quadriceps ligamentoplasty is designed for severe chronic ligamentous laxity of the knee associated with gross anterior and posterior drawer signs and an often complex peripheral laxity. It is well known that none of the palliative reconstructions of the central pivot with various tendinous transplants bears more than a remote similarity to the normal anatomy, since the arrangement of the fibres of the two cruciate ligaments is so complex.

Given this essential preamble, there is bound to be an interest in replacing the entire central pivot with *a single transplant* inserted through *a single access route*, rather than combining several classical procedures for reconstruction of the anterior and posterior cruciate ligaments using several simultaneous incisions.

In addition to reconstruction of the two cruciate ligaments, the procedure proposed here allows stabilization of the lateral condyle by a lateral plasty using the end of the same transplant. Any manoeuvers for stabilizing the medial compartment of the knee seem equally desirable in these complex laxities and could be performed through the same incision according to individual preference.

We shall confine ourselves to indicating our own choice of procedure as an auxiliary to the pivot operation in the strict sense, which is the subject of this technical communication.

Principle of the operation

A long strip excised from the extensor apparatus includes a large patellar fragment in its central portion. This fragment is incorporated in the tibial plateau, the fibres of the patellar ligament replace the posterior cruciate while retaining a bony attachment, and the suprapatellar fibres replace the anterior cruciate, traversing the lateral condyle to be implanted anteriorly at Gerdy's tuberosity.

Operative technique

This comprises the following stages:

1. *A single* anterior vertical incision 18 cm long is required. This is developed somewhat laterally, and further stripping gives easy access to the

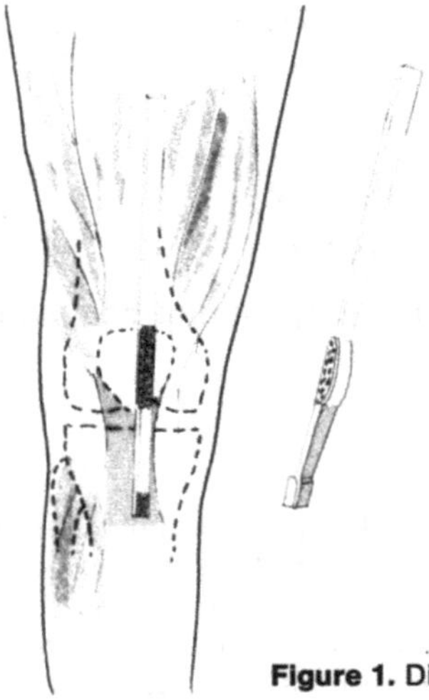

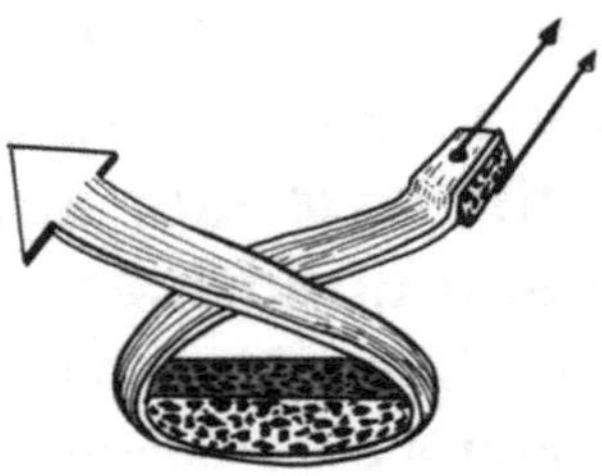

Figure 2. Principle of use of transplant; the two ends of the patellar fragment correspond to the attachments of the two cruciate ligaments

Figure 1. Diagram of transplant excised from extensor apparatus

medial and lateral condyles for performance of peripheral plasties and eventual meniscal reattachment.

2. *Size of transplant.* The transplant includes the medial third of the patellar ligament (10 mm in width) with its bony insertion at the tibial tuberosity, then the corresponding patellar rod (over 5 mm thick), and finally the suprapatellar prolongation with the fibres of the quadriceps and rectus femoris tendons. The total length of this transplant is 28 cm (Figure 1). The patella is marked out with two parallel saw-cuts made with a hand saw with a fine blade up to 5 mm deep, the two cuts then being joined by a wire saw (fretsaw as used in model-making). This yields a regular and very solid rectangular block (Figure 2).
3. *Preparation of the tibia* is performed after division of the transverse ligament and separation of the two anterior meniscal horns (scrupulously repaired at the end of the operation).
   A bony block 1 cm wide by 1.5 cm thick is resected *just in front* of the anterior attachment of the anterior cruciate. (The posterior wall of this fossa is to serve as the point of reflexion of the new anterior cruciate ligament [Figure 3]).

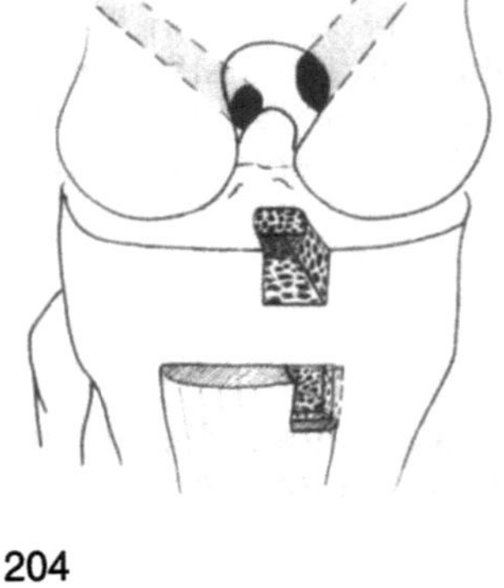

Figure 3. Preparation of the prespinous surface and drilling of the tunnel under the spinous processes

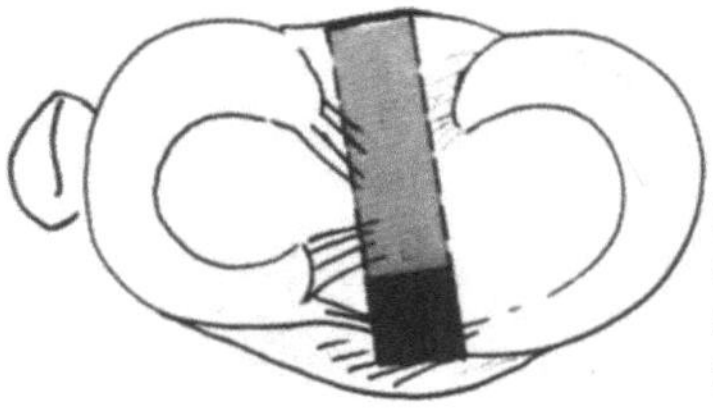

Figure 4. The tunnel under the substance of the tibial spines runs obliquely backward and outward to emerge at the attachment of the posterior cruciate ligament

A tunnel is drilled under the substance of the tibial spines from front to back, 5–6 mm under the surface (Figure 4), carefully adjusted to the dimensions of the patellar rod to be embedded in it. This tunnel starts from the attachment of the anterior cruciate and emerges at the insertion of the posterior cruciate, so that it must be directed slightly outward as well as backward. Forward subluxation of the tibia facilitates the positioning and emergence of the tunnel. At the emergence site inferior fibres of the posterior cruciate still remain, which are stripped backwards with a rugine but preserved. The roughened zone serves as a reflexion pulley for the new posterior cruciate ligament, and the stripped fibres will later attach themselves to the transplant.

4. *Insertion of the transplant* from front to back begins with the bony fragment derived from the tibial tuberosity. It is transfixed with a traction wire and then pulled to the back of the tibia and brought out in front of the notch.
   The patellar rod is forcibly impacted backward into the tunnel. Stability is adequate, but can be improved if necessary by the insertion of fragments of cancellous bone (Figure 5).
5. *The medial condyle is drilled* with an 8 mm box chisel well in front of the normal insertion of the posterior cruciate (in fact, the posterior part of the hole will function as the point of reflexion of the ligament). The bony fragment is transfixed by a metal wire, which is held in tension over a screw above the condyle at the end of the operation (Figures 5 and 6).
6. *The lateral condyle is drilled* using a guide; the entry point is above and behind the attachment of the lateral ligament and the exit at the most posterior part of the normal attachment of the anterior cruciate. The new cruciate ligament thus crosses the lateral condyle, and the whole of its terminal portion serves to stabilize the lateral condyle.

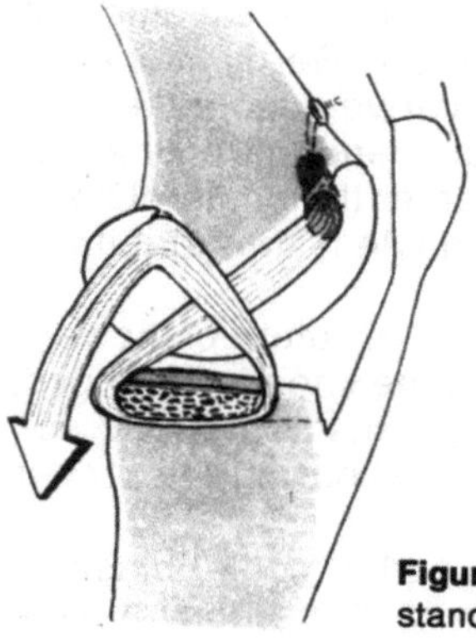

Figure 5. Positioning of the patellar fragment beneath the substance of the tibial spines

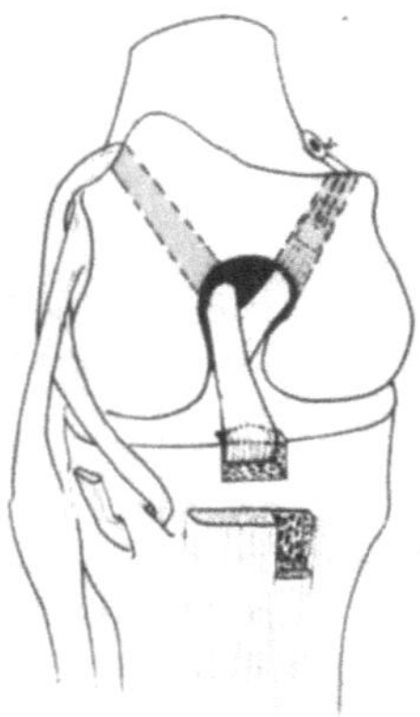

Figure 6. Positioning of the two cruciate ligaments and anterolateral ligamentoplasty via Gerdy's tuberosity

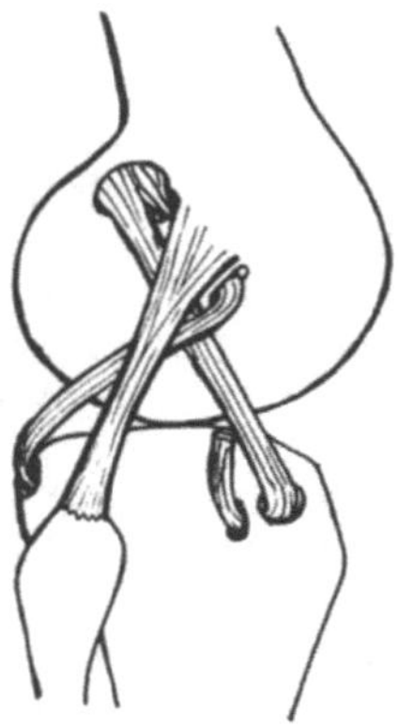

Figure 7. Double lateral ligamentoplasty: anterolateral and posterolateral reinforcement after splitting of the transplant at its emergence from the lateral condyle

7. *Stabilization of the lateral condyle* can be achieved in different ways. In a first variant (Figure 6) the strip is passed under the lateral ligament and then brought through Gerdy's tuberosity via a small tunnel, the transplant being firmly sutured to itself (we use this method to correct anterior laxity, in a procedure derived from the techniques of Jones and MacIntosh).
   In a second variant (Figure 7) the strip is divided in two where it emerges from the lateral condyle. The first strip is taken through Gerdy's tuberosity (as before) and the second is passed in a tunnel driven under the bony attachment of the lateral ligament and the popliteus tendon from back to front and then taken backward and downward to enter the posterolateral portion of the lateral tibial plateau. The lateral condyle is thus stabilized in the anteroposterior direction.
8. *Tensioning of the two cruciate ligaments* and definitive suture of the various peripheral plasties are done at the end, when the knee is extended, which is especially important for good positioning of the posterior cruciate ligament. (Meniscal preservation is cardinal in securing the proper relationship of the femur and tibia in extension.)
9. *A medial plasty* can be performed. We prefer to add a medial plasty of the Lenggenhager type, with upward displacement of the bony attach-

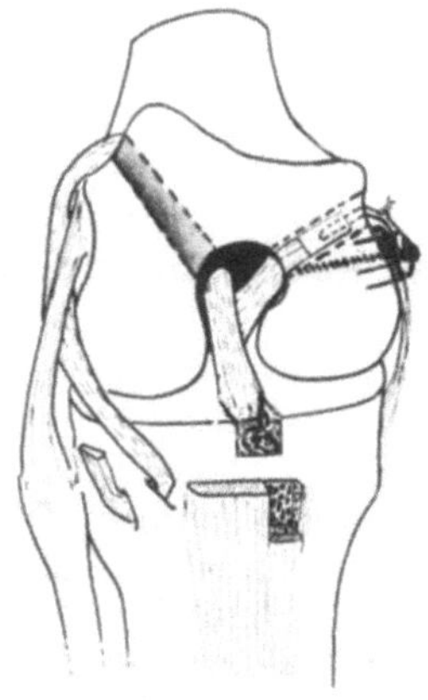

Figure 8. Upward retensioning of the medial ligament with a screwed staple (over which the metal wire of the posterior cruciate ligament is fastened)

ment of the medial ligament using a screwed staple, which controls major valgus laxity. The tunnel in the medial condyle is made to emerge above this attachment, and the metal attachment wire of the new posterior cruciate ligament is held over the screw of the staple (Figure 8). Care is taken with "synovialization" of this metal material.

10. *The operation is completed by replacing the bony block* in front of the spinous processes and the anterior cruciate ligament and by reattaching the two meniscal horns together. All the tunnels are packed with cancellous bone gathered during the various drillings, and Maissiat's strip is carefully closed, as is the medial arthrotomy.

Conclusion

This technique should be reserved for exceptional cases, where the severity of the laxity and major clinical instability often necessitate the use of sticks or a brace. Its advantages can be summarized as follows:

– A single simple access route

– A single transplant derived from the extensor apparatus without noticeable weakening of the latter, as already proved by long experience of this type of excision in the treatment of anterior laxity

– The immediate simultaneous and solid reconstitution of both cruciate ligaments allows a brief period of immobilization and rapid rehabilitation

The procedure offers a step forward in a field where there is nothing very attractive in our current therapeutic arsenal. It should be assessed in medium-term tests and cannot fail to be improved by refinements suggested by such tests.

Radiological analysis of lesions of the posterior cruciate ligament

C. Miremad

Groupe de Chirurgie Orthopédique et Sportive de Paris, Rue de Romainville 67
Paris
France

The severity of instability due to rupture of the posterior cruciate ligament (PCL) varies considerably according to the existence and extent of associated posteromedial and posterolaterla lesions. It is very difficult to assess accurately such associated lesions by clinical examination only. For this reason we have tried to improve radiological examination in order to obtain a perfectly objective diagnosis.

Radiological examination consists of the following:

— comparative lateral and 90° flexion X-ray films, with and without the "drawer" manoeuvre.

— comparative X-ray films in 90° flexion and in forced medial and lateral rotation.

— arthrography, using a radio opaque agent.

Posteromedial or posterolateral lesions may be visualized in this way, and prognosis and treatment of the various types of posterior instability be established on the basis of definite data.

All cases of rupture of the PCL have the common feature of a backward shift of the tibial epiphysis on the lateral film in 90° flexion without any rotation. This shift may be better assessed by precisely identifying the position of the tibial spines.

The rarest variety is isolated rupture of the PCL, without any associated lesion. Backward shift of the tibial spines is moderate, but is accentuated by the posterior drawer manoeuvre. Medial or lateral rotation completely corrects the abnormal position of the tibial epiphysis. This isolated rupture of the PCL is a minor instability, which does not even interfere with continuing sports activity. However, the knee is more vulnerable to a subsequent accident.

The commonest variety is combination of rupture of the ligament with postero medial lesions, lesion of the condylar covering, and, above all, of the posterior oblique ligament. There is a very marked backward shift of the tibial plateau in medial rotation, which is corrected in lateral rotation. This is a type of instability of moderate gravity, very well compensated merely by repairing the postero medial layer.

The most severe cases involved destruction of all the posterior layer. X-ray films show combined postero medial and postero lateral backward shift. This is the most severe form of instability of the knee. It also raises the most difficult surgical problems, and it would seem, in particular, that, in such cases, repair in situ of the posterior cruciate ligament is essential.

Results of primary repair in knee ligament injuries including the posterior cruciate ligament

T. Strand, A. O. Mølster, L. B. Engesaeter, T. S. Raugstad and A. Alho

Haukeland Hospital
University of Bergen
Norway

Introduction

Injuries to the posterior cruciate ligament (PCL) of the knee are relatively infrequent. Most authors recommend primary operative repair, but few larger series with documented results exist. Lately the value of primary operative treatment has been questioned.

The present retrospective study was performed to evaluate the results of primary operative treatment.

Patients and methods

During 1976–1981 all 37 patients with acute PCL injuries diagnosed within 4 weeks were treated by primary repair. Thirty-two could be followed-up after 12–81 (median 45) months, and were included in our series, consisting of 20 males and 12 females with a median age 27 (13–60) years. Twenty-three repairs were performed within 1 week from injury, and only 3 after more than 2 weeks.

By clinical examination in general or epidural anaesthesia prior to operation, a posterior drawer was found in 24 patients, while 19 patients had varus/valgus instability in full extension. Twenty-six patients sustained combined ligament injuries, including both cruciates in 18 cases. All ruptured ligaments, including 11 peripherally detached menisci, were sutured. In five cases an isolated PCL avulsion with a displaced bone fragment from the tibia occurred. The fragments were fixed by screws using a posterior incision. All cases were immobilized in a plaster cast for 6 weeks postoperatively.

At follow-up anteroposterior and medial-lateral instabilities were graded as slight (3–5 mm), moderate (6–10 mm) or severe (>10 mm) compared with the normal knee. Anterolateral rotatory instability was assessed by the Slocum test.

The functional result was evaluated by the Lysholm knee scoring scale, 100 points representing the maximum score. The results were graded according to Odensten et al. (1983) (excellent >90 points, good 77–90 points).

The results were analysed statistically by the Wilcoxen two-sample test and the Fisher exact probability test.

Results

Two wound infections occurred.

A moderate or severe posterior drawer sign was found in 7 patients, and only 14 patients were completely stable in this respect. Five patients had ALRI and one patient significant AMRI.

Two patients had a flexion deficit exceeding 30° and one patient a lack of extension exceeding 10°.

The functional results were graded as excellent in 20, good in 6 and fair/poor in 6 patients. The median score was 92.5 (46–100) points. Seven patients had symptoms of instability (giving-way), four during daily activities. Three of these patients had ALRI, one AMRI and two moderate posterior drawer sign. Thus, five out of seven patients with moderate or severe posterior drawer signs did not have functional instability and obtained excellent functional results. Neither did this group of seven patients have more pain than other patients, and the median score value was 94 points. Of the six patients with ALRI/AMRI only one was graded as excellent. Functional knee score values were significantly ($P = 0.02$) lower in these six patients than in the stable patients (75.5 versus 94 points median score values).

Out of five patients with isolated PCL injuries with a displaced bone fragment, the fragment healed in anatomical position in four patients, all obtaining excellent functional results. In the last patient, the fragment did not heal and was dislocated, resulting in symptoms of instability and a poor functional result.

Discussion

In this series most PCL injuries were combined ligament injuries, half of them being skiing injuries. The isolated PCL injuries were all caused by traffic accidents with a direct blow against the anterior upper tibia.

The functional results were generally good: 80% of the patients obtained good/excellent results. ALRI/AMRI was associated with less satisfying results, indicating the importance of integrity of other ligaments in combined PCL injuries. The relative importance of the PCL repair in combined injuries is difficult to evaluate, but the PCL did not seem to be more important than other ligaments.

In combined injuries including the PCL, no convincing reports of conservative treatment exist. Thus, based on the presented results, we recommended primary repair of all ruptured ligaments.

In isolated PCL avulsions with a displaced bone fragment, the functional results were excellent in all cases in whom the fragment united. In accordance with most authors we recommend primary repair using a posterior incision in such cases.

References

Lysholm J, Gillquist J (1982) Evaluation of knee ligament surgery results with special emphasis on use of a scoring scale. Am J Sports Med 10:150–154

Odensten M, Tegner Y, Lysholm J, Gillquist J (1983) Knee function and muscle strength following distal iliotibial and transfer for antero-lateral rotatory instability. Acta Orthop Scand 54:924–928

Acute tears of posterior cruciate ligament. Results of treatment in 48 cases

H. Seiler, M. Kayser and D. Hager

Chirurgische Universitätsklinik, Abteilung Unfallchirurgie
Homburg/Saar
Federal Republic of Germany

Acute lesions of the posterior cruciate ligament (PCL) are of increasing clinical interest. The results of only a few larger series have been published in the last years. The purpose of this paper is to present the nature of the injury and results of treatment in our own department, obtained in cases where rupture of the PCL was the predominant lesion.

Material and methods

Out of 54, 48 patients and knees could be followed up after a mean time interval of 26 months. 45 had been operated within 2 weeks after the injury. The guideline of the operative treatment was early repair of the ligament with screwing back to bone in tibial bony avulsion, transosseous refixation with sutures in other avulsion tears and intermedial ruptures. The usual approach to PCL, especially in the case of gross valgus opening, was posteromedially as described by Hughston (1980) or anteromedially in femoral tears. Isolated tibial avulsions of the PCL were exposed from posterior (Trickey, 1968). In these cases arthroscopy was usually done before changing position of the patient.

Results

In 11 knees tibial PCL avulsion was the only significant ligament injury. The medial and or lateral compartment ligaments were additional damaged in 12, anterior cruciate ligament, PCL and other ligaments combined in 25 knees. Tibial avulsions (20) were less frequent than femoral ones (28). Isolated tibial tears of the PCL were combined in 7 cases with fractures of the ipsilateral leg; a result of motorcyle accident or dashboard injury. All of the 3 patients with conservative treatment had poor results (results rating: Hughston, 1980). After operation the objective results were good in 18, fair in 16 and poor in 11 patients; subjective results were good in 15, fair in 21 and poor in 9 patients. No fair result was seen after isolated tear of the PCL. Limitations of extension exceeded never 10°.

Discussion

Acute tears of the PCL are still today treated conservatively for various reasons, like missed diagnosis, supposed inaccessibility and difficult technique in repair. Our own results show that surgical repair is efficient, when early and correctly done.

Summary

48 knees with PCL rupture were followed up. The mean time interval was 26 months. The surgical repair was efficient; especially in insolated tears of the PCL.

References

HUGHSTON, J.C., BOWDEN, J.A., ANDREWS, J.R., NORWOOD, L.A.: Acute tears of the posterior cruciate ligament.
J. Bone Jt. Surg. 62—A, 438(1980)

TRICKEY, E.L.: Rupture of the posterior cruciate ligament.
J. Bone Jt. Surg. 50—B, 334 (1968)

Is reefing of the posterior cruciate ligament a worthwhile procedure?

T. Häggmark, E. Eriksson and R. J. Johnson

Section of Trauma, Dpt. of Surgery, Karolinska Hospital
Stockholm
Sweden

Reconstruction of the posterior cruciate ligament is a much debated subject. In some of the patients that have symptomatic posterior drawer and who need surgery for their instability, a remnant of the posterior cruciate can be found. If a remaining prolonged posterior cruciate is found either with arthroscopy or arthrotomography we have operated these cases with reefing of the posterior cruciate. The ligament has been detached from its anterior femoral insertion and pulled out into a hole drilled from the outside of the medial femoral condyle and just anterior to the normal insertion of the posterior cruciate ligament. The ligament has then been fixed with sutures that have been tied over a button at outer opening of the drill hole. The sutures have been tied with the knee in about 20° of flexion. The knee has been kept in a cast in about 20° flexion for 6 weeks and rehabilitation then started.

Material and Methods

All the 20 patients that underwent this type of reefing 2–8 years previously have been reexamined. All patients have been examined clinically and in some cases arthroscopically. The degree of instability has been compared with their preoperative instability and their subjective opinion of the outcome graded. The patients were also asked wheter they had been able to perform vigorous sport after surgey. No one was able to do that before surgery.

Results

Al 20 knees had ++ – +++ posterior drawer sign before surgery. At follow-up 6 were stable without posterior drawer, 10 had a mild instability of + and 4 were unchanged with a ++ – +++ posterior drawer. Subjectively 10 rated the results as excellent, 6 as good and 4 as unchanged. 8 were able to participate in any sport, 5 said they had returned to jogging and 7 said they had not dared to try any sport.

Discussion.

Reefing of the posterior cruciate ligaments is a relatively simple operative procedure that in this material has given good results. In cases of symptomatic posterior instability where an elongated posterior cruciate is found, reefing of this ligament may provide satisfactory results.

Reconstruction for chronic posterolateral rotatory instability of the knee

T. E. Lim and R. K. Marti

Department of Orthopaedic Surgery, Academic Medical Centre
Amsterdam
The Netherlands

Introduction
In recent years attention has been focused on the lateral compartment of the knee in the case of instability. Anterolateral rotatory instability due to insufficiency of the anterior cruciate ligament is nowadays the subject of discussion. Several extra-articular methods of reconstruction have been described for treatment of this instability. Less attention is paid to posterolateral rotatory instability. Hughston et al. (1976) in their classic article about the classification of knee instabilities described this clinical term as an external rotatory subluxation of the tibia around the intact posterior cruciate ligament.

The anatomical structure involved in posterolateral rotatory instability (Baker et al. 1983; DeLee et al. 1983) is the arcuate complex, which consists of the fibular collateral ligament, the popliteus tendon, the arcuate ligament and the lateral gastrocnemius head. The diagnostic features for posterolateral rotatory instability are subtle and frequently misinterpreted. Knowledge of the mechanism of injury, symptoms and clinical findings is required to establish a diagnosis of posterolateral rotatory instability. The mechanism of injury is commonly a varus force to the knee combined with hyperextension. Symptoms consist of giving way and discomfort with long standing and walking. The patient walks with relative knee flexion to avoid hyperextension at the posterolateral aspect of the knee.

The detection of posterolateral rotatory instability is based upon three clinical tests: the posterolateral drawer sign, the external rotation recurvatum test (Hughston and Norwood 1980) and the reverse pivot shift as described by Jakob et al. (1981).

Material and method
Twenty-one patients with a chronic posterolateral instability were reviewed. Eight had a single posterolateral instability and 13 had a combined instability. Anterolateral and posterolateral rotatory instability was diagnosed in five patients. Anterolateral, anteromedial and posterolateral rotatory instability was found in eight patients.

There were 12 male and 9 female patients. The mean age of the patients was 28.8 years (19–44 years).

The primary diagnosis in nine patients was a meniscal injury for which a meniscectomy was performed. A medial instability was diagnosed in six patients and an anterolateral rotatory instability in two patients. In these patients a reconstruction was performed with resultant increased functional disability. Preoperatively all patients had complaints of giving way and discomfort with long standing and walking.

The clinical findings were in all patients a positive adduction stress test at 30° of knee flexion. The posterolateral drawer test was positive in 12 patients and the external rotation drawer test was positive in 6 patients. The definitive diagnosis of posterolateral rotatory instability was made at surgery, where a laxity of the arcuate ligament complex was found.

Surgical method

With an anteromedial arthrotomy the knee is inspected intra-articularly. Any meniscal pathology is treated and medial reconstruction if necessary is performed. On the lateral side a hockey stick incision is made, exposing the iliotibial tract. Dorsal to the biceps femoris the peroneal nerve is identified and freed from its course. This will prevent the nerve coming under tension at its entrance in the fascia behind the fibular head.

Splitting the iliotibial tract longitudinally exposes the lateral and posterolateral capsular structures. A vertical incision parallel to and anterior to the fibular collateral ligament allows exposure of the joint. The lateral meniscus and the popliteus tendon running in its hiatus can be examined. The attachment of the arcuate complex is identified and then isolated with a bone block (Figure 1). More proximal and ventral to the attachment of the arcuate complex on the lateral femur condyle the surface is roughened. The bone block with the isolated arcuate complex is then transferred to the prepared area and fixed with a staple (Figure 2). In the case of a slight posterolateral rotatory instability reefing of the popliteus tendon or arcuate ligament will restore the stability and an advancement of the whole arcuate complex is not necessary. In severe posterolateral rotatory instability reefing of the popliteus ten-

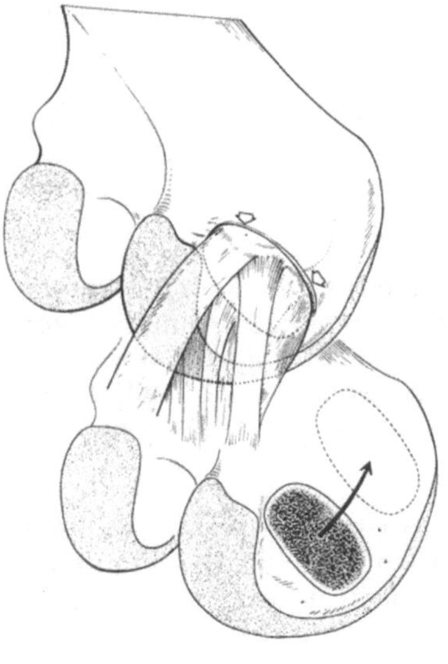

Figure 1. Isolation of the attachment of the arcuate complex (with a bone block)

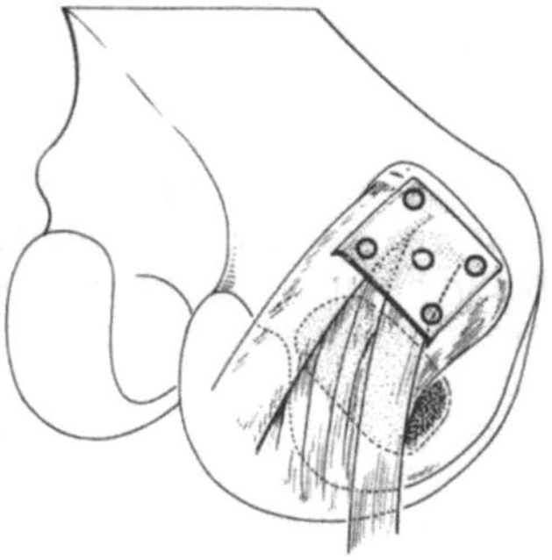

Figure 2. Staple holding the bone block in the prepared area

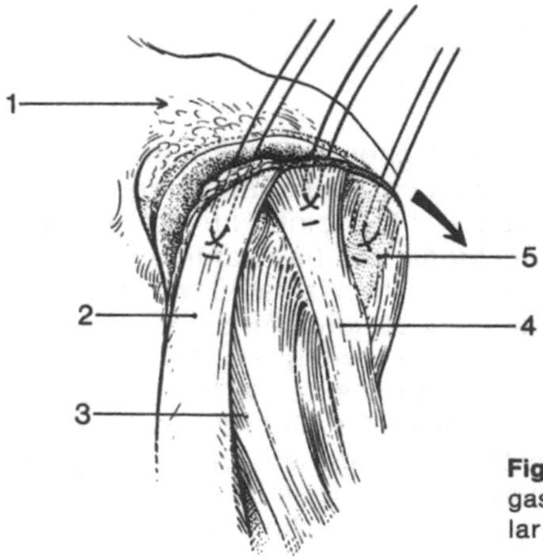

Figure 3. *1*, femur condyle; *2*, tendon of lateral gastrocnemius head; *3*, arcuate ligament; *4*, fibular collateral ligament; *5*, popliteus tendon

don or arcuate ligament in addition to the advancement of the arcuate complex will improve the stability (Figure 3).

In 14 patients the reconstruction for posterolateral rotatory instability was an advancement of the arcuate complex. Reefing of the popliteus tendon was performed in one patient and reefing of the arcuate ligament was done in six patients.

Postoperatively the patient is put in a groin to toe cast with 60° knee flexion for 6 weeks. A pelvic support is applied to prevent posterolateral sagging of the tibia. During rehabilitation the knee is protected with a dial-locked brace. Progressive active extension is gradually allowed. Once the active extension is within 15° of neutral, full weight-bearing in the brace is allowed.

Results

The follow-up period was at least 2 years to allow a rational judgment of the functional results. The mean follow-up was 41.2 months (24–61 months). The postoperative results were graded in three areas: subjective results (Table 1), objective results (Table 2) and functional results (Table 3). Objec-

Table 1. Subjective results

Good
a) No pain
b) No swelling
c) Mild aching after unusual activity
d) No giving way
e) No catching or locking

Fair
a) Pain, non-restricting, associated with prolonged, usual activity
b) Sensation of mild tightness or swelling after unusual activity
c) Moderate aching at rest after unusual activity
d) No giving way
e) No catching or locking

Poor
a) Pain at rest after unusual activity
b) Swelling, moderate, after unusual activity
c) Aching during inactivity or while sitting
d) Frequent giving way
e) Sensation of catching or locking occasionally

Table 2. Objective results

Good
a) Negative posterolateral drawer
b) Negative external rotation recurvatum test
c) No more than a 1+ adduction stress test at 30° flexion
d) Range of motion from at least 10° to 120° flexion
e) Minimum joint changes demonstrable by roentgenograms
f) No swelling

Fair
a) Posterolateral drawer no more than 1+
b) No more than a 2+ adduction stress test at 30° flexion
c) External rotation recurvatum test slightly positive
d) Range of motion from 15° to 120° flexion
e) Mild joint changes demonstrable by roentgenogram
f) Swelling absent or mild

Poor
a) Posterior-lateral drawer 2+ or more
b) A 3+ adduction stress test at 30° flexion
c) External rotation recurvatum markedly positive
d) Range of motion limited: extension lacking 20° or more and flexion limited to 110° or less
e) Moderate to severe joint changes demonstrable by roentgenogram
f) Moderate swelling

tively nine patients were rated good, nine patients fair and three patients poor. Subjectively ten patients had a good result, ten patients a fair result and one patient a poor result.

Table 3. Functional results

Good
a) Able to engage in all recreational sports without limitation and without difficulty or pain
b) Has mild aching following extreme activity
c) Goes up and down stairs and slopes with no difficulty
d) Gets in and out of automobiles without difficulty
e) Squats unconscious of pain or limitation
f) Cuts, pivots or twists without pain or giving way
Fair
a) Can engage in recreational sports with mild limitations
b) Usually has aching after extreme activities
c) Goes up and down stairs and slopes at will, but some slight adjustment is necessary
d) Gets in and out of automobiles without difficulty
e) Is able to squat and to reach filing cabinets and so on, but notes limitation of flexion and discomfort if squatting is continued for an undue length of time
f) Cuts, pivots and twists with some caution and occasional giving way of the knee, but these activities are only mildly limited
Poor
a) Cannot engage in recreational sports; walks with a limp or with a cane or other device
b) Has moderate aching during and after activity
c) Goes up and down stairs and slopes with difficulty and must use some walking aid and/or hold onto a railing
d) Gets in and out of automobiles with moderate difficulty
e) Is unable to squat or has pain while doing so
f) Is unable to cut or pivot and must observe some caution when walking on an incline because of a sensation of the knee hyperextending

Functionally eight patients were graded as a good result, ten patients fair and three patients poor. Of the three patients with a poor functional result one patient had a flexion limitation of 30°, one patient a disabling anterolateral rotatory instability and one patient an infection. Complications were a deep infection in one patient which needed removal of the staple and two superficial wound infections, which healed without further consequences. None of the patients had a problem related to the peroneal nerve.

Of the nine patients with competitive sports activities preinjury, three patients were able to get back to competitive sports postoperatively. Twelve patients were still engaged in recreational sports. None of the patients were limited in their activities of daily living.

Conclusions

The clinical diagnosis of posterolateral rotatory instability of the knee requires a keen awareness and close observation on the part of the examiner. Meticulous performance of specific tests for knee stability and knowledge of symptoms and mechanism of injury are essential to establish the correct diagnosis. Chronic posterolateral rotatory instability causes functional disability of the patient. Surgical treatment by advancement of the arcuate complex gives satisfactory results.

Although the series is relatively small and the follow-up period short, the functional results achieved so far are encouraging.

References

Baker CL, Norwood LA, Hughston JC (1983) Acute posterolateral rotatory instability of the knee. J Bone Joint Surg [Am] 65:614–618

DeLee JC, Riley MB, Rockwood CA (1983) Acute posterolateral rotatory instability of the knee. Am J Sports Med 11:199–207

Hughston JC, Norwood LA (1980) The posterolateral drawer test and external rotational recurvatum test for posterolateral rotatory instability of the knee. Clin Orthop 147:82–87

Hughston JC, Andrews JR, Cross MJ, Moschi A (1976) Classification of knee ligament instabilities: 1 and 2. J Bone Joint Surg [Am] 58:159–179

Jakob RP, Hassler H, Staeubli HU (1981) Observations on rotatory instability of the lateral compartment of the knee. Acta Orthop Scand 191:6–27

Reconstruction of the posterior cruciate ligament

P. M. Karpf, R. Gradinger, H. Hörterer and W. Mang

**Orthopädische Klinik und Poliklinik am Klinikum rechts der Isar
der Technischen Universität München
D-8000 Munich
Federal Republic of Germany**

Introduction

A typical finding for post-traumatic, posterior instability is pathological hyperextension of the knee joint. Because of the close functional relationship of ligamentous and muscular structures, particularly severe functional deficiencies are found in cases of posterior instability.

When looking at the knee joint from a posteromedial direction the semimembranosus complex can be seen. Likewise, the arcuate complex is found on the posterolateral side, consisting of the tendon of the popliteus muscle, the arcuate ligament and the fibular collateral ligament. The posterior dynamic stabilizers are the two heads of the gastrocnemius, the biceps femoris and the semimembranosus and the popliteus. Menisci as well as the posterior cruciate ligament provide additional support to the posterior capsule. The anterior cruciate ligament also limits hyperextension and, according to Kennedy and Grainger, a severe hyperextension of the knee joint includes – besides an obligatory lesion of the posterior cruciate ligament – a simultaneous rupture, or at least an elongation, of the anterior cruciate ligament.

In view of these anatomical facts we also use Kennedy's classification for ligamentous injuries associated with posterior cruciate ligament tears.

Group I "Isolated" posterior cruciate ligament tear
Group II + Anterior cruciate ligament tear
Group III + Major medial or lateral collateral ligament tears
Group IV + Anterior cruciate ligament tear with major medial or lateral collateral ligament tears

Materials and methods

Between 1975 and 1982, 14 acute and 23 chronic posterior instabilities of the knee were operatively treated in our clinic. The interval between injury and surgery in the acute cases averaged 10 days and in the chronic cases 18 months. The age of the patients at the time of surgery ranged from 17 to 60 years, with a postoperative follow-up from 1 to 9 years.

A satisfactory repair is generally possible, by direct suture or reattachment through transosseus drill holes. In contrast to the anterior cruciate ligament, the posterior cruciate ligament is usually avulsed at its tibial origin of femoral insertion and seldom is the rupture interligamentous. On account of the favourable arterial supply, primary healing can be expected after repair of this ligament, with subsequent reconstructive surgery becoming unnecessary. In the case of an eminence avulsion with the anterior cruciate, it is *not* adequate

Table 1. Classification of posterior instabilities according to Kennedy ($n=37$)

	Acute	Chronic
Group I	–	2
Group II	–	–
Group III	5	4
Group IV	9	17
n	14	23

Table 2. Reconstruction of the chronic posterior instabilities ($n=23$)

Posterior cruciate ligament	
Quadriceps and patellar tendon transplant	6
Medial gastrocnemius tendon transplant	5
Reattachment tibial or femoral	7
Extra-articular stabilization	4
Free patellar tendon transplant	1
Anterior cruciate ligament	
Semitendinosus tendon transplant	7
Free patellar tendon transplant	5
Shortening of the anterior cruciate ligament	4

only to replace this fragment because it is possible that the posterior cruciate ligament has been torn as well and will require repair.

Avulsion of the posterior cruciate ligament including a portion of bone is easily reattached with a screw.

Reconstructive procedures for chronic posterior instability are based on two fundamental principles described by Slocum:

1. *Static* stabilization by reconstructing the ligaments
2. *Dynamic* stabilization by musculotendinosus transfer

There is, however, no standard method for applying these principles.

Different surgical methods have to be applied individually, depending upon the type of lesion. Seven chronic cases were successfully treated by reattachment at the tibial or the insertion site. The medial gastrocnemius tendon was used five times, a transplant consisting of the quadriceps tendon and patellar tendon six times; a free transplant of the patellar tendon was carried out once. We performed extra-articular stabilization and simultaneous reconstruction of the anterior cruciate ligament, and in 23 cases extra-articular reconstructive measures were necessary (Tables 1–3).

Results
A follow-up evaluation was performed on patients over 1 year after the operation. Subjective complaints and objective findings were taken into consider-

Table 3. Extra-articular reconstructive measures ($n=23$)

Transfer of the lateral collateral ligament and the popliteus tendon	13
Transfer of the lateral gastrocnemius tendon	13
Lateral stabilization according to James	7
Dorsal stabilization according to O'Donoghue	4
Medial stabilization according to Slocum	3
Reconstruction of the medial collateral ligament	3
Lateral stabilization according to Ellison	2
Reconstruction of the lateral collateral ligament	1
Transfer of the pes anserinus	1

Table 4. Results of reconstruction after posterior ligament tears ($n=21$), with 3–9 years follow-up

Points		Acute	Chronic	Total
Good	160	6	5	11
Fair	120–160	2	5	7
Poor	80–120	1	2	3
Total		9	12	21

ation for evaluation, with 100 points in each category. The analysis was conducted by computer. A result below 120 points was regarded as poor, with 3 patients in this category. The remaining 34 cases had a satisfactory result (Table 4).

Conclusions

1. Severe post-traumatic hyperextension of the knee joint usually includes a lesion of both cruciate ligaments and the posterolateral or posteromedial joint capsule as well.
2. The diagnosis of acute posterior cruciate ligament rupture is essential because the results of primary repair are superior to those of secondary reconstruction.
3. In cases of chronic combined instabilities, both cruciate ligaments and the posterolateral or posteromedial capsule may have to be treated. We recommend the method according to Trillat and Hughston in combination with the transplant of the quadriceps and patellar tendon.
4. Such surgery should only be conducted in patients willing to follow a prescribed postoperative rehabilitation programme.

References

Brückner H (1972) Bandplastiken im Kniebereich nach dem Baukastenprinzip. Zbl Chir 97:65

Clancy WG, et al. (1983) Treatment of knee joint instability secondary to rupture of the posterior cruciate ligament. J Bone Joint Surg [Am] 65:30

Hackenbruch W, Karpf PM (1978) Aktuelle Kniegelenksdiagnostik. Fortschr Med 96:147

Horne JG, Parsons CJ (1977) The anterior cruciate ligament: its anatomy and a new method of reconstruction. J Surg 20:214

Hughston JC, Andrews JR, Cross MJ, Moschi A (1976) Classification of the knee ligament instabilities. J Bone Joint Surg [Am] 58:159

Hughston JC, Degenhardt TC (1982) Reconstruction of the posterior cruciate ligament. Clinical Orthopaedics and Related Research 18:59–60
James StL (1978) Treatment of acute knee injuries. Special reference to the second Scandinavian course on arthroscopy. Skövde, Sweden, 24–28 Sept
Karpf PM (1978) Probleme der operativen Versorgung veralteter Kniegelenksinstabilitäten. Fortschr Med 96:167
Karpf PM, Mang W, Hackenbruch W (1980) Hypermobilität des Kniegelenkes nach dorsalen Kapselbandläsionen. Orthop Praxis 16:154
Kennedy JC, Roth JH, Walker DM (1979) Posterior cruciate ligament injuries. Orthop Digest 7:19
McIntosh DL, Darby TA (1972) Lateral substitution reconstruction. J Bone Joint Surg [Br] 58:142
O'Donoghue DH (1973) Reconstruction for medial instability of the knee. Technique and results in sixty cases. J Bone Joint Surg [Am] 55:941
Slocum DB, James StL (1977) Athletic injuries of the lower extremity. Orthop Digest 15:31
Trillat A (1978) Posterolateral instability. In: Late reconstruction of injured ligaments of the knee. Springer, Berlin Heidelberg New York

Synthetic Ligaments

Mechanical aspects of reconstruction of the anterior cruciate ligament by dacron prostheses in dogs

G. Feldkamp[1], *A. Sandt*[2] *and K.-P. Schulitz*[3]

[1] **Orthopädische Klinik Volmarstein, Wetter, Federal Republic of Germany**
[2] **Institut für Werkstoffe, Ruhr-Universität Bochum, Federal Republic of Germany**
now at Institut CERAC S.A., Ecublens, Switzerland
[3] **Orthopädische Universitätsklinik Düsseldorf, Federal Republic of Germany**

"The fluctuations in technique reflect our present frustration" (J. C. Kennedy 1980).

Our aim in this study has been to create a new ligament by stimulating tissue ingrowth into Dacron prostheses by the homologous fibrin adhesive system (FAS), increasing its strength properties.

A total of 43 sheepdogs were used to study the mechanical properties of 3 different types of Dacron prostheses. The dogs were operated on as follows: the anterior cruciate ligament (ACL) was excised, and the Dacron prostheses were partially impregnated with FAS and inserted by the drill-hole technique (Figure 1). The prostheses were pulled tight and stapled to the bone by barbed staples. Immobilization was carried out by varying methods. We ran three series, each following the other, utilizing the results of the preceding one:

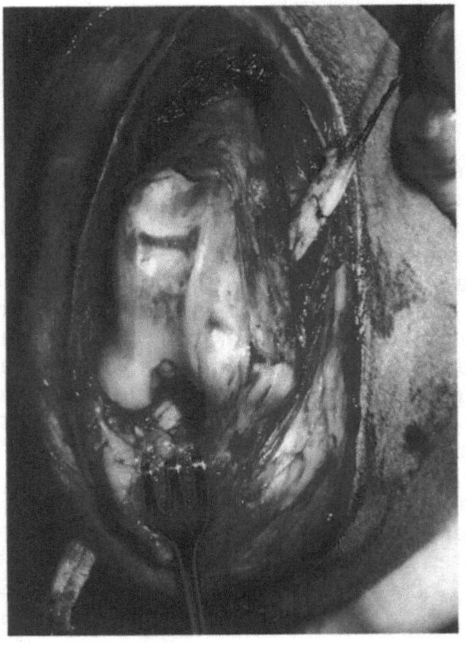

Figure 1. Implantation of the Dacron prosthesis by the drill-hole technique – intraoperative aspect

In series I, consisting of 36 dogs, an original knitted Dacron vascular prosthesis was used with an in vitro maximum load of 230 N and a strain to a maximum load of 60%. Two-thirds of the prostheses were impregnated with FAS and one-third were not. Immobilization was done either by Achilles tendon resection or with a knee-bridging external fixator. The dogs were killed after an interval of 11 weeks.

In series II, consisting of two dogs, a knitted Dacron prosthesis with a tensile strength of 615 N maximum load and a strain of 35% was used. The prostheses were prepared with FAS and immobilized by Achilles tendon resection. The time interval was 11 weeks.

Series III, serving as a long-term test, included five dogs, which had the ACL replaced by a woven Dacron prosthesis with an initial strength of 833 N maximum load and a strain to a maximum load of 70%. The prostheses were left without impregnation of FAS and were partially immobilized by Achilles tendon resection and partially not. The interval before the dogs were killed was 37 weeks (Table 1).

Table 1. Results of the in vitro tensile test of different types of Dacron prostheses

	Tensile test in vitro			
Series	I	II	III	ACL dog
Max. load (N)	230	615	833	686
Strain to m. l. (%)	60	35	70	110
Linear load (N)	Non-measurable			341
Strain to l. l. (%)				49

Finally 14 knee specimens were assigned for tensile test by a Zwick-type testing apparatus. Oscillograph records of load versus time for every knee were taken. The tensile test was performed within 3–4 h of the dogs being killed. The knees were dissected just before the test, removing all structures except for the ACL or the prostheses. The resulting bone-prosthesis-bone preparation was tested, while the intact side served as control. The knees were loaded in a straight position with an extension rate of 2 mm/min. Fourteen out of 43 prostheses failed intravitally and out of these the prostheses of series III failed completely. The breakage happened to the vascular prostheses in nearly all cases at the exits from the bone drill-holes because of abrasive wear and angulation. In a later design of series III failure occurred in the free length of the prostheses.

The load-deformation curves of series I revealed a maximum load of an average of 148 N of the protheses, in series II a mean value of 235 N was recorded and the intact ACLs were measured as 706 N. The corresponding strain to maximum load was calculated as 106% in series I, 87% in series II and 109% in the intact ACLs (Table 2).

Table 2. Results of the tensile test in vivo at an interval of 11 weeks; series III failed totally intravitally

	Tensile test			
Series	I	II	III	ACL
Total	13	1	/	14
Max. load (N)	148	235		706
Strain to max. load (%)	106	87		109

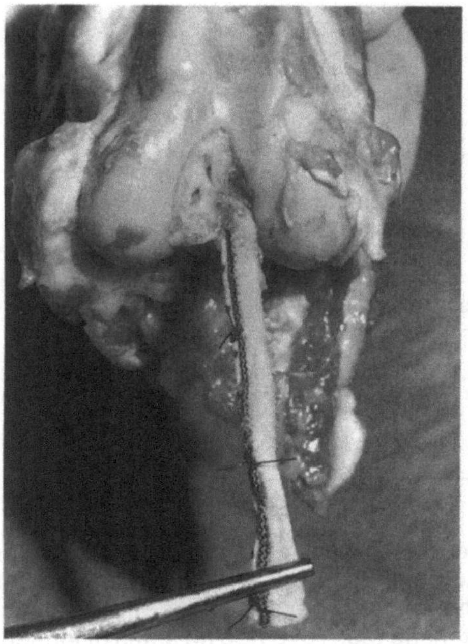

Figure 2. Failure by gliding out of the tibial canal

The most problematic basic parameter to measure in the mechanical analysis is the original length. When testing a bone-ligament-bone system, the original length of the ACL can be more easily estimated than measured, because of the fairly broad insertions. We took the distance from the highest point of the intercondylar notch to the lowest point of the tibial crest (from X-rays) as the original length, considering the two-dimensionel oblique direction of the ACL. Calculating the strain at the maximum load of the prostheses, the determination of the original length is much more difficult or even impossible. The mechanism of failure in testing was different: either disruption occurred at the drill-hole site (Figure 2) or the prostheses slipped out of the tibial anchorage – that means staple plus bone canal (Figure 3). According to the different failure modes, different original lengths that came under stress must be assumed. In cases of failure by sliding out of the tibial canal or rupture under the tibial staple an original length comprising the tibial canal plus

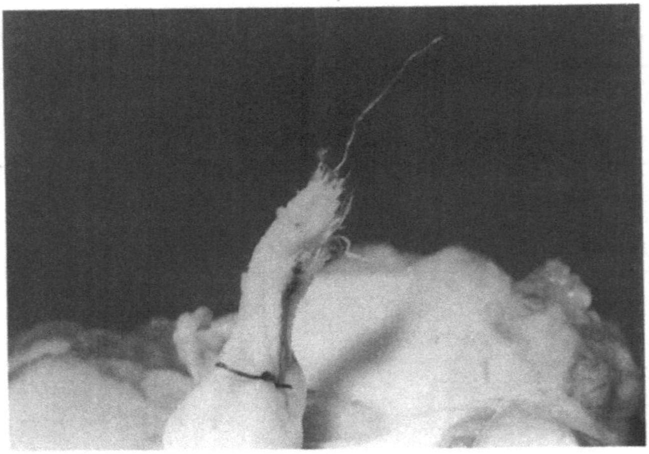

Figure 3. Failure by disruption at the femoral drill-hole site

Table 3. Results of the tensile test in relation to failure mechanism at an interval of 11 weeks

	Tensile test-mechanism of failure	
	Tibial sliding	Drill-hole rupture
Series I N = 13	6	7
Max. load (N)	147.5	148
Strain to max. load (%)	52	152

the intra-articular portion must be accepted. Ruptures at the drill-hole site or in the inner third have to be calculated with an original length adequate for the intra-articular part of the prosthesis only, because these latter specimens, examined histologically after tensile test, revealed no signs of loosening. Thus the mean value of strain to maximum load in series I is calculated as 106% corresponding to 109% of the normal ACL. In relation to the mechanism of failure: the sliding prostheses failed under a strain of 52% and the prostheses with drill-hole rupture had a strain at maximum load of 152% (Table 3). This enormous difference can be understood by the fact that only low stresses with low deformation forces are applied to loosen the "sliding" prostheses out of their tibial anchorage, and conversely higher stresses are necessary at drill-hole failure, which lead to higher deformations.

Concluding remarks

1. In general the mechanical properties, i.e. strength to maximum load and strain to maximum load of Dacron prostheses with low in vitro strength do not increase at an interval of 11 weeks although there was gross appearance of connective tissue ingrowth.

2. The tested materials do not resist the shear stresses at the edges of the drill holes.

3. Prostheses of higher in vitro tensile strength with strain to maximum load similar to that of the normal ACL at intervals of 37 weeks also failed because of intra-articular abrasive wear, which happened because of too high elongation. This high elongation prevents intraosseous tissue anchorage and inhibits an increase of holding properties by bony ingrowth in the bone canals, so that slipping out occurred with time or at the tensile test.

Temporary intra-articular stabilization of the knee joint with a synthetic band: animal experiments and first clinical experience

C. J. Wirth and M. Jäger

Munich Orthopaedic Hospital
D-8000 Munich
Federal Republic of Germany

Replacement surgery of ligaments has so far utilized auto-, homo- or heterologous transplants. The advantage of these materials lies in their acceptance by body tissues, their disadvantage in their need for prolonged immobilization with its inherent problems for bone and soft tissues. Plastic materials, in contrast, have the advantage of immediate joint stabilization with the possibility of early mobilization. Fatigue and wear are disadvantages caused by stress changes. Rupture of the material causes failure of the whole procedure. Therefore the clinical aspect of early mobilization with adequate stabilization especially for the replacement of the anterior cruciate ligament gains importance. Therefore, we undertook to combine both principles – the immediate stabilization of the joint with a synthetic band and the auto-, homo- or heterologous transplant with its subsequent integration into body tissue. After adequate stabilization by the transplant it should be feasible to remove the synthetic band without problems. Therefore, the surface of the synthetic band had to prevent the integration of connective tissue. The fixation of the band had to facilitate its removal through small incisions without opening the joint.
These conditions were first of all tested in animal experiments.

Animal experiments
Thirty Merino sheep between the ages of 1 and 3 years and with an average body weight of 50–60 kg were selected, and the anterior cruciate ligament of the left knee was replaced by lyophilized, gamma-irradiated dura. In 21 sheep, a synthetic band was additionally used for primary joint stabilization. In a control group of nine sheep, a resection of the Achilles tendon was performed for temporary weight reduction. An immobilization was not performed.

As has been customary in humans, the lyophilized dura was fixed by rerouting it through drill holes in the tibial head and lateral femoral condyle, taking care to approximate it to its natural course.

The synthetic band consisted of a bundle of Mersilene strands (polyester, Eticon) with terminal loops. The bundle was pulled through a silicon tube (Silastic) leaving only the terminal loops uncovered. The resistance against tearing of this synthetic band was 810 N on average.

This band was fixed to the lateral side of the distal femoral shaft, slung around the lateral femoral condyle from dorsal through the posterior joint capsule and led out of the joint over the anterior tibial edge to the surface of the medial tibial head. After tightening of the synthetic band it was fixed there by a cortical screw.

The transplants were removed in the first animal test group (replacement of the anterior cruciate by dura and joint stabilization by a synthetic band) after 6, 12, 24 and 40 weeks; in the second group (anterior cruciate replacement by dura only, Achilles tendon resection) after 6, 12 and 24 weeks. The dura transplants were examined macroscopically and microscopically and tested mechanically for their resistance against tearing. The synthetic band was removed through small incisions 33 weeks after implantation.

Six weeks after implantation a tendency for parallel longitudinal orientation of the newly built collagen fibres was already noticeable.

Twelve weeks after implantation the histology showed increasing longitudinal orientation of the collagen fibres of the implanted dura, while the number of cells was decreasing.

Twently-four weeks after implantation microscopically the decreasing cell population and the increasing vasculature dominated within a strictly longitudinally oriented fibrous tissue.

Thirty-three weeks after implantation the synthetic band was removed through small incisions after extraction of the cortical screws and without opening the joint.

Forty weeks after implantation the transformation of the dura implant was complete macroscopically and microscopically.

The *mechanical testing* of the preparations for breaking strength and resistance against deformation showed continual increase when the dura transplant was stabilized by a synthetic band and was almost normal compared with that of an anterior cruciate ligament at the 24th week. Even after removal of the synthetic band a slight increase in breaking strength was noticeable until the 40th week (Figure 1).

So it seemed at least technically possible to achieve primary knee stability by a synthetic band in connection with a suture or replacement of the anterior cruciate also in the human knee.

Mechanical properties of synthetic bands for knee joint stabilization
In a second step the mechanical properties of possible polymer materials were established by static and dynamic testing of about 50 specimens.

Static conditions were a maximal diameter of the synthetic band of 5 mm, a minimal tear stress of 500 N and an elongation lower than 5%. *Dynamic conditions* were a fatigue load of 300 ± 200 N, load cycle of 1.5 million cycles and an angle of deflection between 100° and 130° with respect to the frontal edge of the tibial plateau.

After preselection of commercial artificial materials under static conditions a dynamic test with the dynamic motion simulator was performed. Only a polyester band of about 2.5×5 mm, especially entangled and thermally fixed, could satisfy the requirements. This band was covered with a film of silicone-caoutchouc.

Finally, a suitable solution for bone fixation was found.

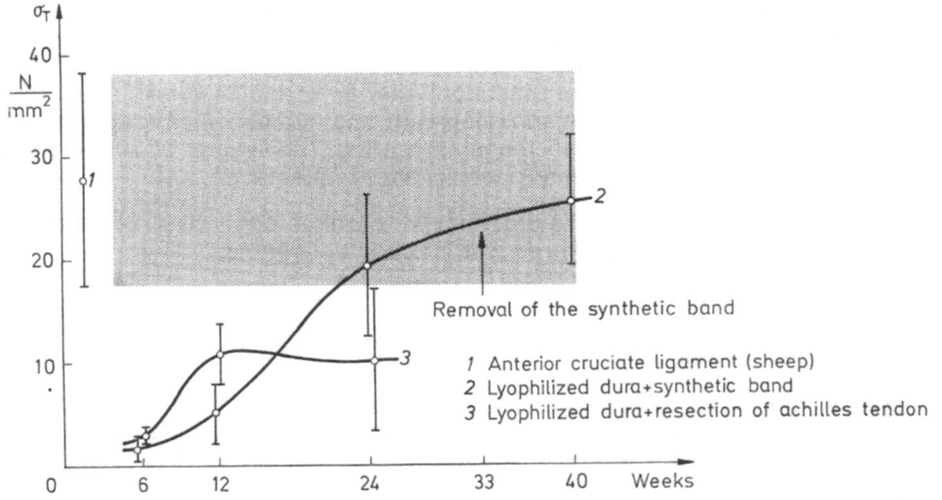

Figure 1. Dependence of breaking strength (N/mm²) of dura implant in the first and second animal control groups in relation to time (weeks) and in comparison with normal anterior cruciate ligaments of sheep

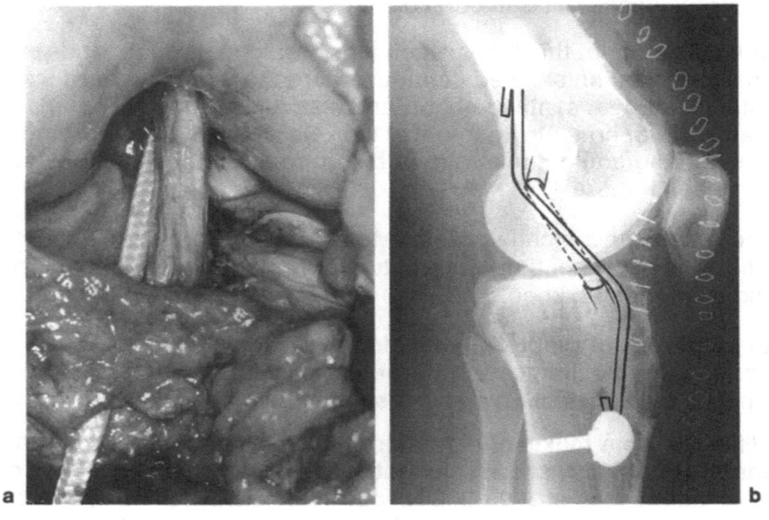

Figure 2. a Replacement of the anterior cruciate ligament in the human knee joint by the middle third of the patellar tendon and the synthetic band lying adjacent. **b** X-ray showing the course of the patellar tendon graft (*dotted lines*) and the synthetic band

Preliminary report of clinical use

In five patients with an old anteromedial knee joint instability grade III the anterior cruciate was replaced with a free patellar tendon graft and the medial structures were stabilized. In addition an often entangled polyester band, coated with silicone, was used for primary knee joint stabilization. This band was brought through the knee joint according to the animal experiments and fixed to the lateral femoral shaft and the medial tibial head (Figure 2). Four days after operation limited motion of the knee was allowed with increasing flexion.

Four months after the operation the synthetic bands were removed through small incisions. Arthroscopic review of the knee joint at this time showed no foreign body reactions and the synthetic band without sheathing by connective tissue. A soft synovialization of the patellar tendon graft was found.

At a first follow-up 6 months after operation no loss of stability after removal of the synthetic band was found. Both the Lachman and pivot shift signs were negative. Knee joint motion was perhaps limited to the final degrees of extension and flexion.

References

Plitz W, Wirth CJ (1981) Dynamische Festigkeitsuntersuchungen an Kunststoffbändern für die temporäre Gelenkführung. In: Jäger M, Hackenbroch MH, Refior T (eds) Kapselbandläsionen des Kniegelenkes. Thieme, Stuttgart

Wirth CJ (1978a) Der Kreuzbandersatz des Kniegelenkes. Thieme, Stuttgart

Wirth CJ (1978b) Experimentelle Untersuchungen zum Kreuzbandersatz am Schaf mit Dura mater in Kombination mit einem synthetischen Band. Z Orthop 116:577

Wirth CJ (1983) Temporary intraarticular knee stabilization with synthetic material (polyester-silicon) in the sheep. In: Burri C, Claes L (eds) Alloplastik ligament replacement. Huber, Bern (Aktuelle Probleme in Chirurgie und Orthopädie, vol 26)

Collagen-coated carbon fibers – a material for ligament replacement. An experimental study on biocompatibility and biomechanical strength

R. Neugebauer, C. Burri and L. Claes

Abt. f. Unfallchirurgie, Hand-, Plastische- und Wiederherstellungschirurgie der Universität Ulm
D-7900 Ulm, Steinhövelstr. 9
Federal Republic of Germany

Carbon fiber strands are used for ligament replacement on knee joints. A big disadvantage of the C-fibers is their low elasticity and a difficult handling in theater, because many fiber fragments will be produced when the strand is cut. To improve these properties we coated a carbon fiber strand of 32 rows, 1000 filaments each with collagen and asked the following questions:

1. Will the elasticity and the handling of C-fiber-strand be improved?
2. Is the biocompatibility of the coated carbon fibers as good as of C-fibers unprotected?
3. Does the collagen disturb the ingrowth of connective tissue around the carbon fibers?

Material and methods

To evaluate these questions we performed the following in vitro and in vivo experiments. Coated and uncoated carbon-fiber-strands were fixed at each end between aluminium tabs with epoxy resin, for testing in a tensile machine (Zwick 1445). Each sample was loaded fifteen times to 100 and 300 Newton and the strain was recorded.

In order to study the biocompatibility the two different types of C-fiber-strands were implanted into the backs of 12 sheep. 4, 8 and 12 weeks later the animals were killed. For histological studies paraffin cuts stained with haematoxylin eosin and van Gieson were made.

Results

For both loads, the carbon fiber strands exhibited a substantial permanent extension during the first five cycles. After 15 cycles however pure elastic deformation was observed. The elasticity of the different strands showed significant variations ($p < 0.01$). The elastic deformation at a tensile force of 100 Newton rose from 0.32 % with the uncoated to 0.86 % with the coated strands. At a force of 300 Newton the values were 0.56 % uncoated and 1.14 % for the coated.

The histoligical preparation revealed a good biocompatibility of the uncoated ligaments with ingrowth of connective tissues around single carbon fibers after all periods. Foreign body giant cells were always present. In the coated samples also no toxic or inflammatory reaction was found. It seemed that the ingrowth of connective tissues is higher and the presence of foreign body giant cells is lower.

Conclusion

The results reveal, that coating of carbon fiber strands with a quick resorbable collagen is of interest because:

1. Handling of carbon fibers is easier because the number of C-fiber fragments is decreased, which are produced by cutting.

2. The presence of collagen gives a significant higher elasticity and decrease in the sensitivity of carbon fibers to shear forces.

3. The collagen will be resorbed completely and replaced by connective tissues, a compound ligament will be produced.

4. The reduced rate of foreign body giant cells indicates a better ingrowth of host tissues and thus a stronger ligament formation.

ACL reconstruction with carbon fibers in animal experiments

A. Górecki, W. Kuś and Z. Salomon

Dept. of Orthopaedics, Academy of Medicine
Warsaw
Poland

The treatment of ACL insufficiency is still an unsolved clinical problem.

The very promising results after the reconstructions of ligamentous structures with carbon fibers have created a new method for ACL substitution. However, several papers deny the value of carbon material in the intraarticular operations.

Material an methods
In 60 rabbits the excised ACL has been substituted with carbon fibers. The bundle of fibers has been pulled through the canals in tibia and femur.

Results
After 8 to 24 weeks the rupture of the implant with an extensive reaction of the synovial membrane was observed.

Histological studies revealed the strong foreign body reaction with the presence of many giant cells and only a few fibroblasts in growing fibrous tissue. Any organization of collagen fibers has been observed. The disintegration of carbon material was of mechanical nature.

Discussion
The well described stimulation of fibrous tissue by carbon fibers has not been confirmed in our experiments. An extensive reaction to the implant from the synovial membrane eliminates the carbon fibers in the use for intraarticular reconstructions. The mechanical properties of fibers are not adequate for such operations.

Further investigations should be carried out to create a new structure of the ACL prosthesis.

We propose to strengthen temporarily the carbon fibers with the elastic rod and to cover the fibers with non-toxic resin separating the carbon material from the synovial membrane. Such a prosthesis would be machanically and biologically adequate for the purpose of ACL substitution, preserving the carbon fibers as a scaffold for the ingrowth of fibrous tissue.

Summary
Because of the existing divergency in opinions the study was designed to assess the value of carbon fibers in the reconstruction of the ACL. The reconstruction was carried out in 60 rabbits.

After 8 to 24 weeks a rupture of the implant with an extensive reaction of the synovial membrane was observed. Histological studies revealed a foreign body reaction.

The results imply that carbon fibers have no use in the intraarticular reconstruction of ligaments of the knee.

Experimental investigations on the biomechanics of carbon fiber replacement of the knee ligaments in animals

L. Claes, C. Burri and R. Neugebauer

Department of Traumatology, University of Ulm
7900 Ulm
Federal Republic of Germany

From the biomechanical point of view in vivo ligament replacement has to have a sufficient utimate rupture strength and fatigue strength, as well the elastic properties similar to the normal ligament. These properties were tested in a braided carbon fiber ligament prosthesis used to replace the MCL and ACL in sheep knees.

Material and methods

Woven carbon fiber ligament prostheses made of 96000 high-strength graphite fibers (diameter 7 um) were implanted into 38 sheeps knees. In group I 30 MCL were replaced using 3 different anchorage techniques (Fig. 1). In group II an ACL-MCL combined replacement was performed for a period of 1 year in 8 sheep (Fig. 1d). After explanting the knees all the structures except the replaced ligaments were resected. A tensile test of the intact replaced ligament was then performed.

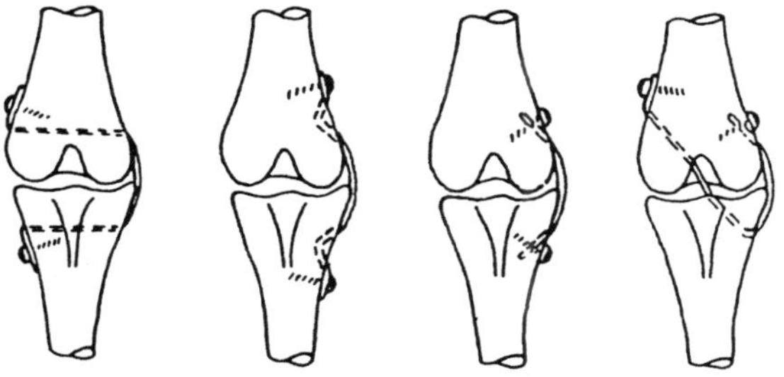

a b c d

For group II an osteotomy through the femoral condyle was performed, so that the MCL and ACL could be testet separately.

Results

All carbon fiber ligaments were surrounded by connective tissue. Signs of broken carbon fibers were seen in 4 ACL but in none of the MCL. After 3 months the rupture strength of the MCL was 625 ± 218N for group Ia, 291 ± 57N for group Ib, 291 ± 142 for group Ic and after 1 year 650 ±239N (group II). The average value for the ACL was 280 ±60N. All collateral ligament prostheses were pulled out of the anchorage, whereas the ACL group in 4 cases ruptured in the substance of the prosthesis. The stiffness and elasticity of the carbon fiber ligament replacement achieved 50-100 % that of natural ligaments, depending on the anchorage type.

Discussion

MCL replacement: 3 months ultimate rupture strength is mainly influenced by the anchorage type. The anchorage 1a showed the highest strength corresponding to 107 % of the rupture strength of the natural MCL (590 ± 204N). The anchorage strength increases with time. Type 1c anchorage increased from 291N after 3 months to 650N after 1 year. The rupture strength was still far from the ultimate strength of the ligament prosthesis itself (2461 ± 238N).

ACL: For the ligament replacements which showed some broken carbon fibers rupture of the ligaments at the entrance into the drill hole was seen, whereas the other specimens without broken carbon fibers pulled out of the anchorage. The reason for the fiber breakage was felt to be insufficient preparation on the drill hole. The sharp edge was not always rounded enough to avoid shear stress on the carbon fibers.

These animals experiments showed that with good operating technique carbon fiber ligament replacements can reach biomechanical properties similar to natural ligaments.

Preliminary report on the use of bovine xenograft in knee instability problems

E. P. Abbink and F. J. K. Kramer

Carolus hospital, Willem-Alexander hospital
's-Hertogenbosch
The Nederlands

Instability fo the knee proposes serious concerns for correction. Although many materials — including autogenous tissues and synthetics — have been proposed, results in general leave concerns about the adequacy of the management of these problems.

Recently, the bovine Xenograft has been introduced which is prepared with 0,2 % buffered glutar aldeyde. The reported animal and biomechanical studies of these grafts by William Mc Master were encouraging. We have begun initial human use of these materials.

Material and methods

This report is an initial evaluation of experience with our flrst 80 patients. Average follow up is 30 months. We have treated 63 males — average age 25 years and 17 females — average age 26 years. The indications included 68 ACL, 17 PCL and 18 medial ligament complexes. Additional extra-articular procedures were often required to correct complex rotational instability. A double bony tunnel with staple fixation was used.

Results

The early results indicate the following:
No infections.
Re- operation because of mechanical graft failure, due to trauma, incorrect position of the bony tunnels, or too much residual laxity of the knee — ligaments and capsule was needed in 21 patients. An unspecific synovial reaction causing pain, effusion and restricted range of motion was observed in 5 patients.

Discussion

Biopsy material has been collected and shows hostinvasion with vessels and fibroblasts, producing host collagen along the scaffolding of the passive graft; but progress is slow.

Early results have encouraged us to continue the use of bovine Xenografts. It appears that bovine Xenografts are acceptable and may provide a useful means of restoring stability.

Reabsorbable ligament plastic: animal experiments and first clinical results

K. H. Schultheis, K. E. Rehm, P. Bopp, D. Kölzer, R. Holzheimer and H. Ecke

Zentrum für Chirurgie, Abt. Unfallchirurgie
Gießen
Federal Republic of Germany

Nowadays various alloplastic ligament materials are inserted successfully as substitute ligaments. The meaning of these substitute structures consisting of heterogenous materials is simply the function of a guide rail. Therefore we examined the reabsorbable suture material PDS (poly-dioxanon-suture) in experiments with animals.

Material and methods

Series I: PDS ligaments were paravertebral subcutaneous implanted in 28 male rats in anaesthesia. 42, 56, 70, 84 and 112 days later histological evaluation followed after autopsy.

Series II: 20 rabitts received a resection of the medial collateral ligament and the anterior cruciate ligament. The ligaments were replaced by a continuous PDS plastic with the initial breaking load of 1.80-200 Newton. After 9, 12, 19 weeks the animals were killed and the ligament plastics were tested for tensile strength.

Results

Series I: The PDS plastic was replaced by collagenic-fibrous connective tissue in the course of the test time. This connective tissue accumulates concentric around the PDS monofilaments which were totally reabsorbed at the end of the test.

Series II:
First there was a drop in the breaking load to 112 $\pm$ 4 Newton with a following rise of the breaking load in the 12th and 19th week. Beginning with the 19th week the starting point of 185,5 $\pm$ 11,5 Newton was obtained. There was a continuous drop in the breaking load of the anterior cruciate so that no mechanical functions were fulfilled.

Discussion

In the area of adjacent connective tissue structures the reabsorbable ligament plastic is highly qualified for alloplastic replacement. This is not effective in structures without contact to connective tissue — like the anterior cruciate ligament — with the consequence that the ligament plastic should be enveloped in fascia as it is done with nonreabsorbable alloplastic materials. First clinical results with 10 patients provided with PDS Fascia lata plastic due to isolated rupture of the anterior cruciate ligament assured the results of experiments with animals. Arthroscopic, CT and histological documentations is presented.

The usage of a textile band prosthesis for the operative correction of chronic knee ligament instability

J. Mockwitz and H. Contzen

Berufsgenossenschaftliche Unfallklinik
6000 Frankfurt am Main
Federal Republic of Germany

Since 1980 a total of 73 patients were operatively treated at the BUK Frankfurt for chronic instability of the knee ligaments. Of these, a total of 33 had undergone previous-usually multiple-unsuccessful operations, so that autologous replacement material was either no longer present or not of adequate quality. In addition, all these patients had, without exception, refused alternative modes of treatment (e. g. arthrodesis, conservative orthopaedic measures).

For these 33 patients, then, alloplastic ligament replacement was a last resort treatment. On the basis of materials science information we chose a textile band made of Polyethyleneterephthalate in these patients for the alloplastic replacement of isolated ligamentous structures in the presence of chronic combined knee ligament instabilities.

The initial problem of tight durable anchoring was solved through the development of a new technique. This will be explained and demonstrated.

Finally, the results of treatment after alloplastic knee ligament replacement will be conveyed. The criteria chosen for knee joint stability after band-plastic measures were the clinical, functional and radiological results with regard to mobility of lateral ligament structures, drawer phenomenon, total mobility, muscle wasting and eventually radiological changes. These criteria then provided the basis for an overall assessment with five different grades.

We found that, with regard to ligament stability, the results achieved after Polyethyleneterephtalate were noticeably superior to those achieved with autologous transplants, and that the overall function achieved was comparable.

After approx. three years of using alloplastic ligament prostheses made of Polyethyleneterephthalate, it is already becoming clear, that the well-known problems in treating chronic capsule and band instabilities of the knee joint amenable only to plastic procedures can very probable be substantially — but not completely — reduced by using textile synthetic bands.

Prosthetic replacement of cruciate ligaments of the knee

C. Chaix, M. Dive, G. Legre, J.-M. Aubaniac, C. Mailaender and J.-P. Franceschi

Our experience of the prosthetic replacement of cruciate ligaments of the knee began in a strange way 2½ years ago.

Observations

A 29-year-old man presented with posterior luxation of the knee, with a wound of the popliteal artery. The restoration of the arterial axis was carried out quickly 6 h after the injury, but the surgical stabilization of his knee was delayed by numerous complications: renal, septic and digestive. A tibial extension, put in on the 10th day, reduced the displacement, but on removal of this extension a repetition of the luxation took place. The scars healed, but poorly; they did not allow a wide-range articulation. As we were encouraged by vascular surgeons, we used shoulder Dacron, presented recently, to repair the coracoclavicular lesions. In the 3rd month, by a narrow anterior-internal arthrotomy, on the route of the posterior cruciate ligament we grafted double shoulder Dacron clasped to both ends. The immediate good stability, still present 2½ years later, and the perfect tolerance of this ligament have led us to adopt this material. During these last 2 years we have grafted 390 prosthetic ligaments, but our study is limited to the first 258 cases, all of them dating from more than 6 months ago. Only shoulder Dacron, double, treble or quadruple thickness, and knee Dacron have been used in this series of 258 patients.

Histological Study

We carried out an animal test, grafting some Dacron fibres into the hip bone of a sheep weighing 25 kg, in contact with the bone, the periosteum and the soft tissues. It was technically impossible to graft this transplant intra-articulary. In the 3rd month, the Dacron fibres were invaded by a fibroblastic reaction with giant cells; we noticed numerous capillaries and no inflammatory granuloma. In the 4th month, the fibroblastic reaction intensified and the osseous tissue grew, circumscribing the Dacron fibres. Then a homogeneous whole formed: bone-fibroblasts-Dacron. This animal test was completed with the observation of broken ligaments; the open knee investigation has always revealed the perfect intra-articular tolerance of the neoligament. In its intra-bone course, we traced back the fibroblastic reaction which interposes between the Dacron and the bone. In its intra-articular course, the synovial lining of the Dacron fibres presented no inflammatory reaction. On the whole, the velvety Dacron tied into the bone by a collagenic reaction which appeared distinctly in the 3rd or the 4th month. There was no synovial reaction in the contact of the prosthesis in its intra-articular course.

Surgical technique
We will only consider the replacement of the anterior-external cruciate ligament, which is the most frequent operation on the central pivot (149 cases, as opposed to 9 cases with surgery to replace the posterior internal cruciate), this replacement being made according to two methods: the direct method or the MacIntosh method.

Direct method
In the direct method the aim is to substitute the prostethic ligament for the normal anterior-external cruciate ligament as anatomically as possible. As far as possible, the Dacron is placed in the synovial remainder or associated with the reinsertion of the cruciate ligament; thus is called the "reinforced cruciate ligament". The orientation of the neoligament is made easier by the use of a sighting tube. At present, we use a modification of our own of the AO sighting tube. The incision is double: anterointernal arthrotomy and an external incision facing the condyle. The tibial and femoral tunnels are dug out with a 4-, 5- or 6-mm drill bit. The pulling wire is led from the condyle to the tibia and the prosthetic tendon passed form the tibia to the condyle. It is stretched while the knee is inflexed to 30°; it is fixed at two ends with toothed clasps. Most of the time the reinserted ligament or the synovial sheath conceals the Dacron in the opening.

Postoperative measures are simple:

- Splints for 48 h
- Walking with sticks has been shortened to the duration of stay in hospital, i.e. 8 days and no longer 21
- Resumption of sports is possible in the 3rd month
- The articular amplitudes are usually normal by the end of rehabilitation.

MacIntosh method
The MacIntosh method uses two routes: direct, into the opening and an external return. The incision is also double, but the external incision is wider in order to reach down to the Gerdy tubercle. The direct route is subsynovial; the external route runs from the condyle to the Gerdy tubercle. This external segment must be measured precisely in order to avoid a limitation of mobility. The postoperative measures are the same as those after the direct method, but extension is often recovered less quickly.

Results
In our series of 258 patients, 2 developed sepsis, which of course limited the mobility of the knee, and in these patients the Dacron had to be removed. Our patients were re-examined according to the criteria of the Arpege card; the examination was completed by testing the articulation, and performing the drawer test (Lachmann) and the jerk test (Lemaire) to give three categories:

1. Stable: drawer = 0 or + jerk = 0
2. Doubtful: drawer = + + jerk = 0
3. Lax: drawer = + + jerk = +

Direct method
With double shoulder Dacron (122 cases/117 re-examined) there were 86 (73%) good results, 22 (22%) average results and 9 (7%) poor results. Articulation was stable in 74 (63%), doubtful in 11 (9%) and lax in 33 (28%). The double shoulder Dacron inserted by the direct method is not sufficient to stabilize the knee perfectly (28% are lax). The high figure of 73% good results should not make us forget that these are short-term results. Nevertheless, if we differentiate between recent and chronic laxities, we notice that stability improves when the Dacron strengthens the reinserted cruciate ligament. In 82 cases of chronic laxities, articulation was stable in 48 (58%), doubtful in 9 and lax in 26. These cases included 62 good results (70%), 17 average results and 4 poor results. In 35 cases of recent laxities articulation was stable in 26 (75%), doubtful in 2 and lax in 7. These cases included 24 (70%) good results, 5 average results and 5 poor results.

With treble or quadruple shoulder Dacron inserted by the direct method (37 cases), the percentage of stable knees was the same as with the MacIntosh method. There were 29 good results, 6 average results and 2 poor results. Articulation was stable in 32, doubtful in 3 and lax in 2. The two lax knees were both chronic. With double shoulder Dacron (28 cases) there were 21 good results, 5 average results and 2 poor results. Articulation was stable in 14, doubtful in 11 and lax in 3. With treble shoulder Dacron there were 31 good results, 7 average results and 4 poor results. Articulation was stable in 25, doubtful in 15 and lax in 2.

The percentage of good results was the same for each setting, i.e. three times out of four, although the number of lax knees, and consequently of ruptures, was reduced when the setting was strengthened.

With knee Dacron (29 cases) there were 23 good results, 3 average results and 3 poor results. Articulation was stable in 25, doubtful in 4 and lax in none. The use of knee Dacron, which can carry up to 270 kg, improves the stability of the knee remarkably (86% knees are stable). We have not noticed any rupture of this material, though it is worth remembering that this good stability hardly modifies the functional result.

Conclusion
Dacron, although not the ideal ligament, is an excellent material which sets on the bone and induces no synovial reaction. Shoulder Dacron must be at least treble, or better still quadruple. The direct method is sufficient; the external return of the MacIntosh method does not improve the stability of the knee at all.

An operative procedure for reconstruction of the anterior cruciate ligament

V. Pietrogrande

Milan
Italy

The surgical procedures for reconstruction of the A.C.L. are numerous, because the difficulty is to have a strong reconstructed ligament and a solid anchorage, not resulting in an excessive stiffness of the joint.

Method

A strip of Tensor of fasciae latae aponeurosis from the opposite side is converted into a cylinder of 25 cm of length holding inside a plait of nylon or carbon fibers, for an adequate resistance against strains.

This new formed ligament is passed through a hole in the external femoral condyle and the inner tibial condyle according to the direction of the A.C.L. and fixed to the external and internal collateral ligaments, in order to provide an elastic anchorage; stiff in extension and enough relaxed in flexion.

Results

15 patients are controlled after a follow-up longer than 5 years, and late results are tested with clinical, radiographic and mechanical evaluation.

This method seems to provide a stable and good reconstruction.

Summary

A new method for reconstruction of A.C.L. was proposed: the originality of this method is the armed aponeurotic transplant in order to increase its mechanical resistance, and the anchorage of the strip to the collateral ligaments, for a better dynamic function of the reconstructed A.C.L.

Patello-Femoral Joints

The correlation between patello-femoral joint pathology and the patella syndrome

U. E. P. Lindberg, J. Lysholm and J. Gillquist

Department of Orthopaedic Surgery, University Hospital
Linköping
Sweden

A poor correlation between intra-articular pathologic findings and patello-femoral pain, the so-called patello-femoral arthralgia syndrome (PFA) has been reported (DeHaven, 1980). This alleged lack of correlation has often been poorly supported, but nonetheless with nothing said about the intra-articular pathology. PFA has been given as the indication for different surgical reconstruction of the patello-femoral joint, which is often discouraging, possibly indicating that a more specified diagnosis would be of value (DeHaven, 1979).

For analyses of different types of intra-articulare patello-femoral joint pathology and its correlation to the patella-femoral arthralgia (PFA) syndrome all patients with patello-femoral joint pathology on arthroscopy were selected from a consecutive series of 1156 arthroscopies in 1078 patients (702 men and 376 women). 175 patients (88 men and 87 women) filled the criteria of patello-femoral joint pathology and were included in the study. All data concerning the arthroscopic findings were continually computerized, details concerning the case history, especially the presence or absence of PFA and clinical findings were collected retrospectively from the patients' records. Three different types of patello-femoral pathology were identified. 53 patients showed chondromalacia of the patella, with no signs of patella subluxation. This was seldom an isolated injury, but was frequently associated with a generalized osteoarthrosis or meniscus lesions. In these patients other symptoms than PFA were predominating. 42 patients showed a subluxation of the patella without chondromalacia. This was also rarely an isolated finding, although infrequently associated with osteoarthrosis. The most common associated pathology was ligament and meniscus tears. Also in this group other symptoms than PFA were the common complaint. 47 patients showed subluxation of the patella in combination with chondromalacia. This was commonly a single pathologic finding, and it was frequently associated with complaints of PFA. In this group, in patients with a longer case history, the chondromalacia was more pronounced and observed in all parts of the patella. In patients with a short history (less than 1 year) the chondromalacia was mostly limited to superficial fibrillation or soft areas in the cartilage, and was predominantly located in the central and lateral parts of the patella.

The aetiology of chondromalacia and peripatellar pain

L. Weh, W. Eickhoff and R. Prahl

Orthopaedic and Neurological Clinic of the University
Hamburg
Federal Republic of Germany

Introduction

The origin of spontaneous peripatellar pain is still open to discussion. Many authors still assume a primary cartilage problem. Some names of the syndrome, such as "jumper's knee", suggest a high-pull stress aetiology. The aim of this study was to show the primarily functional character of the spontaneous peripatellar pain and subsequent chondromalacia.

Methods

Selection and clinical investigation. More than 100 patients with spontaneous peripatellar pain had been examined (Weh and Eickhoff 1983). Patients with previous trauma or operations had been excluded. The patients complained of characteristic pains under weight bearing of the flexed knee. A typical pressure pain at the lower patellar pole was found in almost all cases, sometimes also at the medial or lateral quadriceps insertion, though less pronounced. The pressure pain at the patella apex was classified into three categories of intensity.

Electromyography

All patients underwent electromyographic investigations of the vastus medialis and lateralis as well as the paravertebral lumbar muscles. In almost all cases the electromyography of the quadriceps muscle showed neurogenic lesions, mostly with the characteristics of older changes: prolongation of the mean potential duration, an enlargement of the amplitudes and also complete lack of electromyographic activity in some periods. Only in a few patients could polyphasic potentials with reduced amplitudes and long duration be seen, which can be interpreted as signs of fresh nerve root lesions. In some cases the signs of anterior horn cell damage could be found, as giant motor units. In patients with nerve root lesions, changes in the corresponding paravertebral muscle segments could also be seen. The details of this part of the study have been published previously (Weh and Eickhoff 1983).

Analysis of quadriceps tension

An analysis of the quadriceps tension was performed in 45 of these patients with spontaneous peripatellar pain (mean age, 24.9 years; range, 16–53 years) and 16 healthy control subjects (mean age, 27.6 years; range, 16–40 years). The patella was marked percutaneously with three thin injection needles. The leg fixed in an extended position, radiographs were taken with and without contraction of the quadriceps muscle. Rotation and lateral/medial displacement of the patella were calculated by means of a computer programme (B. Ebens, Basis 108; Computer with Apple Graphics Tablet).

Results

1. Innervation disorders in the quadriceps muscle in young adults are common, especially in combination with lumbar hyperlordosis and hypermobility.
2. In spontaneous peripatellar pain syndrome, asymmetrical innervation disorders of the third and fourth lumbar nerve roots are frequently found.
3. The pain at the patellar poles can be regarded as an insertion tendinitis, caused by shear forces. The intensity was a function of the patella rotation due to quadriceps tension. The pressure pain increased, parabolically deviating from normal rotation (Figure 1) (mean of the control group: 3.97°; mean of the patellar pain group: 3.06° elevation of the medial pole).

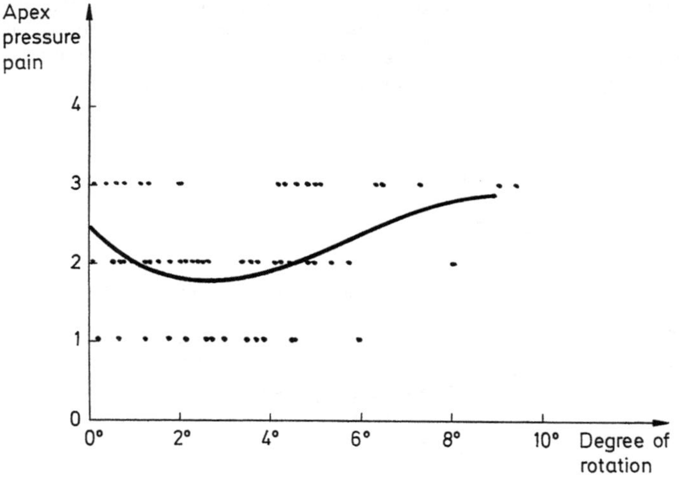

Figure 1. Apex pressure pain of the patella and degree of rotation under quadriceps tension, measured radiologically. The minimum is close to the average value of the healthy control group (3.97°). The pressure pain increases with the rotation angle deviating from normal. $a(3) = -8.5107E\text{-}3$, $a(2) = 0.14787$, $a(1) = -0.5951$, $a(0) = 2.4732$, $n = 65$, $r = 0.384$

4. The normal patella movement in healthy control subjects under quadriceps contraction was dependent on the varus/valgus position. In varus knees we found an elevation of the medial pole and a medial translation. In the valgus position there was an elevation of the lateral pole and a lateral transposition (Figure 2).
5. In patients with spontaneous peripatellar pain an abnormal patella movement could be found.

   a) Contrary to the control group, in cases with varus knees the patella under contraction moved laterally. In valgus knees the lateral transposition was less than in normal kness (Figure 3).

   b) Decrease of third and increase of fourth lumbar innervation disorders lead to an elevation of the medial pole under tension. There was only a poor correlation between the lateral dominant innervation disorder and the malrotation (Figure 4).

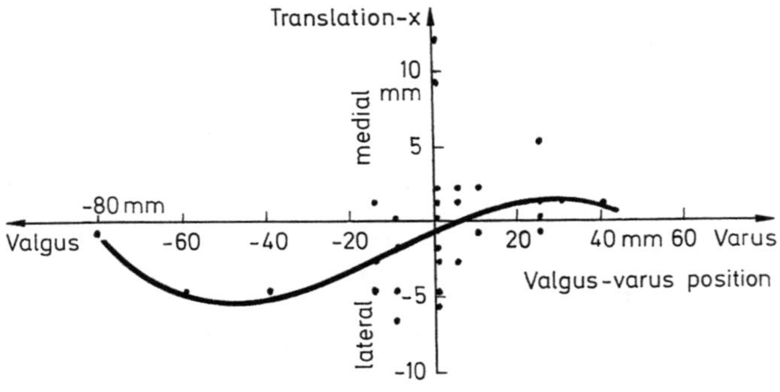

Figure 2. Translation of the patella under quadriceps tension in the healthy control group. Correlation to the varus/valgus position of the knee joint. The valgus malaglignment is measured by the ankle and the varus by the condyle distance. (millimetres). Coming from the rest position there is a lateral movement of the patella in the valgus and a medial movement in the varus position under quadriceps contraction. $a(3) = -3.10498E\text{-}5$, $a(2) = -8.5812E\text{-}4$, $a(1) = 0.12993$, $a(0) = 0.8888$, $n = 43$, $r = 0.41$

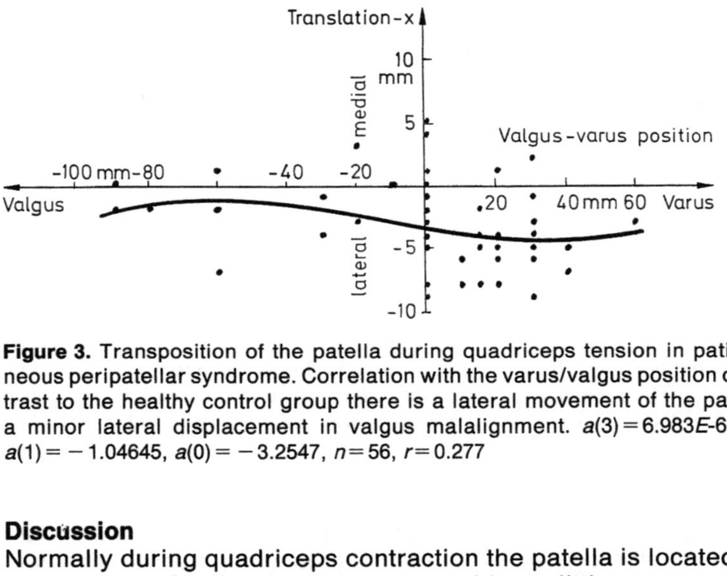

Figure 3. Transposition of the patella during quadriceps tension in patients with spontaneous peripatellar syndrome. Correlation with the varus/valgus position of the knee. In contrast to the healthy control group there is a lateral movement of the patella in varus and a minor lateral displacement in valgus malalignment. $a(3) = 6.983E\text{-}6$, $a(2) = 2.5825E\text{-}4$, $a(1) = -1.04645$, $a(0) = -3.2547$, $n = 56$, $r = 0.277$

Discussion

Normally during quadriceps contraction the patella is located exactly above the trochlea. Coming from the rest position a little movement to the lateral side in valgus knees and to the medial side in varus knees is necessary before the knee starts to bend (Figure 5).

The painful tendinitis at the patellar poles is a consequence of malposition of the patella, leading to a kinking upon moving into the trochlea. This malrotation and deviating occurs under high quadriceps tension. Strong shear forces at the patella apex due to forced rotation and transposition occur.

In addition high pressure on the cartilage results, inducing chondromalacia over the course of time. In these cases pressure-induced pains at the trochlear margin can be found.

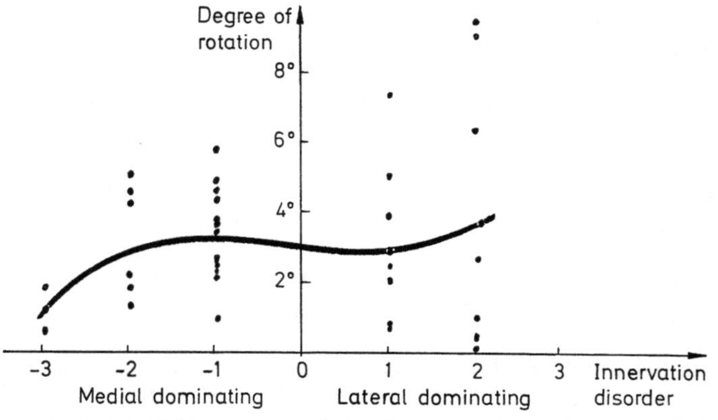

Figure 4. Rotation of the patella under quadriceps tension and difference between medial and lateral quadriceps innervation disorder in spontaneous peripatellar pain syndrome (third and fourth lumbar nerve segments). With relative increasing lateral innervation disorders a slight increasing medial pole elevation could be found. The correlation was poor. $a(3) = 0.12119$, $a(2) = 0.05853$, $a(1) = -0.2798$, $a(0) = 2.9991$, $n = 41$, $r = 0.271$

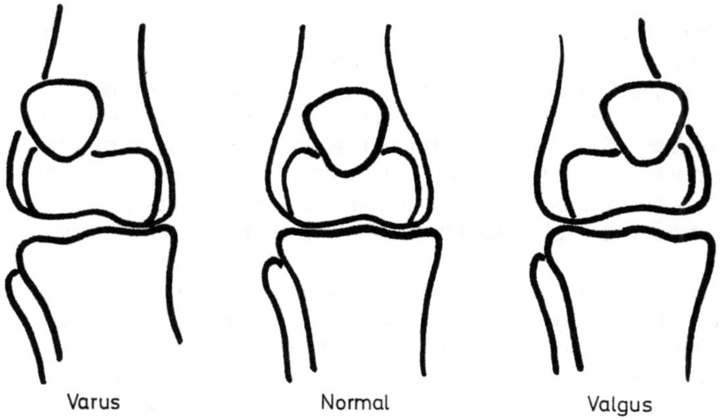

Figure 5. Resting position of the patella in varus, normal and valgus knee axis. In varus knees the resting position of the patella is lateral, in valgus knees medial to the trochlea. For the entry of the patella into the trochlea in knee flexion, a lateral movement in the valgus and a medial movement in the varus knee are necessary. In spontaneous peripatellar pain syndrome the position of the patella deviates from its normal position above the trochlea, induced by muscular dysbalance

Several reasons for this discrepancy between muscular forces and the preformed femoropatellar joint position exist. Usually there is a combination of different causes. Predisposing and triggering factors can be assumed.

Very important predisposing factors are unstable interaction of muscular forces, varus/valgus position of the knee, the torsion of femur and tibia and the resulting direction of the trochlea. An unstable, imbalanced interaction can be assumed in all kinds of malalignments of the lower extremity, the pelvis and the lumbar spine.

Changes in athletic activity in young adults, either greatly increasing or decreasing in amount, are important factors leading to imbalance.

Since the studies of Johnson et al. (1980) the varus-directed forces on the knee during walking are known.

In athletes these must be counteracted by high medial muscular forces. To keep the system in balance, a varus axis position develops.

Assuming this determinig influence of muscular tension on skeletal development, abrupt changes of athletic activity must lead to imbalance.

In a period of inactivity the weakened force of the vastus medialis can no longer sufficiently elevate the medial pole or initiate medial movement of the patella before gliding into the trochlea when coming from the resting position. An analogous mechanism for valgus deviation or rapidly increasing power of the vastus medialis is likely.

Our group of patients, consisting of athletes with rapidly increasing or diminishing sport activity, corresponds with this theory.

The innervation disorder can be regarded as a triggering factor of the peripatellar pain syndrome. The nerve root lesions can be partly explained by lumbar hyperlordosis and hypermobility. The segmental hypermobility between the third, fourth and fifth lumbar vertebrae can be shown radiographically (Weh and Eickhoff 1983). We found these changes especially in young girls active in sports in which forced hyperlordotic movements are common, e.g. volleyball, jazz dance and gymnastics. So far there has been no satisfactory explanation for the high incidence of anterior horn cell lesions.

In addition to this investigated spontaneous peripatellar pain, secondary apex pain occurs frequently. In these cases a reflex mechanism induces the weakening of the quadriceps segment. Almost every disorder of the knee joint is capable of causing this reflective pathway. The mechanism of subsequent abnormal gliding of the patella and resulting tendinitis and chondromalacia corresponds with the described spontaneous peripatellar syndrome.

The position of the femoropatellar joint is a consequence of forces during skeletal development. The gliding of the patella is a function of the balance between the vastus medialis (nerve supply mainly by the third lumbar root) and the vastus lateralis (mainly innervated by the fourth lumbar nerve root). Peripatellar pain syndrome and chondromalacia result from a discrepancy between the femoropatellar joint position and muscular forces.

Therapeutic aims

The therapeutic aim in the peripatellar syndrome is to achieve normal patella gliding. This is possible by strengthening of the weakened quadriceps segment. Only in very severe cases should surgical therapy, e.g. transposition of the tibia tubercle, be considered. There is no indication for an elevation of the patella tendon insertion (Maquet/Bandi).

Acknowledgment. This study was supported by the Deutsche Forschungsgemeinschaft (We 9443/1-2)

References

Johnson F, Leitl S, Waugh W (1980) The distribution of load across the knee. J Bone Joint Surg [Br] 62:346

Weh L, Eickhoff W (1983) Innervationsstörungen des M. quadriceps bei Chondropathia patellae. Eine kritische Revision des gültigen Chondropathie-Konzeptes. Z Orthop 121:115

The patello-femoral syndrome

F. A. J. van Hussen

Stichting R.K. Ziekenverpleging
Hilversum
The Netherlands

Introduction

The patellofemoral syndrome is a very complex syndrome because it encompasses a number of clinical pictures which are similar in presentation but different in aetiology. It has become more and more apparent in recent years, however, that these clinical pictures can be differentiated by careful investigation.

Classification

The patellofemoral syndrome can be divided into four clinical pictures. The first is that of the *hypermobile patella.* This is a result of increased primary laxity of the extensor apparatus, which is one of the expressions of the lax morphotype.

The clinical symptoms of increased primary laxity of the extensor apparatus are:

1. Hypermobility of the patella in a lateral as well as in a medial direction
2. Genu recurvatum
3. An anterior drawer phenomenon
4. An increased range of lateral rotation

The principal general manifestations of the lax morphotype are hyperextension of the elbow, passive mobility of the thumb to the volar aspect of the forearm, hyperextension of the fingers and wrist, and increased dorsal flexion of the ankle.

It is to be noted that this clinical picture should be differentiated from precisely defined systemic diseases such as Marfan's disease, the Ehler-Danlos syndrome and osteogenesis imperfecta.

The clinical picture of a hypermobile patella is encountered in young patients, usually about 14–15 years old, and shows a female predominance. It is nearly always localized bilaterally. Conventional radiography as a rule reveals no changes other than pseudoelevation of the patella. Arthroscopy reveals changes in the cartilage of the medial facet of the patella. These chondral changes often show pseudotumorous features.

In aetiological terms the clinical picture of hypermobile patella is a histological condition. The associated chondral changes are possibly caused by the shearing forces which impinge on the patellar cartilage.

The second clinical picture of the patellofemoral syndrome is that of an *anatomical abnormality of the patellofemoral joint*, which may have the following anatomical localizations:

1. Dysplasia of the femoral trochlea
2. Dysplasia of the patella
3. Deviation of the long axis of the lower extremity (genu valgum)
4. Deviation of the axis of rotation
5. An abnormality of the lateral retinaculum or of the fascia lata

The mechanical morphology of the patellofemoral joint is less than optimal as a result of one or several of these abnormalities. In some cases this mechanical abnormality leads to subluxation of dislocation of the patella. The anatomical abnormality can usually be diagnosed clinically and radiologically, and measured with the aid of conventional radiography or CT scan.

The third clinical picture of the patellofemoral syndrome is that of an *osteochondral fracture.* This results from a trauma and can sometimes be diagnosed radiologically. An arthroscopic diagnosis is nearly always possible. Chondral fractures should be distinguished from osteochondral fractures.

The fourth clinical picture is that of *patellofemoral arthrosis.* This is generally encountered in older patients. It can be diagnosed on the basis of conventional radiography, which reveals the characteristic features of arthritis deformans such as narrowing of the joint space, sclerosis and osteophyte formation. These changes are generally localized laterally but may also sometimes be found medially.

Therapy

Dissatisfaction about the poor results obtained in the treatment of the patellofemoral syndrome has led to the introduction of many different therapies over the years. This survey shows the various possibilities of conservative and operative treatment.

Patients with a patellofemoral syndrome based on hypermobility of the patella should preferably be treated conservatively. This conservative therapy consists of exercises aimed at enhancing the active muscular stability. A versatile exercise programme is used in an effort to improve the arthrokinetic reflex mechanism of the knee. Another important objective is to restore the balance of the forces which impinge on the patellofemoral joint and to ensure adequate coordination of these foces. Only very rarely are the chondral changes so severe that operative therapy is required.

An anatomical anomaly of the patellofemoral joint can be treated by operation. Surgery aims specifically at improvement or abolition of the anatomical cause of the mechanical abnormality. For example, dysplasia of the femoral trochlea and patella leading to subluxation or dislocation is preferably treated by realignment procedures such as capsulorrhaphy, myotendinous procedures and patellar ligament procedures. Deviations of the longitudinal axis and axis of rotation are treated by osteotomy. Release of the lateral retinaculum can be indicated in patients with a patellofemoral syndrome based on rigidity of the lateral retinaculum.

The problem encountered in the choice between conservative and operative therapy is that some patients with anatomical abnormalities of the patellofemoral joint also show features of the lax morphotype. Conservative therapy is to be preferred in this group. In determining operative indications it should be carefully assessed whether the anatomical abnormality is sufficiently severe to justify operative therapy.

The treatment of osteochondral fractures largely depends on early diagnosis. Treatment aims at refixation of the osteochondral fragment. In a later stage it may be necessary to remove a foreign body and to treat a cartilage ulcer. Patients with arthrosis of the patellofemoral joint can be treated either conservatively or by operation. In the latter case the Maquet procedure is to be preferred.

Patient discussion

A retrospective study was performed in an effort to gain some impression of the distribution of patients with a patellofemoral syndrome over the four groups. The case records of a continuous series of 100 patients seen during the period 1979–1981 were examined (Table 1).

Table 1. Case records of a series of 100 patients seen during the period 1979–1981

1979–1981			n=100	
			♀	♂
I	63	23 > 29	43	20
II	21	6 > 29	12	9
III	4		1	3
IV	12		9	3

Some evidence of anatomical abnormalities of the patellofemoral joint was present in 23 of the 63 patients in group 1. In group 2, six of the 21 patients showed features of the lax morphotype. This means that 29 patients in groups 1 and 2 formed a transitional group.

Failures

A follow-up was performed on all patients with a patellofemoral syndrome treated by operation during the period 1973–1980. The total number was 235, but in view of the available time I shall discuss only the 19 patients (14 females, 5 males) in whom the operative result was a failure. I define a failure on the basis of three criteria:

1. After one or several operations the patient has more complaints than before the first operation, and these complaints clearly affect his or her daily functioning.
2. If the patella is still present, its chondral condition as assessed arthroscopically is classified as Outerbridge stage 3–4.
3. Conventional radiography reveals signs of arthrosis of the knee joint.

Fourteen of these 19 patients were females and 5 were males. The average age at the first operation was 15 (14–21) years. Of the 19 patients, 12 had had three operations, three had had two and four had had one. The total of 46 operations included: release of the lateral retinaculum in 19 cases, a Hauser procedure in 12 cases, chondrectomy with cancellous bone graft in 10 cases and patellectomy in 5 cases.

It is quite striking that these 19 patients were all more or less clearly classifiable in the group with a hypermobile patella due to increased primary laxity of the extensor apparatus. Since we have separated this group of patients, to treat them by operation only in exceptional cases, our overall results in the operative treatment of the patellofemoral syndrome have improved very much.

Our analysis of the operative results over the period 1973–1980 has led to the conviction that, in patients with a hypermobile patella as manifestation of the patellofemoral syndrome, operations such as capsulorrhaphy, myotendinous procedures and patellar ligament procedures only cause the pathological mobility of the patella to increase. Such an increase in pathological patellar mobility is disastrous for the patellar cartilage.

Consequently these patients have in recent years been treated conservatively. This conservative therapy consisted of enhancement of muscular stability by therapeutic exercises. The initial results were disappointing. Making use of information supplied in reports by Lieb and Perry, Mariani and Caruso, Geneste, and in a later stage Reynolds and co-workers, we developed an exercise programme described in a booklet of which each patient is given a copy. This booklet contains information about the syndrome, a description of the exercises and a page to be used for notes on the exercises performed.

The programme focuses on the following aspects:

1. Strength training, in particular of the vastus medialis and lateralis muscles.
2. Improvement of strength and endurance by brief dynamic contractions.
3. Stretching of muscles which are or tend to become shortened.
4. Restoration of coordination and defence reflexes, more in particular those of the vastus medialis muscle and the medial rotators.

Before the exercise programme is started muscular strength is measured with the isokinetic Cybex apparatus. The 30 exercises of the programme are performed daily, with a physiotherapist in attendance three times a week during the first 8 weeks. After 8 weeks new Cybex measurements are obtained and the programme is adjusted accordingly. At that time it is usually possible to switch emphasis to training of coordination and defence reflexes. Final Cybex measurements are obtained after 4 months.

Although I cannot yet give quantitative data on the results of this therapy in this preliminary report, it is my strong impression that this exercise programme can be very effective in the treatment of patients with a patellofemoral syndrome in the hypermobile patella category.

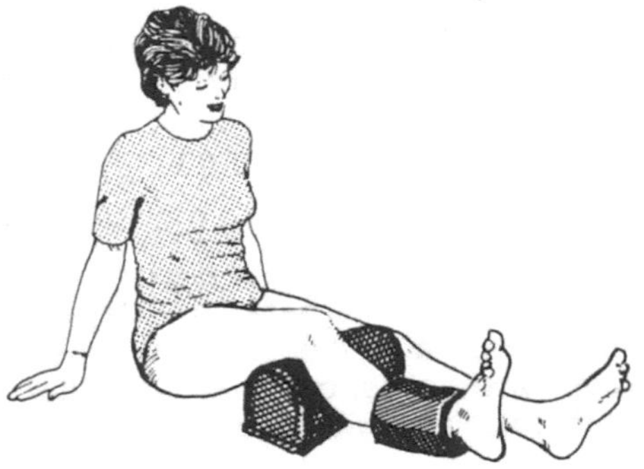

Fig. 1. Exercise (III) performed in sitting position with a large roll under the affected knee

Repetitions	Duration of contractions (s)	Resistance during 1st and 2nd treatments	Resistance during 3rd and 4th treatments	Resistance during 5th and 6th treatments etc.
16 ▻ 50	1	3 kg	3½ kg	4 kg
17 ▻ 30	7	3 kg	3½ kg	4 kg
18 ▻ 10	10	3 kg	3½ kg	4 kg
19 ▻ 50	1	3 kg	3½ kg	4 kg

Conclusions

1. The patellofemoral syndrome encompasses four clinical pictures of identical presentation (patellar pain).
2. To improve therapeutic results, the first two clinical pictures should be differentiated. The first is characterized by patellar hypermobility due to increased primary laxity of the extensor apparatus (lax morphotype) and the second by a changed relation between patella and femoral trochlea due to anatomical abnormalities.
3. The first mostly requires conservative therapy.
4. The second can be treated by operation, provided this focuses specifically on the causative abnormality and there is no pronounced laxity.
5. The results of conservative therapy of patients with patellar hypermobility can be improved by means of an exercise programme performed under careful supervision and controlled by Cynex measurements.

Increased medial torsion of the knee joint producing chondromalacia patellae

G. Janssen

Orthopädische Abteilung, St. Bernhard Hospital
Kamp-Lintfort
Federal Republic of Germany

Terminology

"Torsion" means a twisting of a lengthy body around its longitudinal axis or a twisting in itself. The word describes both the process of twisting and its result (Kummer 1962). It is still unknown whether the long bones show real or only apparent torsion.

Torsion of the distal femur

Three-dimensional position

The transverse axis of the proximal end of the femur has a normal outward or lateral torsion of 6°, and that of the distal end of the femur has a normal inward or medial torsion also of 6° (Figure 1). If the medial torsion of the distal femur is increased the angle is larger than 6°. In relation to the position of the distal femur the osseous shape of the patellofemoral joint varies distinctively. There is a direct correlation with the anteversion and retroversion of the proximal femoral end.

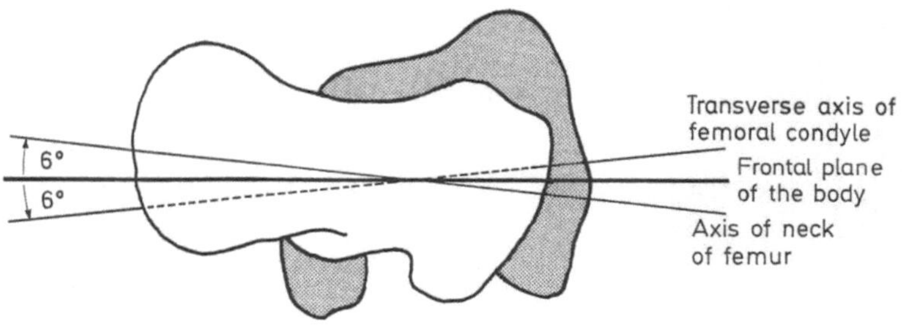

Figure 1. Normal position of the transverse axes of the proximal and distal end of the femur in relation to the horizontal plane of the body

Clinical findings

With increased medial torsion of the distal femur the knee joint is twisted inwards (kneeing in) and the patella is located medially (Figure 2). The lower limb, at least the leg, shows a varus deformity depending on the medial torsion. The proximal end of the fibula is shifted ventrally (Figure 3). The torsion on the distal tibia decreases, and the feet are turned toward the knees, giving the situation of toeing in (Janssen 1981).

Radiographic findings

In the A-P view the medial condyle of the femur looks small and the lateral one large (Figure 4). The position of the patella is medial with the intercon-

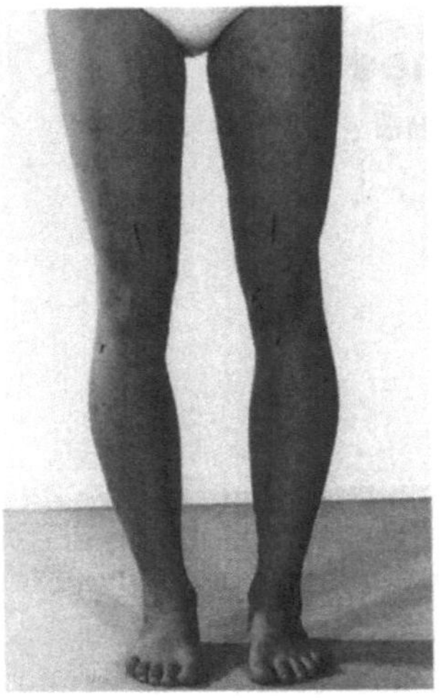

Figure 2

Figure 3

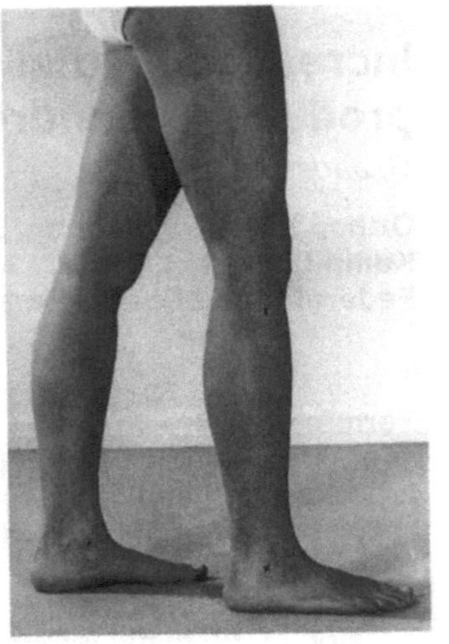

Figure 2. Increased medial torsion of the knee: Medial position of the patella (kneeing in) and torsion-related varus deformity (toeing in)

Figure 3. Increased medial torsion of the knee: Ventral shift of the fibular head and minor torsion of the malleoli in habitual position (same patient as in Figure 2)

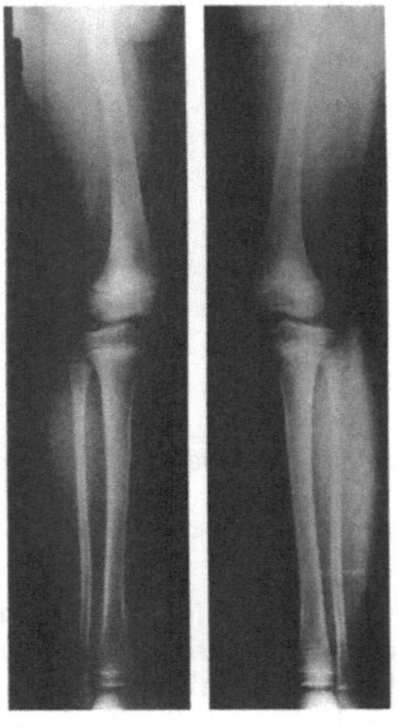

Figure 4. Increased medial torsion, habitual position: torsion-related varus of the leg, recognizable from the lateral contours of the calf muscles, but mild valgus of the lower limb. Free projection of the tibiofibular syndesmosis by decreased torsion of the malleoli

dylar groove distorted medially. The head of the fibula is projected next to the tibia. The lateral contours of the calf muscules show the varus of the leg produced by medial torsion. The lateral X-ray view shows the posterior condyle margins with increased distance to each other. The tangential view, at least, correlates with dysplasia of the patellofemoral joint.

Materials and methods
A radiological method for measurement of the distal femoral torsion has been described (Janssen 1978). The angle of torsion was measured in 250 knee joints. There were three groups of patients, the first with normal knee joints, the second with minor medial torsion of the distal femur, and the third with severe medial torsion.

Results
Measurement of the angle of torsion in 120 knee joints with increased medial torsion proved that the torsion might range from a nearly normal position to severely increased medial torsion (torsion from 6 ° to 25 °). Furthermore, we found that dislocation of the patella was mostly combined with increased medial torsion.

Subluxation and luxation of the patella by increased medial torsion are normally accompanied by dysplasia of the patellofemoral joint. Adjacent laxity and hypermobility of the joints were found in more than 80% of the patients, and in many further cases some degree of muscular weakness was present. In all these cases examination revealed chondromalacia patellae which was improved by the surgical procedure described below.

Aetiology of dysplasia
With increased medial torsion of the distal femur the patella is located medially and the tibial tuberosity laterally, a situation designated as malalignment. This basic situation can persist or undergo further changes.

One essential change is lateralization of the patella. Lateralization is produced if there is concomitant ligamentous laxity and muscular weakness, as is found in the majority of cases. With forced contraction of the quadriceps muscle, when the patient starts to bend the knee joint loosening of the medial retinacula might arise in the presence of malalignment.

The lateralization of the patella is only *one* result of the torsion-related development, for increased medial torsion is generally a congenital disturbance and present as long as growth continues, moulding the osseous shape of the femoral condyles under functional conditions.

Thus the *other* result of growth is dysplasia of the patellofemoral joint. With increased medial torsion of the distal femur the anterior aspect of the lateral condyle is turned forward, crossing the frontal plane of the body ventrally (Figure 5).

The medial condyle, in contrast, faces in a dorsal direction. Under these conditions the proximal lateral condyle puts the lateralized patella under pressure, while the medial condyle and medial facet of the patella lose contact with each other. The increasing pressure on the main weight-bearing area of the lateral condyle, in the starting phase of flexion, seems to be the growth-related reason for the flattening and broadening of the lateral condyle, while the medial condyle is in fact dysplastic (Janssen 1978). This is what we find in any joint with subluxation and recurrent or habitual dislocation of the patella (Figure 6).

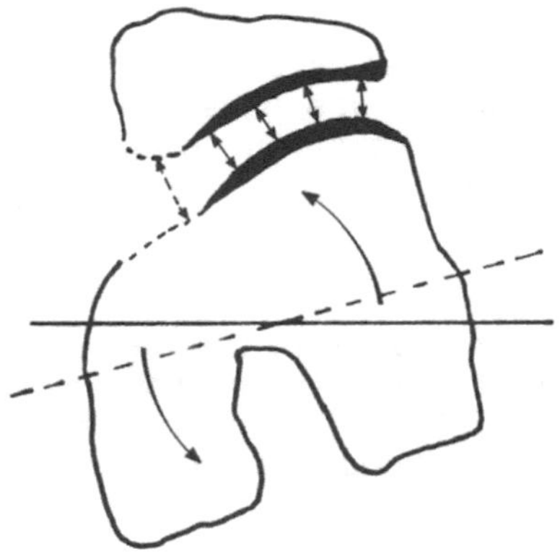

Figure 5. Development of dysplasia of the patellofemoral joint related to increased medial torsion: forward eversion of the anterior aspect of the lateral condyle and lateralization of the patella induce dysplasia during growth

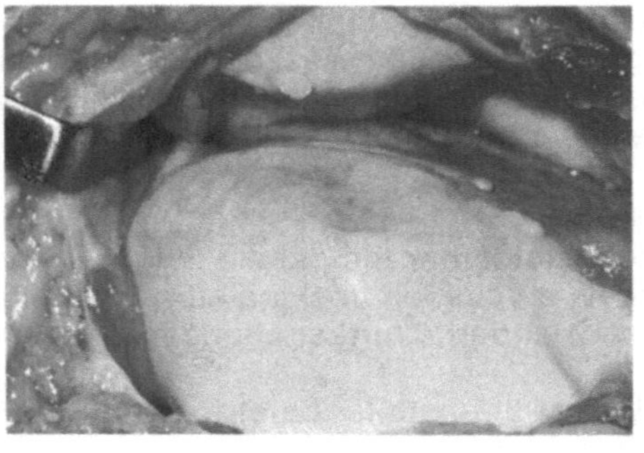

Figure 6. Recurrent dislocation of the patella in a 14-year-old girl: Large lateral condyle, over it the patella. Small, distally displaced articular surface of the medial condyle. Proximally elongated surface of the lateral condyle by patella alta. Functional disorder with chondromalacia

In the last analysis, the degree of medial torsion and the extent of malalignment are responsible for the degree of dysplasia. The consecutive biomechanical result of growth is a varied shape of the patellofemoral joint influenced by ligamentous laxity. Precisely definable types of the patella in Wiberg's sense (1941) do not exist.

Aetiology of chondromalacia

Hehne (1983), in his work on the patellofemoral joint, recommends a restriction of the concept of dysplasia, specifically to Wiberg's type III. Thus, the question arises as to why the radiological feature of dysplasia is correlated to chondromalacia.

Dysplasia and associated chondromalacia in subluxation and recurrent dislocation of the patella are well known. Here the traumatic process is thought to lead to chondromalacia. Are there any other mechanisms?

With reference to the adaptation during growth it should be accepted, first, that the dysplastic patellofemoral joint is provided with congruent articular surfaces depending on the different degrees of flexion. Why do we find that chondromalacia is nevertheless frequent in increased medial torsion of the knee joint, in cases with minor dysplasia without any dislocation of the patella?

As an attempt at explanation we might cite the ligamentous laxity seen in 80% of the patients with increased medial torsion. First, laxity occurs as a biomechanical disorder; secondly, when ligamentous laxity is present it is possible that the cartilage itself may be of poor quality owing to a metabolic disorder of the soft tissues (Beighton et al. 1983).

Conclusions

Under normal conditions the clinical phenomenon of increased medial torsion of the knee and the correlated radiological sign of dysplasia of the patellofemoral joint seem to be the result of growth; that is to say it is predominantly influenced by ligamentous laxity and muscular imbalance (malalignment).

If the common concept of dysplasia is restricted, we consider a biomechanical disorder produced by ligamentous laxity as one explanation for frequent chondromalacia with increased medial torsion of the knee.

In addition to a primary, nutritionally induced lesion of cartilage, chondromalacia is also interpreted as the result of poor quality of the cartilage related to ligamentous laxity.

References

Beighton P, Rodney G, Bird H (1983) Hypermobility of joints. Springer, Berlin Heidelberg New York

Hehne AJ (1983) Das Patellofemoralgelenk. Enke, Stuttgart

Janssen G (1978) Das Ätiologie der Patellaluxation. Z Orthop 116:656

Janssen G (1981) Der Innentorsionsfehler des Kniegelenkes. Orthop Praxis 3:227

Janssen G, Prüssner P (1978) Eine Methode zur Messung der distalen Femurtorsion. Z Orthop 116:270

Kummer B (1962) Torsionsprobleme an den unteren Extremitäten. Z Orthop 96:115

Wiberg G (1941) Röntgenographic and anatomic studies on the femoropatellar joint. Acta Orthop Scand 12:319

Chondropathia patellae, arthroscopic findings and early detection of cartilage changing

H. Buehlmann

Falkenstraße 4
Zürich
Switzerland

The chondropathia patellae (CP) can be recognized earlier with arthroscopy. This paper describes clinical and arthroscopic findings of all stages of CP and presents a new photographic method to recognize early stages of cartilage damage.

Material and methods

From a collection of 2000 diagnostic arthroscopies 320 cases with a typical isolated retropatellar finding have been studied. Arthroscopic, radiological, clinical and laboratory findings are compared. A new photographic technique demonstrates, that damage of the cartilage can be recognized in a very early stage.

Results

Diagnostic arthroscopy is absolutely essential in assessment of retropatellar cartilage damage. Especially in the early stages the arthroscopic findings are helpful in considering the treatment. If clinical signs of a CP are present, the retropatellar cartilage should be checked very carefully, otherwise the arthroscopy will be negative. In about 10% of early stage of CP with clinical symptoms a beginning alteration of the cartilage is demonstrable only by infrared pictures.

Summary

An early proof of a retropatellar damage or alteration of the cartilage is very important and can only be detected by arthroscopy. In a controlled group of 320 patients with clinical symptoms the arthroscopic appearance of CP is demonstrated by a new method.

"Chondromalacia" and recurrent subluxation of the patella – an EMG study of V. L. and V. M.O. before and after physiotherapy

G. Cerulli[1], *V. Gallai*[2] *and G. Mazzotta*[2]

[1] **Orthopaedic and** [2] **Neurological Clinics – University of Perugia
Perugia
Italy**

Several EMG studies exist and some of these are correlated with the pathologies (Mc Leod et a., Mariani-Caruso) and with the rehabilitation (Wild) of the extensor mechanism of the knee.
We carried out a clinical, radiographical and electromyographical evaluation of extensor mechanism.

Material and methods
An EMG investigation was performed in 50 normal knees (control group), in 60 "Chondromalacia" and in 48 recurrent subluxation (the diagnosis was clinical and radiographical).

A Medelec-MS-6 with two channels was used; the activity of vastus laterals (V.L.) and vastus medialis obliquus (V.M.O.) were studied simultaneously using superface electrodes with the knee bent at 90, 60 and 30 degrees of flexion and in extension. All cases of "Chondromalacia" and recurrent subluxation were treated with straight-leg isometric exercises for six months. After this we performed again an EMG investigation.

Results
In the control group: no difference between V.L. and V.M.O.

In the "Chondromalacia": the activity of V.L. (1283 $\pm$ 473 micro V.) was higher than V. M. O. (851 $\pm$ 367 micro V.) with a significant difference ($P < 0{,}0005$), the difference was more in the cases with Q angle > 20°.

In the recurrent subluxation: the activity of V.L. (1224 $\pm$ 355 micro V.) was higher than V. M. O. (831 $\pm$ 293 micro V.) with significant difference ($P < 0{,}0001$). The difference was more in the cases with a congruence angle > + 10° after treatment.

In 50 cases of the "Chondromalacia" treated: no significant difference between activity of V. L. (1235$\pm$ 329 micro V.) and V. M. O. (1145 $\pm$ 307 micro V.).

In 40 cases of the recurrent subluxation treated: no significant difference between activity of V.L. (1245 $\pm$ 214 micro V.) and V. M. O. (1151 $\pm$ 383 micro V.). All these cases became asymptomatic.

Discussion
We did not find high electromyographical difference between "Chondromalacia" and recurrent subluxation. It therefore seems to strengthen the hypothesis that these are the quantitative expression of the same pathology: malalignment of the extensor mechanism. The physiotherapy is a valid treatment in most of "Chondromalacia" and recurrent subluxation.

Summary
The authors carried out a clinical, radiographical and electromyographical study of extensor mechanism of the knee. The EMG investigation performed in the pathological cases before and after physiotherapy showed that this treatment was effective in 80% of "Chondromalacia" and in 75% of recurrent subluxation.

Treatment in patello-femoral arthralgia. Lateral release or conservative treatment?

U. E. P. Lindberg, J. Lysholm, and J. Gillquist

Department of Orthopaedic Surgery University Hospital
S-581 85 Linköping
Sweden

46 consecutive patients with complaints of patellofemoral arthralgia were examined with standardized physical examination and arthroscopy of the knee joint. Function was measured with the Lysholm kneescore and quadriceps torque with a Cybex II isokinetic dynamometer. 23 patients were randomly selected for lateral release and 23 for conservative treatment.

Lateral release was done percutaneously at the arthroscopy. Postoperatively a compression dressing with a lateral pad was worn for 14 days. All patients were seen two weeks postoperatively. They were then put on a quadriceps rehabilitation program guided by a physiotherapist. Follow-up with Lysholm score and Cybex test at 10 and 18 weeks postoperatively. There was no difference in success rate in the two groups. We found good or excellent results only in approximately 40%. In patients with severe problems neither conservative treatment nor lateral release gave good results.

The Elmslie-Trillat procedure for recurrent subluxation/dislocation of the patella

A. Leyshon and E. L. Trickey

The Royal National Orthopaedic Hospital
Stanmore
United Kingdom

Dissatisfied with the results of the Hauser procedure for recurrent subluxation/dislocation of the patella we have used the Emslie-Trillat procedure for the past six years.

Material and methods

Twenty-two knees in 20 patients were followed up retrospectively at a mean interval of 36 months from surgery (range 15-72 months). The mean duration of symptoms was 44 months and all patients had typical symptoms and signs of patella instability.

Radiographic measurements showed all patients to have patella alta according to the criteria of Blackburne and Peel (1977).

The operative procedure consists of two stages. An open, radical, lateral patella retinacular release is performed. The patella articulation is inspected and any lesion of the articular cartilage dealt with by excision and/or drilling as required. The tibial tubercle with its attached patella tendon is mobilised on a long, distally based, osteo-periosteal flap, transposed medially by 11 mm and fixed with a screw, after checking for normal patellar tracking. The wound is closed over a suction drain and the knee immobilised in a cylinder cast in extension for six weeks.

Results

The symptoms of instability were cured in all but two knees. Nineteen patients were able to return to their former employment and sporting activities. Of six patients with pain pre-operatively, only two were relieved. The remaining four patients had gross articular cartilage lesions which had been excised and drilled.

Complications of superficial wound infection, deep vein thrombosis and stiffness requiring manipulation under anaesthesia each occurred once in separate patients. Three patients required late removal of the screw for persistent tenderness.

Discussion

The Emslie-Trillat procedure results in reliable correction of extensor apparatus malalignment without the disadvantages inherent in the Hauser procedure. The tibial tubercle is not recessed which may increase patellofemoral compression forces and give rise to pain. The cosmetic result, particularly in women, is better, for the normal prominence of the tibial tubercle is retained. The procedure does not allow distal advancement of the tubercle and thereby eliminates possible problems of patella baja.

The operation can be recommended for symptoms of patella instability. If there are secondary degenerative changes in the patello-femoral joint, associated with pain, then the procedure will not alter this sympton.

Osteotomy

Indications for osteotomy in the treatment of osteoarthritis of the knee

P. Maquet

25 Thier Bosset
B-4070 Aywaille
Belgium

In order to establish the indications for osteotomy in the treatment of osteoarthritis of the knee, the concepts on which this surgical solution is based must be known. During the single support period of gait, each knee alternately supports the mass of the body minus the loaded lower leg and foot. Through its mass and accelerations this mass acts on the knee eccentrically with the force *P* (Figure 1). Force *P* is counterbalanced by a muscular force *L*, acting successively anterolaterally, laterally and posterolaterally during the single support period. The resultant *R* of forces *P* and *L* is transmitted across the knee by weight-bearing surfaces which decrease in size and move posteriorly during flexion. Meniscectomy decreases the weight-bearing surfaces of the joint by about 50%. Force *R* evokes compressive stresses in the femorotibial joint. These compressive stresses are materialized by the subchondral bone densities underlining the tibial plateaux. In a normal knee, the subchondral densities are of the same width and appear symmetrical beneath the medial and lateral plateaux. Since the quantity of bony material depends on the magnitude of the stresses (Pauwels 1980), the subchondral bone densities in a normal knee mean that the compressive stresses are distributed evenly in the joint and that the resultant force *R* must act at the centre of the weight-bearing surfaces of the knee.

In osteoarthritis affecting predominantly the medial aspect of the knee, which is then usually deformed into varus, a dense triangle underlines the medial plateau of the tibia and the medial joint space becomes narrower and narrower. Finally the femur is subluxated on the tibia. Simultaneously, the subchondral density beneath the lateral plateau decreases and moves towards the tibial spines, and the structure of the cancellous bone beneath the lateral plateau becomes less and less easily visible. The X-ray picture shown in

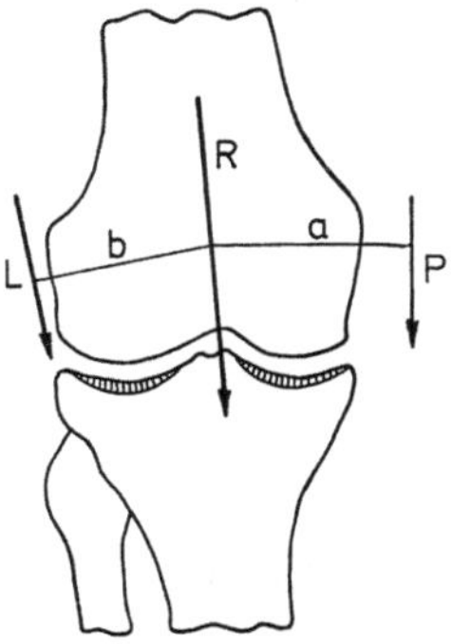

Figure 1. Normal knee. *P*, force exerted eccentrically on the knee by the partial mass of the body; *L*, muscular force counterbalancing force *P*; *R*, resultant of forces *P* and *L*; *a*, lever arm of force *P*; *b*, lever arm of force *L*

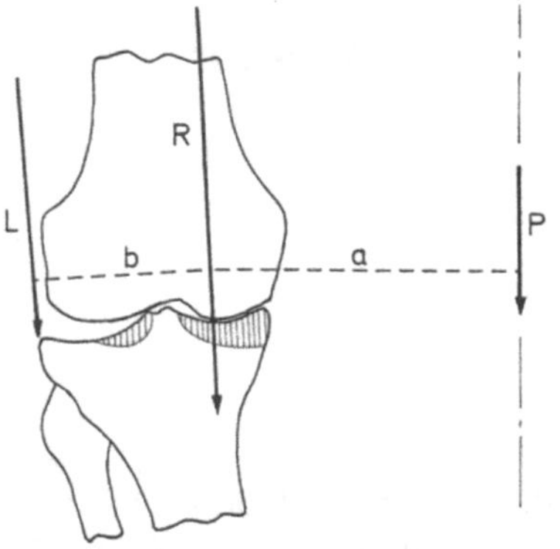

Figure 2. Osteoarthritis with a varus deformity. Medial displacement of resultant *R*. Same abbreviations as in Figure 1

Figure 2 suggests a medial displacement of the resultant *R* with increased compressive stresses in the medial aspect of the joint

In osteoarthritis affecting predominantly the lateral aspect of the knee the limb becomes deformed into valgus, the subchondral density underlining the lateral plateau increases and moves towards the intercondylar eminence, the lateral joint space disappears, and the femoral condyle penetrates into the lateral plateau. The X-ray picture suggests a lateral displacement of the resultant force *R* with increased compressive stresses in the lateral aspect of the knee (Figure 3).

In the lateral view, a normal knee is underlined by a subchondral density of even width, suggesting an even distribution of the compressive stresses in the joint. When there is a flexion contracture, a dense triangle appears beneath the posterior aspect of the plateaux. This picture corresponds to a posterior displacement of the resultant *R*, with a considerable increase of the articular compressive stresses. When the knee is maintained in flexion the weight-bearing surfaces are permanently decreased and, consequently, the articular compressive stresses are increased.

Osteoarthritis thus results from a disturbance of the balance which normally exists between the resistance of the articular tissues and their mechanical stressing, i.e. the articular pressure. This balance may be restored by a suf-

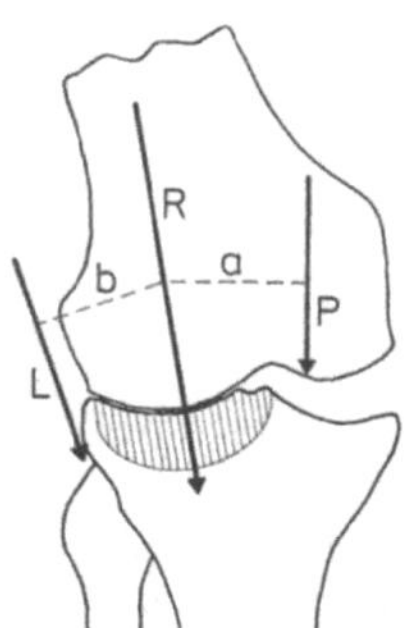

Figure 3. Osteoarthritis with a valgus deformity. Lateral displacement of resultant *R*. Same abbreviations as in Figure 1

ficient decrease of the articular pressure. An efficient way of decreasing the articular pressure consists in enlarging the weight-bearing surface of the joint. This is possible by bringing the resultant force *R* back to the centre of gravity of the articular weight-bearing surfaces. Recentering of force *R* can be achieved either by a proximal osteotomy of the tibia overcorrecting the varus deformity, or by a distal osteotomy of the femur, slightly overcorrecting a valgus deformity. As a very first step, the deformity of the knee must be measured as precisely as possible. To this end, an anteroposterior X-ray showing the whole leg, with the patient standing, is necessary. In a normal individual, the centre of the femoral head, that of the knee and that of the ankle lie on the same straight line.

When the leg is deformed into varus, a line is drawn from the centre of the femoral head to the mid-point of the transverse diameter of the tibia at osteotomy level and another line from this point to the centre of the ankle. The angle formed by these two lines corresponds to the varus deformity. An exact correction of the deformity would bring the knee back to the mechanical conditions which provoked osteoarthritis to appear and develop. To compensate for the weakness of the muscles, which is the usual cause of osteoarthritis with a varus deformity, overcorrection of the deformity is necessary, thus creating some valgus (3°–6°). Overcorrection of a varus deformity is achieved by a tibial osteotomy. After sufficient overcorrection of the deformity, the resultant force *R* acts at the centre of the weight-bearing surfaces of the joint at right angles to the plane tangential to the plateaux (Figure 4a). If the varus deformity was corrected by a femoral osteotomy, the resultant force *R* would be inclined to the plane tangential to the tibial plateaux and the articular stresses would not be distributed symmetrically over the plateaux (Figure 4b). An osteotomy of the proximal end of the tibia thus rep-

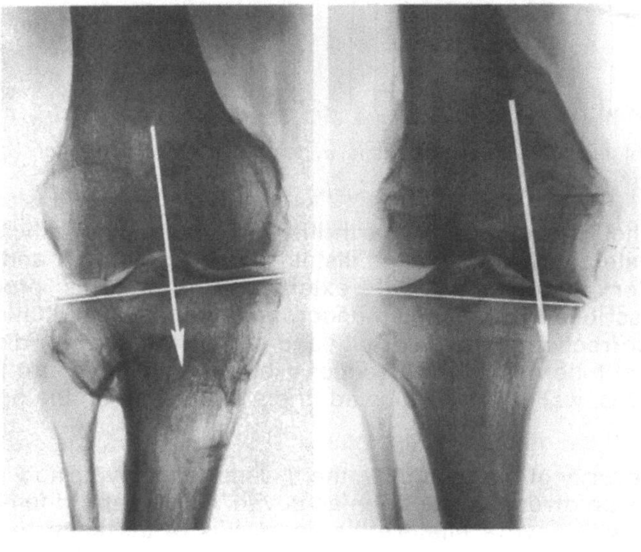

a b

Figure 4a, b. Overcorrection of a varus deformity: **a** through a tibial osteotomy; **b** through a femoral osteotomy

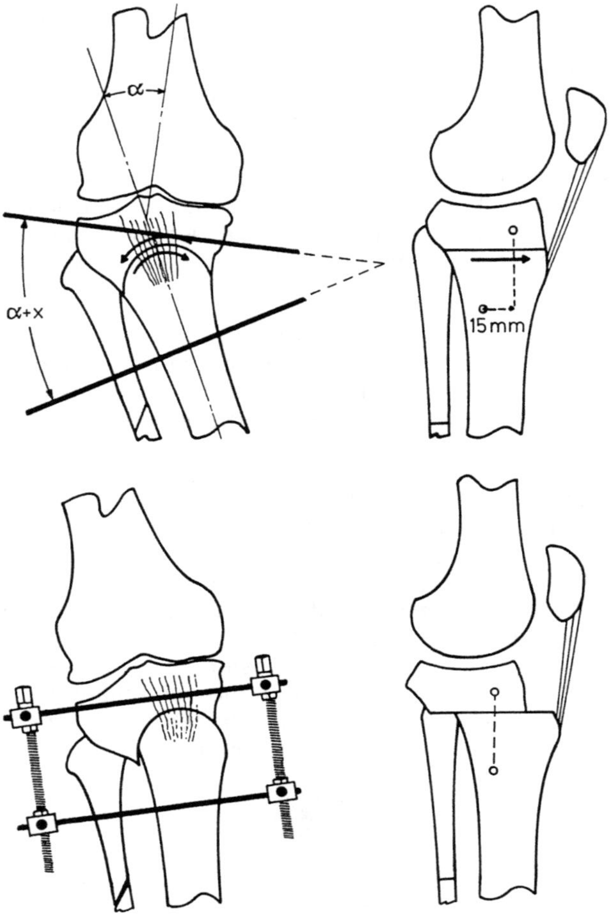

Figure 5. The barrel-vault osteotomy of the tibia. α, deformity; x, overcorrection

resents the method of choice in osteoarthritis with a varus deformity. We use a barrel-vault osteotomy, displace the distal fragment anteriorly and fix the fragments under compression with external fixators. This procedure (Figure 5) is described in detail in a monograph (Maquet 1983). It allows for a precise overcorrection of the deformity and permits an anterior displacement of the tibial tuberosity, which reduces the articular pressure further. The patient moves, walks and is allowed to put full weight on the operated knee immediately.

Whatever the severity of the deformity, the tissues react favourably as long as a sufficient overcorrection has been achieved. A 69-year-old female patient presented with severe bilateral osteoarthritis of the knee as a consequence of deformities due to rickets in infancy and childhood. In both knees the medial joint space had disappeared and the medial plateau was underlined by a triangular sclerosis. The subchondral density beneath the

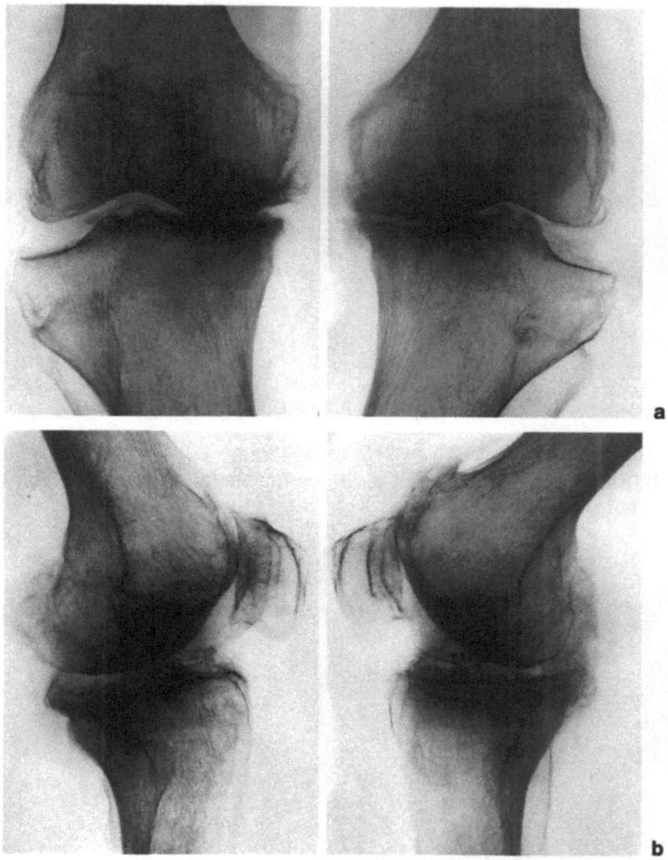

Figure 6. a Sixty-nine-year-old female patient with severe osteoarthritis with bilateral varus deformities. **b** Thirteen years after a bilateral barrel-vault osteotomy of the tibia, overcorrecting the varus deformity

lateral plateau was thinner than normal and displaced towards the intercondylar eminence (Figure 6a). On both sides the angle of the thigh and lower leg axes was changed by 37 ° through a barrel-vault osteotomy. Thirteen years after the barrel-vault osteotomies, the clinical and cosmetic result remains excellent. In the X-rays taken with the patient standing and putting full weight on the examined knee, the tibial plateaux are underlined by subchondral densities of even width throughout. The cancellous structure is more clearly visible beneath the lateral plateau. A joint space has reappeared in the medial aspect of the knees (Figure 6b). The postoperative X-ray picture demonstrates an even distribution of the compressive stresses over the largest possible articular weight-bearing surfaces.

As shown by this example, advanced age is no contraindication. The tissues react favourably to a decrease in the articular pressure up to the end of life. Once achieved the good result persists as demonstrated by the long follow-up.

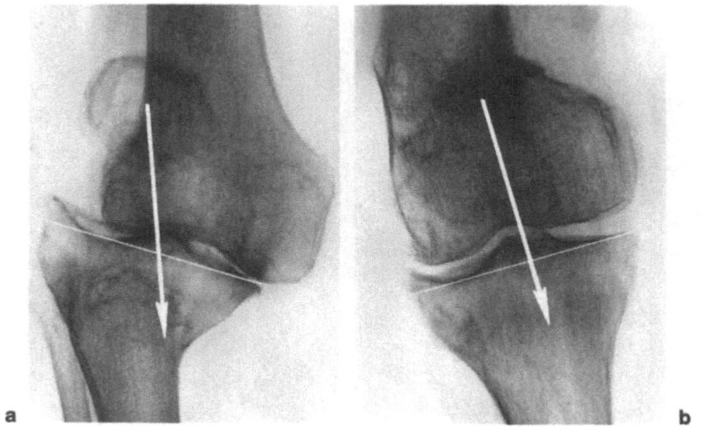

Figure 7 a, b. Slight overcorrection of a valgus deformity: **a** through a tibial osteotomy; **b** through a femoral osteotomy

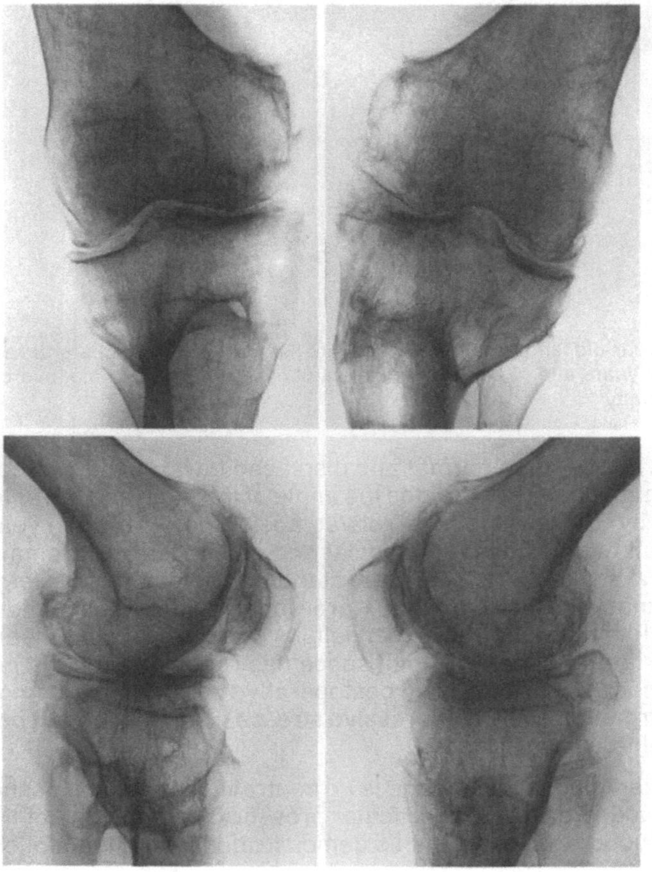

'igure 7c

Considerable destruction of the medial plateau of the tibia has not deterred us from carrying out a barrel-vault osteotomy, overcorrecting the varus deformity with an amazingly good result.

Osteoarthritis with a valgus deformity constitutes a somewhat different problem. The deformity must also be measured in an anteroposterior X-ray showing the whole leg with the patient standing and putting full weight on the affected knee. A line is drawn from the centre of the femoral head to the midpoint of the transverse diameter just proximal to the femoral condyles. Another line is drawn from this point to the centre of the ankle. The angle formed by these two lines shows the amount of the valgus deformity. This must be overcorrected slightly (1 °–2 °) in order to avoid putting the knee in the same mechanical conditions under which osteoarthritis appeared and developed. If the deformity is overcorrected through an osteotomy of the proximal end of the tibia the resultant force *R* is inclined to the plane tangential to the tibial plateaux and, as consequence, is increased further and remains concentrated on the lateral aspect of the joint close to the intercondylar eminence (Figure 7a). This aggravates the condition. The resultant force acting on the knee becomes perpendicular to the plane tangential to the tibial plateaux and can be moved to the centre of the joint only after a supracondylar osteotomy of the femur overcorrecting the deformity (Figure 7b). The femoral osteotomy is carried out through a 5-cm-long incision on the medial aspect of the condylar region. The two fragments are forced into each other and fixed under compression with four Steinmann pins and external fixators (Figure 8) (Maquet 1983). The patient moves the knee and is encouraged to walk with weight-bearing immediately.

A 72-year-old female patient presented with severe osteoarthritis with a valgus deformity. The lateral plateau of the tibia was underlined by an exaggerated subchondral sclerosis and the cancellous structure was hardly visible beneath the medial plateau underlined by a thinned subchondral density. The lateral joint space was narrowed considerably (Figure 9a). A change of 25° in the angle between the axes of the thigh and that of the lower leg was

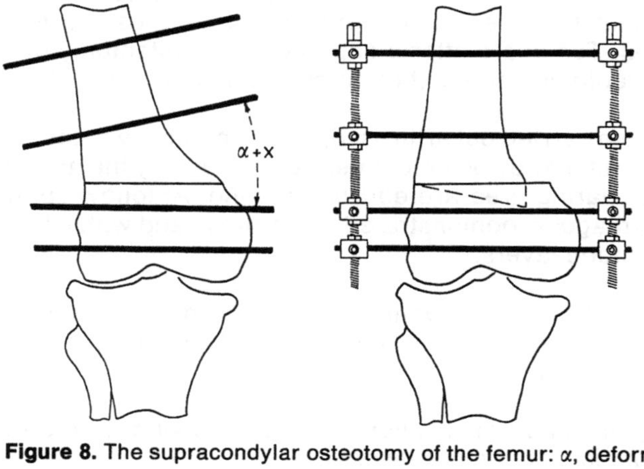

Figure 8. The supracondylar osteotomy of the femur: α, deformity; x, overcorrection

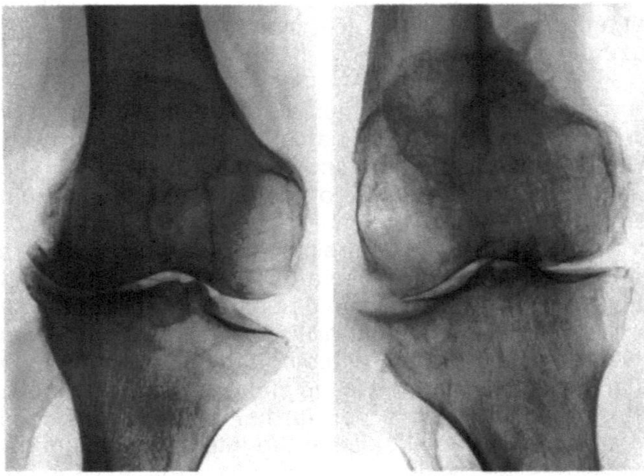

Figure 9 a, b. a Seventy-two-year-old female patient with severe osteoarthritis with a valgus deformity. **b** One year after a supracondylar osteotomy of the femur overcorrecting the valgus deformity slightly

carried out, resulting in an overcorrection of 2°. One year after the operation, the clinical result is excellent. In the X-ray taken with the patient standing a large joint space has reappeared in the lateral aspect of the knee. The subchondral bone densities and the cancellous structure tend to become symmetrical beneath the two tibial plateaux (Figure 9b). This surgests an even distribution and a diminution of the articular pressure. As shown again in this example, advanced age is not a contraindication to an appropriate osteotomy even if the condition is severe and degeneration far advanced.

As long as the overcorrection has been sufficient, the good results last. We demonstrated this lasting effect of the osteotomies in a review of several hundred knees operated on (Maquet 1983). A last example will illustrate this. A 65-year-old female patient was operated on for severe lateral osteoarthritis of the knee (Figure 10a). Ten years after a supracondylar osteotomy of the femur, the clinical and radiological result remains excellent (Figure 10b).

Fujisawa et al. (1979) have carried out arthroscopy systematically before and some months and years after knee osteotomies. Before surgery the articular surfaces in the weight-bearing area are eburnated bone. At follow-up they are covered by fibrocartilage as demonstrated at histology and with islets of hyaline cartilage in the deep layers.

In conclusion, in the treatment of osteoarthritis of the knee osteotomy is usually indicated and has nearly no contraindication. However, in order to achieve good and lasting results:

1. The varus deformity must be frankly overcorrected; the valgus deformity must also be overcorrected but more discretely.

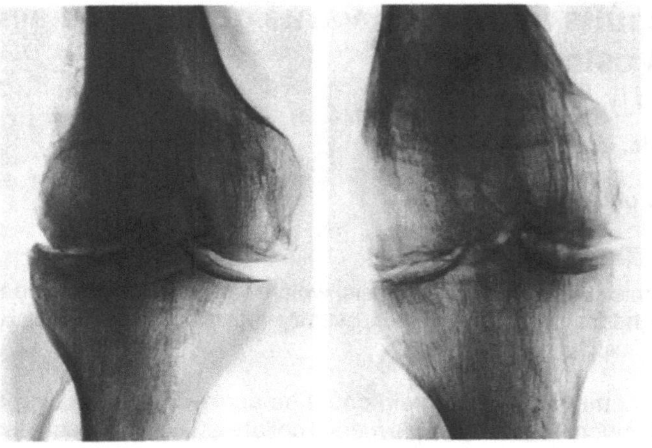

a b

Figure 10. **a** Sixty-five-year-old female patient with severe lateral osteoarthritis. **b** Ten years after a supracondylar osteotomy of the femur overcorrecting the valgus deformity slightly

2. As a rule, the varus deformity must be overcorrected by an osteotomy of the proximal extremity of the tibia, the valgus deformity by an osteotomy of the distal extremity of the femur.

References

Fujisawa Y, Masuhara K, Shiomi S (1979) The effect of high tibial osteotomy on osteoarthritis of the knee. An arthroscopic study of 54 knee joints. Orthop Clin North Am 10:585–608

Maquet P (1983) Biomechanics of the knee, 2nd edn. Springer, Berlin Heidelberg New York

Pauwels F (1980) Biomechanics of the locomotor apparatus. Springer, Berlin Heidelberg New York

Mid-term results in treating varus gonarthrosis with a high tibial osteotomy

M. A. Schmidt and W. R. Hepp

Orthopaedic Clinic, University of Kiel
2300 Kiel
Federal Republic of Germany

Of 152 patients with severe varus gonarthrosis, which were operated between 1973 and 1982 with a high tibial osteotomy in the Coventry-technique, modified by Blauth, 130 were examined clinically and by X-ray.

In 82% a great or complete relief of pain could be achieved, the walking ability could be improved much. The laxity of the medial collateral ligament decreased, as did the joint effusion.

There were no remarkable X-ray improvements of degenerative joint alterations, although there was an increase of height of the medial joint line in some cases.

Patients with persisting pain showed in general a too little correction of the axis of the leg, in addition there were mostly severe degenerative alterations of the joint.

A sufficient correction has to be considered very important for the success of a high tibial osteotomy in varus gonarthrosis (at least 5° more valgus than the physiological axis of the leg).

Differentiated operation technique and results of osteotomies in the region of the knee-joint

K. H. Müller and J. Müller-Färber

Chirurgische Universitätsklinik und Poliklinik
Hunscheidtstr.
D-4630 Bochum 1
Federal Republic of Germany

The complex anatomy, the differentiated static and dynamic strains, the traumatic predisposition, and the topography between the large leg joints combine to cause a very sensitive reaction of the knee joint to axial deviations [1, 4, 5, 9]. On the basis of the specific numbers of cases seen in a hospital for accident cases it is opportune to go into the particulars of the posttraumatic malpositions (Figures 1–8) [9]. Even more persistently than idiopathic axial defects, traumatic axial defects necessitate especially adapted operation techniques. But even then, a successful operative intervention only remains successful if the patient is cooperative. The biomechanics of the knee joint are described by the vector sum of alternately influencing strains. In this area we are particularly indebted to Maquet [1, 4, 5, 10]. The proof of the accuracy of such perceptions is the fact that the correction osteotomy is the most important basis for the biological recovery of the wrongly strained knee joint (Figure 2) [13]. The main indications for osteotomies near the knee joint are subjective complaints, inadequate stability of the ligaments, an extension deficit and the remaining range of movement, the condition of the traumatically damaged epicondyle and condyle, and pathologic findings in the adjacent and contralateral joints. *Correction osteosynthesis* is possible as long as the fragments can still be mobilized. Consequently, correction osteosynthesis is a causal correction. In cases of osseous healing in malposition the rule is that the osteotomy must be carried out as early as possible, but only after training for muscular strength, ligamentous stability and optimal function (Figures 6–8) [5, 9, 11, 13]. Early correction osteotomy prevents secondary damage and encourages repair processes (Figure 8). A late correction osteotomy can no longer aim to avoid joint detrition, but only to slow it down.

Planning and differentiated operation technique
With the help of long X-rays of the legs the numerical correction angle in relation to the particular level of the osteotomy and localization of the correction can be precisely determined (Figures 5–7) [3, 6–8, 10, 12]. Careful consideration of preoperative drawing allows decisions on the course of the operative processes, the individual osteotomy with removal of a wedge or cleft interposition, the size of the interponate, and the method of osteosynthesis and determines the result of the axial correction. Preoperative recognition of any difficulties is helpful as the operation time can be shortened and the likelihood of success enhanced: they should be adequately dealt with in the patient information interview [9]. Generally removal of a wedge with its base on the convex side of the malposition causes first, a shift of the resulting main force to the centre of the joint, and secondly rotation of the axis of the articular surfaces [1, 4, 10]. Accordingly, the correction must not only consist in

a b

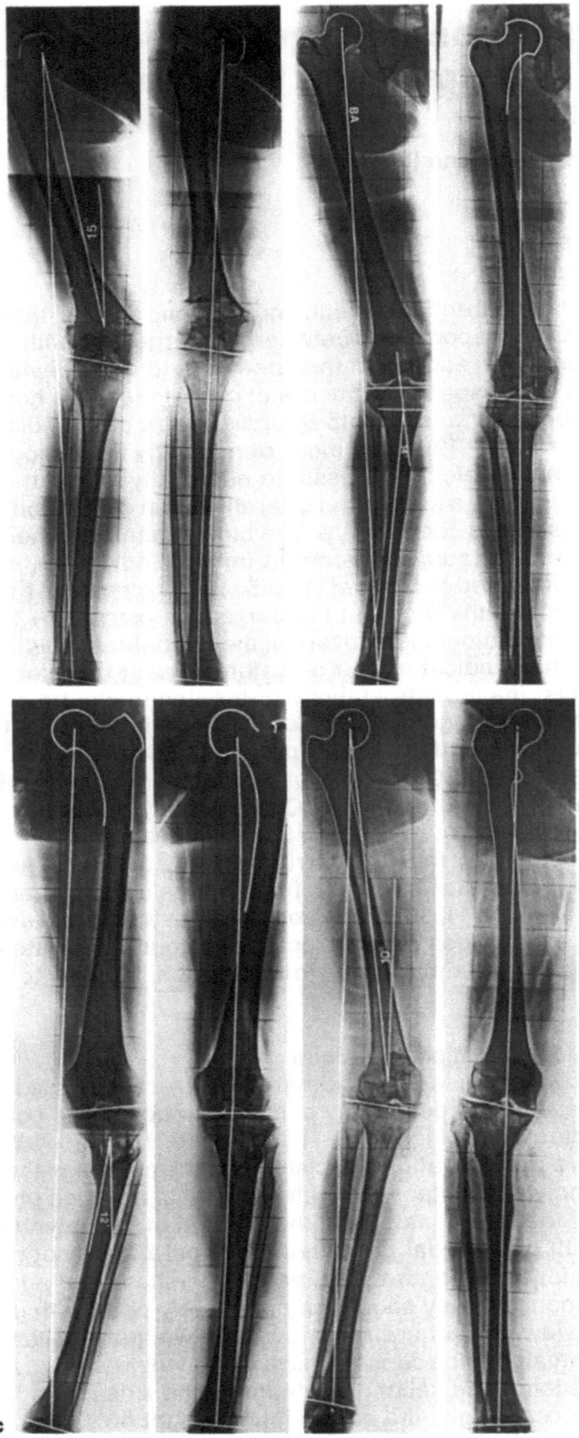

c d

Figure 1 a–d. Planning of an operative correction of malpositioned knee-joints by long X-rays of the leg in the frontal plane. **a** Supracondylar correction osteotomy after post-traumatic false position of 15 ° (subtractive wedge osteotomy). **b** Infracondylar correction osteotomy after intra-articular fracture of the head of the tibia healed in a valgus deformity of 14 °; correct axial position of the leg after subtractive correction. **c** Osteotomy of the head of the tibia after post-traumatic juxta-articular valgus deformity (15 °) of the tibia; subtractive correction with correct axial position. **d** Badly planned correction osteotomy close to the knee joint; the supracondylar valgus deformity of 10 ° was corrected at the head of the tibia leading to slanting axis of the knee and ankle joints despite a centric axis of the main force, exacerbating symptoms

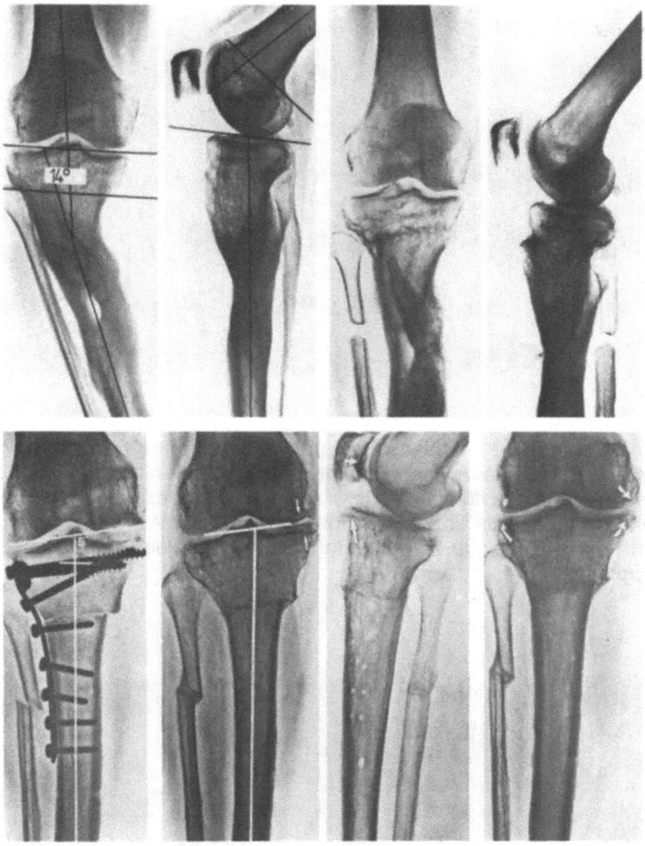

a

b

Figure 2a, b. Late radiological results of biomechanically correct and badly planned correction osteotomies in the head of the tibia. **a** 42-year-old man, 3 years after juxta-articular fracture of tibial after post-traumatic varus deformity; 9 years after biomechanically correct osteotomy there has been no progress of arthrosis and there is free flexibility of the knee joint. **b** falsely indicated tibia head osteotomy of a valgus deformity in a 76-year-old woman. The axis of the knee-joint which takes a slanting course towards the axis of the main force leads to a bayonet-like displacement of the osseous parts of the knee-joint: the unphysiological situation of the axis of the joint essentially intensifies the arthrosis 7 years after operation despite the central position of the axis of main force

centering of the force. At the same time the osteotomized part of the joint with its articular surface must be adjusted vertically to the resulting force [5–9]. Only then do mere pressure forces have an effect, and the strains are then distributed among the remaining supporting surfaces. Badly planned osteotomies with slanting clefts and bayonet-like displacement of the femoral condyles and the tibial plateau lead to an unstable knee joint, and they are doomed to failure even in the planning stage (Figures 1 d, 2 b) [7–9]. After defects due to a fracture or traumatically deformed juxta-articular shaft the localization for a supra- or infracondylar correction osteotomy is nearly always fixed [7, 9]. Furthermore, the principal differentiation to be made is that between subtraction procedures, which involve taking out a wedge, and osteo-

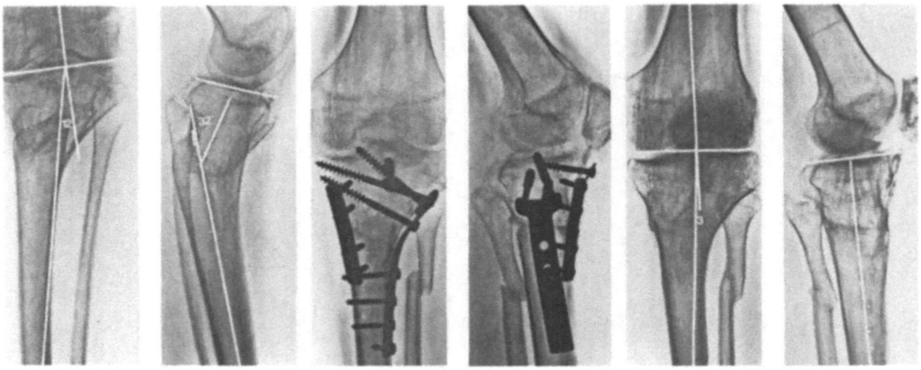

a b c

Figure 3a–c. Correction osteotomy of the head of the tibia in two planes with internal fixation in a 19-year-old man after a motorcycle accident. **a** X-ray 11 months after accident, showing the necessary correction of a tibial head deformity in two planes. **b** Tibial head osteotomy in correct axial position and stabilization by internal fixation. **c** At 4 years after correction, correct axial conditions in two planes, insignificant arthrosis, free functioning of the knee, no subjective symptoms

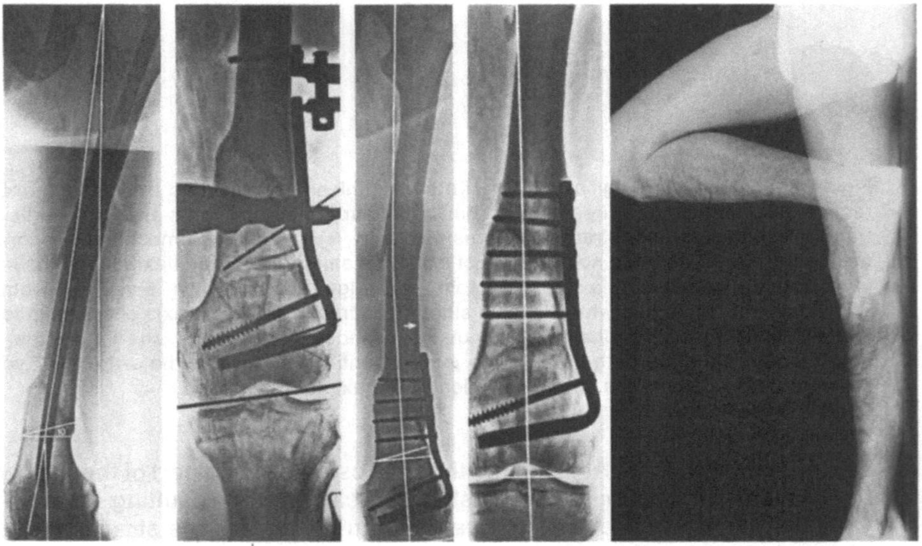

a b c d

Figure 4a–d. Example of a supracondylar correction osteotomy for traumatic malposition. **a** Supracondylar valgus deformity of 10 ° after intramedullary nailing in another hospital of a fracture in two layers of the femur. **b** Intraoperative X-ray to check the axial position after lateral interposition of a cancellous bone graft, stabilization by internal fixation with condylar angle plate and interfragmentary compression. **c** Correction in right axial position 2 months after operation. **d** Radiological and clinical result with correct axial position of the legs and free function 2 years after operation

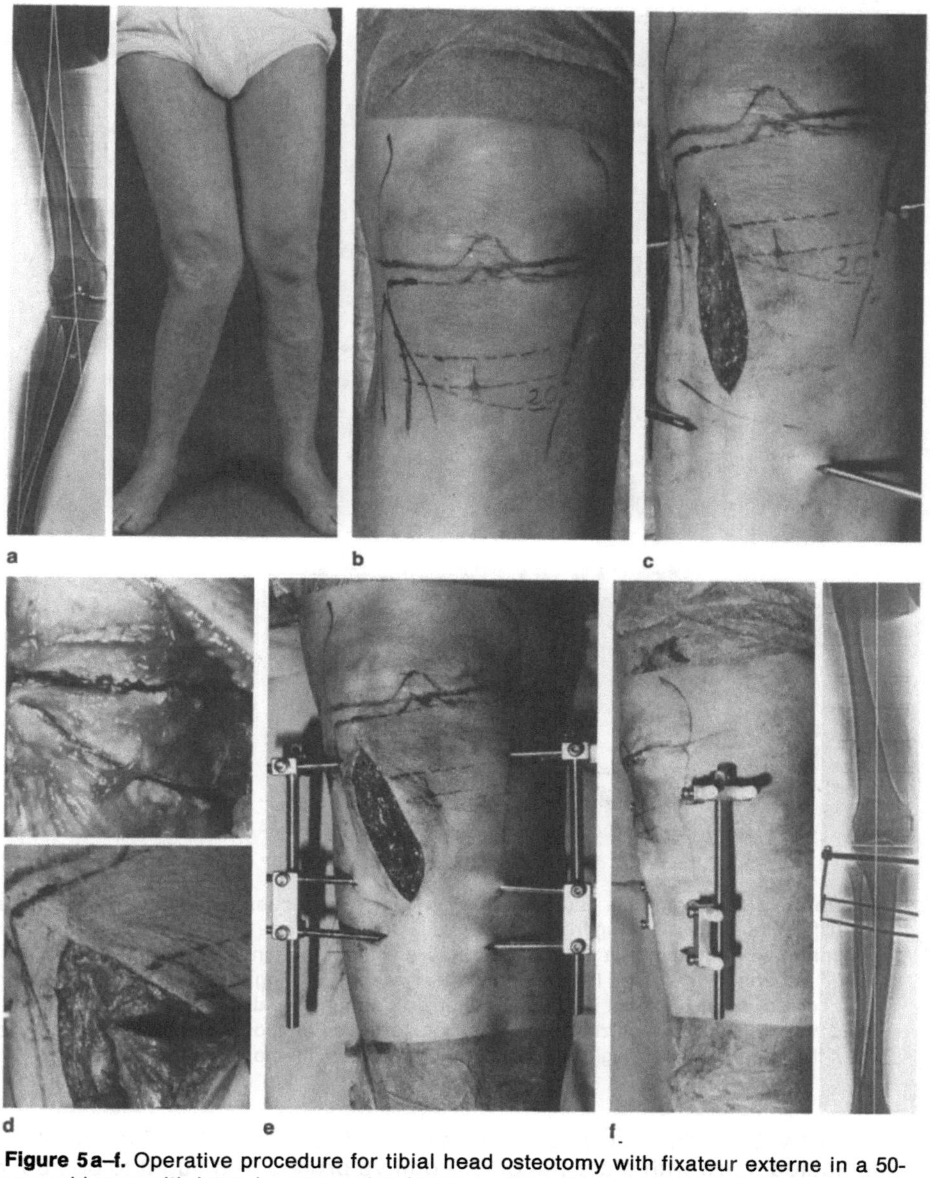

Figure 5a–f. Operative procedure for tibial head osteotomy with fixateur externe in a 50-year-old man with lateral compression fracture of the tibia after trivial distortion 4 years before start of treatment. **a** Long X-rays of the leg and clinical presentation of the valgus deformity of 20 °. **b** X-ray image converter allows joint cavity and positions of Steinmann nails to be marked with a coloured pencil. **c** The Steinmann nails are inserted proximal to the osteotomy, parallel to the articular surface of the head of the tibia and distal to the osteotomy according to the valgus deformity measured during the preoperative planning. **d** After lateral incision, periosteal marking of the size of the wedge and osteotomy with subtraction of the wedge. **e** Changing the position of the shaft distal to the osteotomy, correction of the deformity, and positioning the fixateur externe with medial compression. **f** Postoperative X-ray with axial conditions and the correct position of the fixateur externe maintained

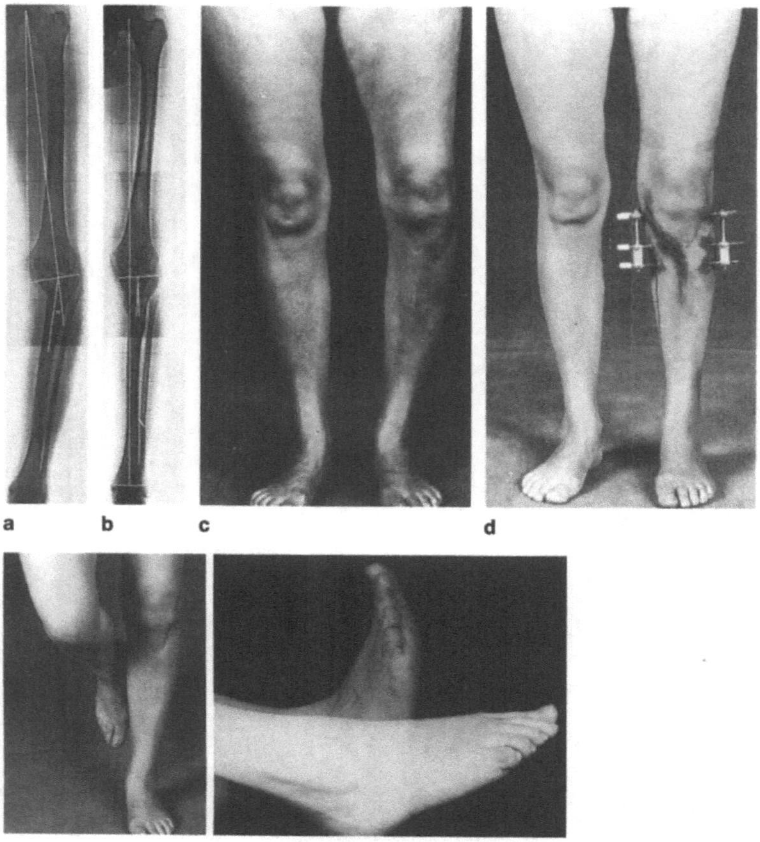

a b c d

e

Figure 6a–e. Example of a causal therapy by early correction osteotomy of a post-traumatic false position resulting from a bicycle accident at the age of 44 years. **a** 7 months after conservative treatment of a tibial head fracture without joint involvement, varus deformity of 15 °. **b** Long X-rays of the leg 9 months after osseous healing of the correction osteotomy with correct axial position. **c** Clinical picture on admission. **d** Clinical picture after tibial head osteotomy and stabilization by fixateur externe. **e** Functional picture with free flexibility of the knee joint, firm leg and no subjective symptoms 9 months after operation

tomies with wedge interposition (Figures 4, 5, 8) [9, 11, 13]. The former are indicated more with older patients. Additive procedures ought to be applied with adolescents, especially if leg shortening is already present. Juxta-articular correction of a diaphyseal axis rotation disturbance is necessary in cases of local defects of the soft tissue or bone infections which inhibit an adjustment in the referring region of the shaft [9, 13]. It must be borne in mind that in contrast to idiopathic false positions, correction operations for a deformation caused by a trauma are often very serious and complex [9]. Thus, on account of the injuries to the knee joint and intra-articular lesions an approximate adjustment of the strain axis can be considered as the therapeutic aim.

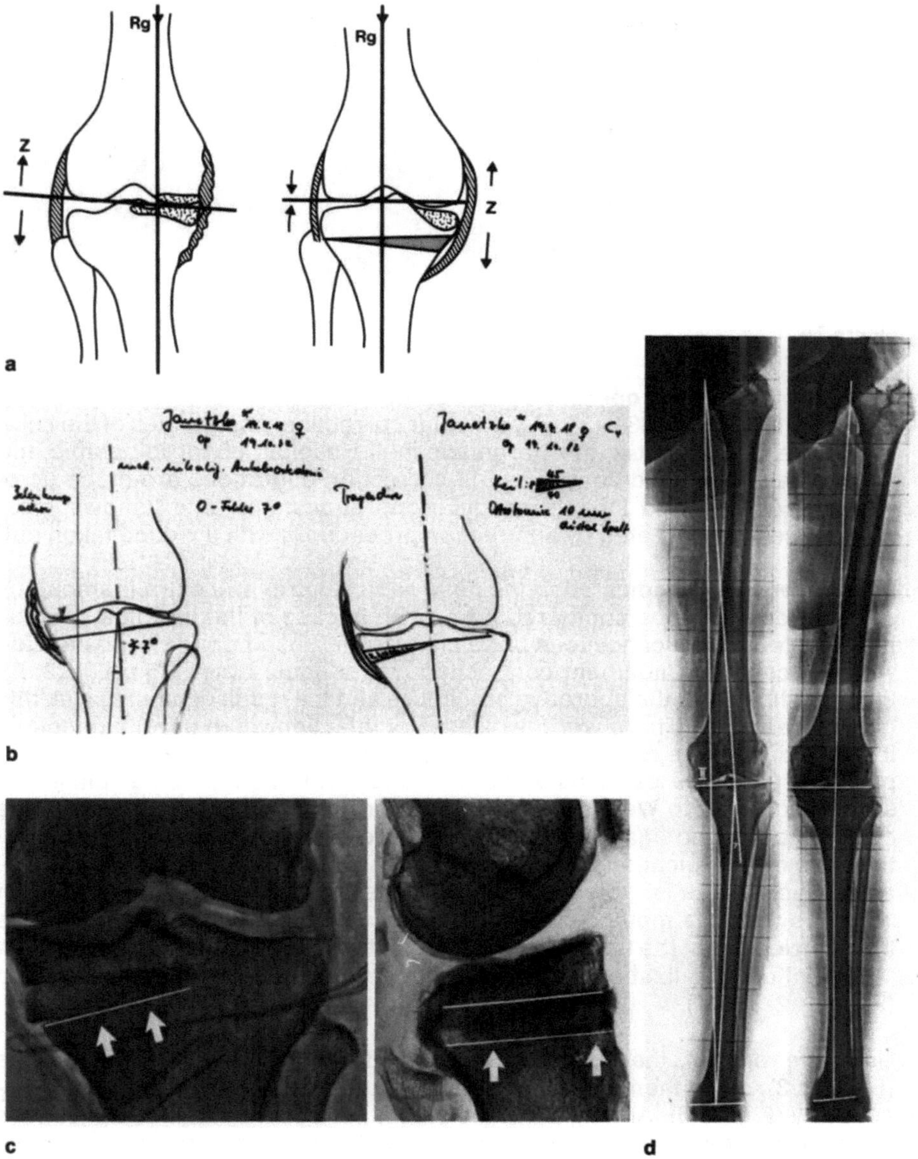

Figure 7 a–e. Radiological planning and planning of the drawing of a tibial head osteotomy using the fixateur externe after malposition in two planes in a 49-year-old man with closed intraarticular fracture of the head of the tibia after falling from scaffolding. **a** Preoperative X-ray showing a valgus deformity of 12° and pathologic inclination of the tibial articular surface of 8° at 7 months after the accident. **b** Planning of the drawing for correction in 2 planes, with marking for the Steinmann nails to be inserted and the size of wedge to be removed. **c** X-ray with fixateur externe, 2 months after operation. **d** Radiological X-ray of the healing with moderate arthrosis owing to post-traumatic deformation of the medial tibial head plateau. **e** Clinical and functional picture with undisturbed flexibility and no symptoms 1 year after operation

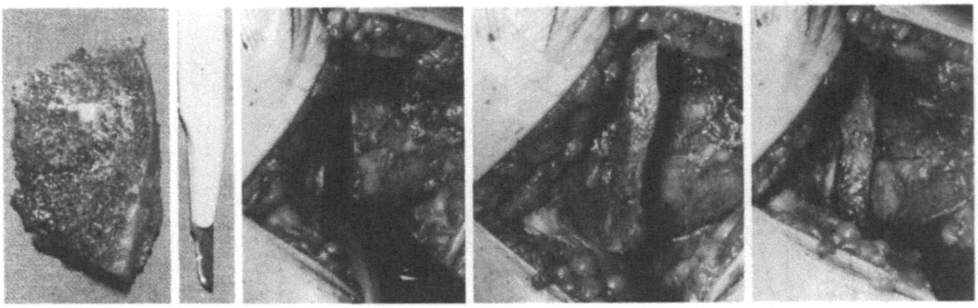

Figure 7e

Number of cases and operation procedures
Between 1972 and 1983 213 juxta-articular correction osteotomies of the knee joint were carried out in the Bergmannsheil Hospital, 86 for idiopathic and 127 for traumatic conditions. The 213 correction operations are made up of 59 supracondylar and 115 infracondylar operations. As Table 1 shows, most of the cases were treated by subtraction procedures with a wedge taken out.

If the *osteotomy* is indicated *in the tibial region*, intra- and extraligamentous procedures should be compared [2, 3, 5–8]. In case of the intraligamentous linear osteotomy a cancellous bone cleft is interposed on the concave side with the collateral ligament contracting at the same time (Figure 8) [2, 9]. Figure 8 illustrates the operative procedure and the result of healing with this type of treatment. There were two cases of infection when intraligamentous interpositions were carried out; in one case the infection progressed to empyema articuli. We use tension band fixation with a semitubular plate and screw according to Weber to make a further procedure unnecessary in the case of contracted ligaments; this procedure is juxta-articular, but subtractive. The main indication is varus gonarthrosis of the head of the tibia [2, 11], and its advantage is the simple operation technique. We have operated on 14 cases with this method. The second main type of tibial osteotomy is the type carried out at the tibial head very close to the tuberosity of the tibia [6–8, 11, 13]. For stabilization internal and external instruments can be used (Figures 2, 3, 5–7).

Until the end of the 1970s we preferred internal fixation with plates (Figures 3), since then the small external fixator was generally applied successfully (Figure 5). Among 54 cases of fixation treatment the complications encountered were peroneal lesions (2 cases), knee joint empyema (1), controllable irritation of the Steinmann nail canals (8), and canal osteomyelitis (1). Fixation with plates is more ambitious with regard to the operation technique; it does not allow any postoperative correction, and healing is more likely to be problematic. In this collective of 47 cases we had the following complications: local wound healing disturbances (10 cases), knee joint empyema (1) and tibial head osteomyelitis (1), which led to an amputation in 1977.

Osteotomies of the supracondylar femur necessitate a very delicate operation technique and particularly careful handling of the soft tissue

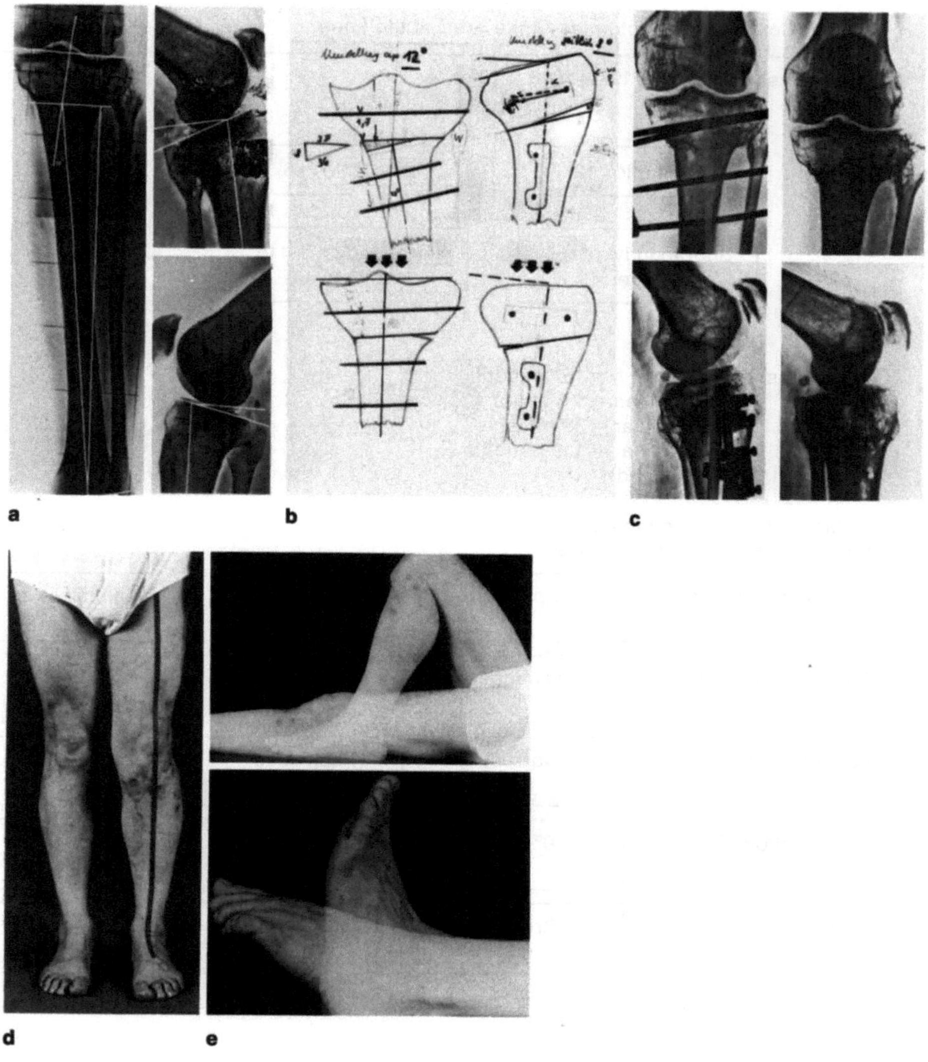

Figure 8 a–e. Planning of the drawing and radiological planning of an intraligamentous linear osteotomy in a 62-year-old woman after an accident. **a** The principle of the intraligamentous linear osteotomy presented in a diagram showing the interposition of a wedge on the concave side and simultaneous tightening of the unstable ligaments. **b** Preoperative drawing of the individual case. **c** Postoperative X-ray in two planes after interposition of the wedge, which is previously exactly determined concerning its size and shape, no osteosynthesis. **d** Pre- and postoperative long X-rays of the leg; reconstruction of the physiological axial positions, free flexibility, tightning of the inner longitudinal ligament. **e** Site of the operation in steps: taking out and preparing the wedge, intraligamentous osteotomy 1 cm distal to the medial tibia head console, cautious opening of the osteotomy cleft, interposition of the prepared cancellous bone graft and advancement of the wedge to its final impacting position

Table 1. Correction osteotomies in the area of the knee

Bergmannsheil Hospital 1972–1983: 213 cases

Traumatic: 127	Idiopathic: 86
Supracondylar: 59 Additive: 19	Infracondylar: 115 Additive: 68

a

Follow-up
Bergmannsheil Hospital, $n = 157$ patients
Mean = 5.6 years after operation
Supracondylar = 38 patients
Infracondylar = 119 patients
(Tibial head)

b

Results of tibial osteotomies[a]
Bergmannsheil Hospital, $n = 119$

Subjective patients:	Optimal 73	Satisfactory 25	Unsatisfactory 21
Gait (Distance normal):	Unchanged 81	Limping 27	Limping + aid 11
Axis on X-ray:	Correct 94	Fault ⩽ 10° 10	Fault > 10° 5
Joint function:	0°–0°–> 120° 77	0°–10°–< 120°–90° 24	0°–20°–~ 90° 12
Arthrosis:	Grade I 66	Grade II 33	Grade III + IV 20

(Figures 1a, 4) [9, 13]. Consistent physiotherapy prevents functional impairment. A medial access route is often selected for supracondylar correction of a valgus disturbance, but is unfavourable because of its proximity to the vessels and the traumatic and scar pain on the extremely sensitive inner side of the femur, but also because of adipose soft tissue susceptible to poor healing [13]. These difficulties were also encountered with valgus disturbance when lateral approach and lateral positioning of the implant were selected, which meant that a wedge was taken out on the medial side by a supracondylar open wedge osteotomy (Figure 4) [9]. The complications seen with this procedure were wound healing disturbances (4 cases), osteomyelitis without empyema articuli (1 case), pseudarthrosis (4 cases). Overall, the most serious complications among 213 knee joint osteotomies were an empyema rate of 1.9% and the amputation mentioned above.

Table 1 (continued)

c

Results of suprakondylare osteotomies[b]
Bergmannsheil Hospital, $n=38$

Subjective (patients):	Optimal 31	Satisfactory 5	Unsatisfactory 2
Gait (Distance normal):	Unchanged 29	Limping 7	Limping + aid 2
Axis on X-ray:	Correct 18	Fault ⩽10°	Fault >10° 11
Joint function:	0°–0°–>120° 25	0°–10°–<120–90° 8	0°–20°–~90° 5
Arthrosis:	Grade 0–I 8	Grade II 22	Grade III + IV 8

d

The character of the hospital meant that traumatic axis deformities predominated, most of which were corrected at the tibial head and by subtractive wedge osteotomy.
Follow-up examinations performed up to early 1984 have been taken into account.
[a] Late results were subjectively assessed as optimal by only 61% of patients, and gait and walking distance as unchanged in 68%. The axis of main force was correct in 79%, and function of the knee joint was largely free in 65%, though severe gonarthrosis followed post-traumatic damage in 17%.
[b] Late results were subjectively assessed as optimal by 80% of patients and the walking distance as unchanged in 76%. In contrast, perfect correction of the axis was achieved only in 47%, the joint functioned freely in 66%, and gonarthrosis recognizable on X-ray as severe was present in 21%.

Results

At the beginning of 1984, after an average postoperative interval of 5.6 years, we re-examined 157 patients, of whom 38 had undergone supracondylar and 119 infracondylar surgical correction (Table 1b). As we expected, the traumatic lesions generally had a worse final outcome. In the case of *tibial head osteotomies* (Table 1c) the result was subjectively assessed as optimal by 73 patients and as satisfactory by 25. The gait was reported as unaltered and the distance it was possible to walk as scarcely reduced by 81 patients. Of the remaining 38 patients, 11 needed a walking aid. Radiological examination indicated that 94 extremities had been adjusted to the correct axis, but 5 patients had a postoperative axis disturbance of more than 10 °. Free extension and flexion up to 120 ° or more were achieved by 77 patients. An unsatisfactory proportion of patients (12) had reduced maximum extension up to 20 °. After tibial osteotomy the arthrosis frequently became worse in spite of clinically continuous subjective and objective improvement. Among the patients who had undergone *supracondylar correction* (Table 1d), 31 of 38 were satisfied, and 29 expressed their satisfaction with an unlimited walking distance. After supracondylar correction osteotomy flexion was good in all cases; only 5 patients had reduced extension of 20 °. Postoperative axis disturbances by more than 10 ° resulted in 11 cases, including 9 with post-traumatic treatment.

References

1. Debrunner AM (1970) Die operative Behandlung von Gonarthrosen. In: Nicod L (ed) Die Gonarthrosen. Huber, Berne
2. Dolanc B (1973) Die Behandlung des instabilen Kniegelenkes mit Achsenfehlstellung durch intraligamentäre Anhebe-Tibiaosteotomie. Arch Orthop Unfallchir 76:280–289
3. Frank W, Oest O, Rettig H (1974) Die Röntgenganzaufnahme in der Operationsplanung von Korrekturosteotomie der Beine. Z Orthop 112:344–347
4. Maquet P (1976) Biomechanics of the knee. Springer, Berlin Heidelberg New York
5. Maquet P (1979) Korrekturosteotomien in der Behandlung der Kniearthrose. Orthopade 8:296–308
6. Müller KH (1979) Prinzipien kniegelenknaher Umstellungs-Osteotomien – gestern und heute. Acta Traumatol 9:127–133
7. Müller KH, Biebrach M (1977 a) Korrekturosteotomien und ihre Ergebnisse bei kniegelenknahen posttraumatischen Fehlstellungen. Unfallheilkunde 80:359–367
8. Müller KH, Biebrach M (1977 b) Korrekturosteotomien und ihre Ergebnisse bei idiopathischen kniegelenknahen Achsenfehlstellungen. Unfallheilkunde 80:457–464
9. Müller KH, Müller-Färber J (1984) Indikation, Lokalisation und Planung knienaher Osteotomien nach Traumen. In: Hierholzer G, Müller KG (eds) Korrekturosteotomien nach Traumen an der unteren Extremität. Springer, Berlin Heidelberg New York
10. Müller ME (1970) Posttraumatische Achsenfehlstellungen an der unteren Extremität. Huber, Berne
11. Müller W (1976) Die Tibia-Osteotomie in der Therapie posttraumatischer Arthrosen am Kniegelenk. Hefte Unfallheilkd 128:175–181
12. Oest O (1978) Die Achsenfehlstellung als präarthrotische Deformität für das Kniegelenk und die röntgenologischen Beinachsenbeurteilung. Unfallheilkunde 81:629–633
13. Wagner H (1976) Indikation und Technik der Korrekturosteotomien bei der posttraumatischen Kniegelenkarthrose. Hefte Unfallheilkd 128:155–174

A blade plate for high tibial osteotomies

G. Giebel and H. Tscherne

Unfallchirurgische Klinik d. Medizinischen Hochschule Hannover
3000 Hannover
Federal Republic of Germany

Introduction
Jackson reported in 1961 on a large series of successful osteotomies of the upper tibia. Since that time the high tibial osteotomy has become an established procedure for the treatment of idiopathic and post-traumatic valgus and varus deformities of the lower extremity. Boitzy, Coventry, Engelhardt, Haas, Insall, and Rutt state that the wedge-resection osteotomy should not be carried completely through the opposite cortex so that the cortex-periosteal envelope will be preserved on one side as a stabilizing structure. In that way it can act as a hinge for closing the osteotomy. The associated tension-band effect provides additional stability.

Weber stabilizes his osteotomies with a semitubular plate and a cortex screw. The semitubular plate is flattened, driven into the bone laterally above the osteotomy site, and anchored distally with a lag screw to exert compression across the osteotomy.

Material and method
Because it has been our experience that the semitubular plate is not easily driven into bone and does not stabilize the osteotomy securely enough for early postoperative function, we developed an implant designed to give greater stability. The device is a blade plate with two screw holes placed closely adjacent to each other to conserve space (Figure 1). The limb is not placed in a cast postoperatively and can bear full weight at 8–10 weeks.

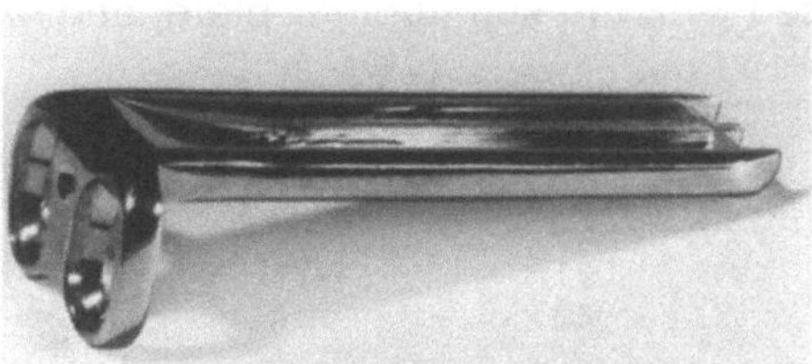

Figure 1

Operating technique
An anterolateral skin incision is made with the knee flexed 90 ° (Figure 2). The peroneus nerve is exposed, and the seating chisel is driven in through the lateral cortex, parallel and close to the tibial articular surface.

An incomplete bony wedge is removed, leaving the medial cortex intact, and the osteotomy surfaces are apposed. The posterior cortex is osteotomized

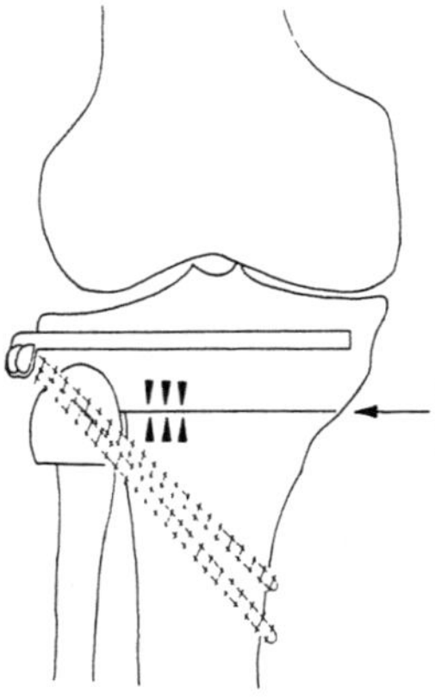

Figure 2

distally but not proximally and thus overrides the cortex of the distal fragment. A Bandi effect is created by advancement of the tibial tuberosity.

The blade plate is driven into the prepared bed and anchored with two long cortex screws that are angled distally.

Clinical material

Of the 72 patients who underwent high tibial osteotomies, 63 were available for follow-up. The average patient age at operation was 58 years (Table 1).

Table 1. Clinical material

Operated	73 knee joints
Followed	63 knee joints
Age at operation	Average 58 years (22–81 years)

Twenty-one osteotomies were stabilized with the semitubular plate, and 42 with the blade plate (Table 2).

Table 2. Distribution of internal fixations

Semitubular plate	21 ×
Blade plate	42 ×

Three hematomas had to be evacuated postoperatively in each group. Three infections and two nonunions in two unstable fixations resolved after revisionary fixation was carried out.

Results

At follow-up we were struck by the numerous cases of recurrent varus deformity following use of the semitubular plate (Table 3). The incidence was 16 times greater than with the blade plate.

Table 3. Recurrent varus deformity at follow-up

	Patients	%
Semitubular plate (n=21)	7	33
Blade plate (n=42)	1	2

Seventy-six percent of the patients treated with the blade plate rated their result as excellent or good, as opposed to 67% of those treated with the semitubular plate (Table 4).

Table 4. Rating of results by the patients

	Group 1 (n=21)	Group 2 (n=42)
Excellent or good	14 (67%)	32 (76%)
Fair	4 (19%)	6 (14%)
Poor	3 (14%)	4 (10%)

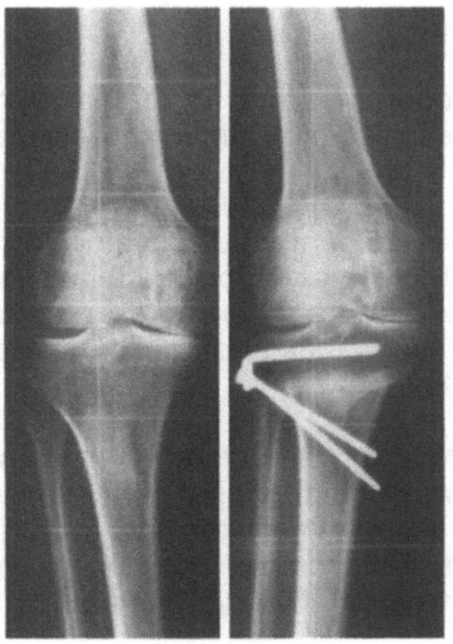

Figure 3. High tibial osteotomy stabilized with the blade plate in a 62-year-old man. Radiographic appearance before and after surgery

Discussion

The blade plate, in contrast to T plates, double plates and metal brackets, does not interfere with joint motion when used on the supratubercular corrective osteotomy. Once the osteotomy has united, the implant loses its biomechanical effect and function and causes no stress protection.

Only a small part of the implant is extraosseous. This is consistent with the dimensional constraints of the lateral aspect of the upper tibia and with its thin soft-tissue covering.

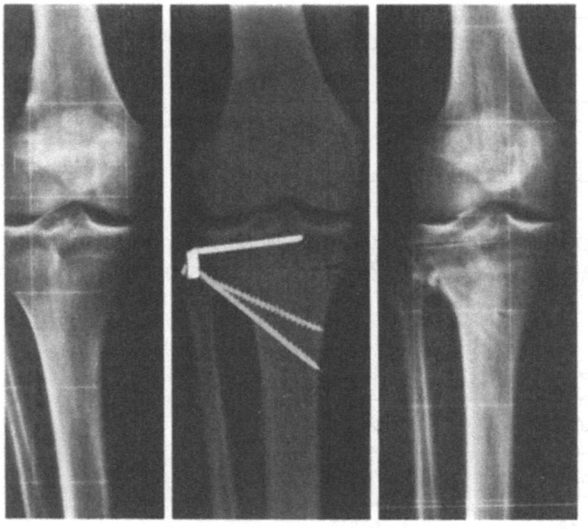

Figure 4. Ten-degree valgus correction stabilized with the blade plate in a 22-year-old man. Appearance before, immediately after, and 22 months after surgery. The final radiograph shows a physiologic degree of valgus

Older patients in particular are better able to cope with this internal, motion-stable fixation than with an external fixation device, which also requires special nursing care.

The blade plate is easier to drive into bone than the semitubular plate, which is not designed for that purpose. It can compress the osteotomy with two lag screws. Casting is not needed postoperatively to maintain the correction. The blade plate provides a strong and dynamic stabilization of the supratubercular closed wedge osteotomy.

It will be noted that the blade is positioned away from the osteotomy line and parallel to the articular surface. The lag screws should be angled as far distally as possible. Tightening of the screws should be moderated only in cases where compression is so strong that the lateral distal cortex impacts into the cancellous bone of the overriding proximal fragment. Overtightening in this case would lead to valgus deformity.

We recommend this technique because it combines technical simplicity with reliable and effective stabilization, it obviates the need for plaster fixation, and its results are good.

The V-shaped diacondylar osteotomy of the femur

G. Korisek

Unfallkrankenhaus Kalwang
Kalwang
Austria

The V-shaped osteotomy in the plane of the "true angle" has proven in our hands to be a very easy and safe technique to correct deformities of long bones. Encouraged by the good results, we developed the technique of diaconylar V-shaped osteotomy for the correction of knee deformities, to treat or to prevent gonarthrosis.

Technique
A longitudinal skin incision of 8 cm is done in correspondence to the distal end for the femur – medially in case of genu valgum, laterally in case of genu varum. The dissection of soft tissues is done along the intermuscular septum, and the distal femoral metaphysis is protected by two Hohmann levers. With the oscillating bone saw a V-shaped cut is performed through the mass of the condyles. The ridge of the osteotomy has to be placed in the plane of the true deviation and towards the epiphysis. Once the bone, is dissected the position wanted can easily be obtained by simply swinging the fragments; osteosynthesis is not necessary. After drainage without suction and skin closure, a plaster tutor is given. 8 days after surgery the patient has to walk fully weightbearing, and 6 weeks after the operation the plaster is removed (Figures 1, 2).

Material and results
Since 1968 we performed 36 diacondylar osteotomies; in 27 of those we corrected a valgus deformity, in 9 a varus deformity. In 25 of our cases the deviation was subse-

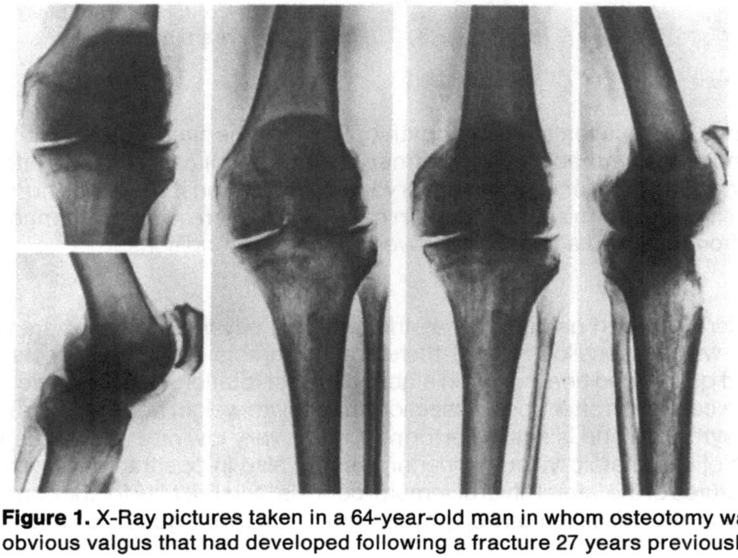

Figure 1. X-Ray pictures taken in a 64-year-old man in whom osteotomy was performed for obvious valgus that had developed following a fracture 27 years previously

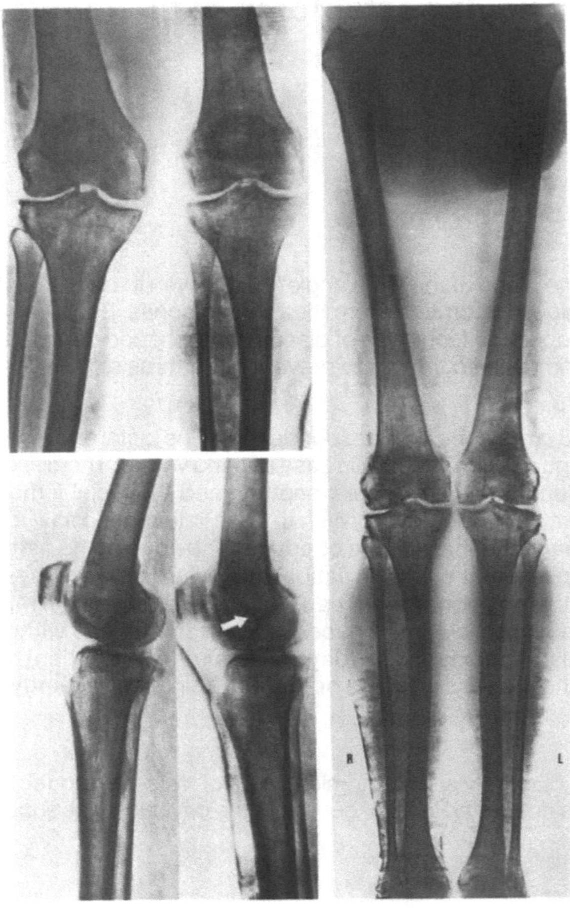

Figure 2. X-Ray pictures taken in a 74-year-old woman in whom osteotomy (*arrow*) was performed for painful genu valgum that had developed following fracture of the lateral tibial condyle 4 years before

quent to trauma, in 11 cases it was idiopathic. Besides the first 4 cases with K-wire fixation, no osteosynthesis was performed. In none of our cases had we either an infection or a non-union, or vascular or nervous complications. There was no loss in the range of motion. Contrarily we found in cases with severe arthritic changes a good release from pain and a notable improvement of joint conditions.

Conclusions

The diacondylar V-shaped osteotomy has the following advantages: great area of bone contact within cancellous bone, therefore favourable biological effects of osteotomy and quick bone healing, good stability against rotation, but free choice of the angle of the correction after bone dissection, immediate weight bearing, does not require osteosynthesis and is easily performed with a very low rate of risks. Especially in cases of rheumatoid valgus gonarthrosis, but also in posttraumatic genua valga after fractures of the lateral tibial or femoral condyle, and likewise for the correction of deviations after distal femoral epiphyseal arrest, there is a good indication for this method.

Bone scintigraphy of the knee after valgus osteotomy

V. Pietrogrande[1,2], *F. Motta*[1], *M. Ulivi*[1], *S. Cusimano*[1], *E. Savoldi*[2], *L. Recanatini*[2], *and L. Tosca*[2]

[1] **Institute of Clinical Orthopaedics, University of Milan, Italy**
[2] **Department of Nuclear Medicine, Istituti Clinici di Perfezionamento, Milan, Italy**

Introduction

Bone scintigraphy with [^{99m}Tc]methylene-diphosphonate (MDP) is conventionally used in orthopaedics in different situations (Subramanian 1971; Bauer 1968; Lull 1983). Its optimal use is to search for metastatic or neoplastic lesions of the bone that cannot be detected by radiography, in cases of osteonecrosis and infections of various kinds, and in the study of fracture healing processes and pseudoarthrosis evolution.

The recently introduced diphosphonates bind with the bone's hydroxyapatite crystals direct (Jung 1973). In 1973, Yano evidenced their direct relationship with local vascularization, while Kayen (1975) and Rosenthall (1975, 1976) demonstrated that diphosphonates bind with the organic matrix of the bone, for which they appear to have strong affinity.

Independently of its clinical applications, bone scintigraphy with [^{99m}Tc]-MDP is always positive in high metabolism zones, and a positive scintigraphic response is found where the bone tissue is active.

In the light of these considerations, we decided to use [^{99m}Tc]MDP scintigraphy to investigate the biomechanical imbalances of the knee, and specifically to study the overload zones before and after tibial valgus osteotomy.

An excess load causes the bone's local metabolism to increase; when applied gradually and progressively, it induces the apposition of new mineral, which coincides with radiographic sclerosis, while when localized it leads to bone reabsorption phenomena.

In 1970, Koscino evaluated how the formation of a bone callus after tibial valgus osteotomy is affected by a specific axial deviation of the knee. Koscino writes that pressure on the bone accelerates the formation of bone tissue; therefore, when valgus osteotomy does not fully correct a varus condition, the bone callus will form earlier medially, while an excessive valgus condition will cause it to grow laterally.

On this basis we submitted to scintigraphic examination some varus or valgus knees that were characterized by typical overload zones. Excess uptake always occurred medially, in the subchondral condylic zone of a varus knee and laterally in a valgus knee (Figures 1–3).

We found that the more biomechanically effective tibial valgus osteotomy is in correcting the knee's axial deviation, the more negative is scintigraphy,

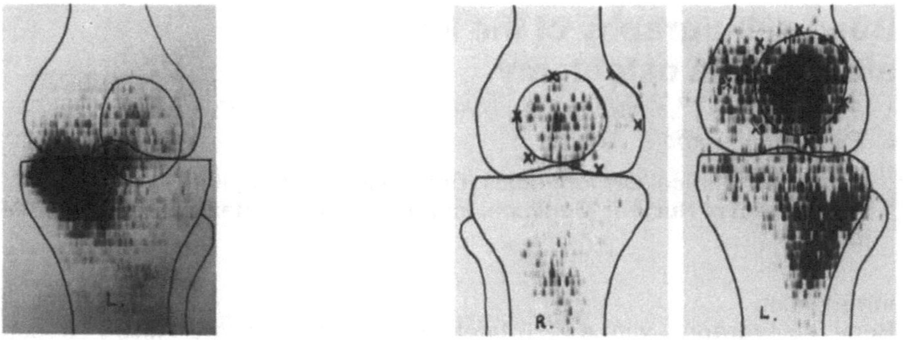

Figures 1. Sixty-three-year-old woman. Severe varus condition in the left knee: 12 ° at the radiographic measurement of the femoral-tibial axis. Evident gonarthrosis with subchondral sclerosis and medial joint space narrowing. Sharp gonalgia also at rest. Bone scintigraphy with [^{99m}TC]MDP shows evident medial uptake, especially on the tibial condyle. Scintigraphic image of a varus knee

thereby proving that the medial overload has disappeared. Similarly, excessive valgus correction causes the overload to shift from a medial to a lateral position, as clearly shown by external pathological uptake, thereby reversing the problem.

We maintain that [^{99m}Tc]MDP bone scintigraphy detects overload-caused lesions which remain radiographically and clinically undetected; it can therefore be greatly useful for the diagnosis and prognosis of such lesions.

The examination may turn out as positive earlier than the radiographic data or clinical picture, as bone hypervascularization and the initial formation of organic matrix can make scintigraphy positive before the build-up of a radiographically detectable mineral deposit (sclerosis). Moreover, a positive scintigraphic report does not necessarily correspond to a clear-cut clinical picture, instead of which it can precede this.

We scanned the knees of 20 patients who had undergone tibial valgus osteotomy, to assess the change of femoral-tibial loads resulting from the operation.

With the same angle we also investigated the patello-femoral joint, as this too, when overloaded, exhibits typical, scintigraphically visible build-up.

Materials and methods

Twenty patients who had undergone valgus osteotomy for varus knee were examined, all of them after a minimum of 1 year and 8 years from the operation. This was done to prevent identification by scintigraphy of any metaphyseal excess uptake due to the onset of bone callus, which could hide the excess uptake caused by biomechanical overload on the condylar bone.

Having delayed the examination by at least 1 year after the operation, the knee load distribution had time to adjust from varus to postoperative conditions.

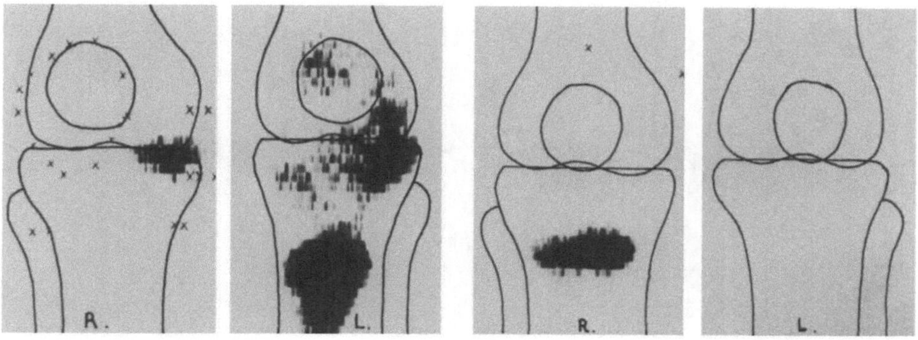

Figure 2. Seventeen-year-old woman. Bilateral valgus knee condition, more severe (8 °) on the left knee. Positive [^{99m}Tc]MDP bone scintigraphy with external excess uptake area, chiefly on the tibial condyle. Scintigraphic image of a valgus knee. Patellofemoral uptake due to displacement of the extensor apparatus

Every patient was also assessed by radiography of the knee and lower limbs under load and by the measurement of the femoral-tibial axis. A detailed clinical evaluation was also performed. The scintigraphic protocol involved the use of [^{99m}Tc]MDP intravenously, with imaging performed 3 h later; all the knees were imaged by linear scanner. For 80% of the patients the clinical picture after the operation had decidedly improved. However, radiography showed satisfactory correction of the mechanical axis in only 50% of the operated knees; the other 50% still suffered from a varus condition albeit slighter.

In the latter cases, scintigraphy was consistently positive with a pathological medial uptake, while it was negative for the radiographically correct cases.

In the knees we observed, the valgus condition was more frequently associated with secondary disaxation of the extensor apparatus. However, when the patellofemoral joint was affected, scintigraphy showed significant local excess uptake. The seriousness of the clinical picture does not seem to correspond to the positivity of the scintigraphic report. Hereunder are three clinical cases:

Case 1. Twenty-five-year-old male, affected by bilateral varus knee, submitted to right valgus osteotomy 2 years ago and to left osteotomy 1 year ago. At present pain is absent and the lower limbs are radiographically in axis. The scintigraphic examination of both knees was negative and confirms the success of the operation. Excess uptake in the right tibial tuberosity is justified by intolerance to recently removed staples.

Case 2. Sixty-six-year-old women, suffering from severe (11 °) bilateral varus knee. Left tibial valgus osteotomy performed in 1979. At present, there is 11 ° varus condition in the right knee and 9 ° in the left knee: insufficient surgical correction. Scintigraphy of January 1984: bilateral pathological uptake at the medial tibial condylic level; note the scintigraphic confirmation of the right knee varus condition and persistent varus condition in the left knee. Slight

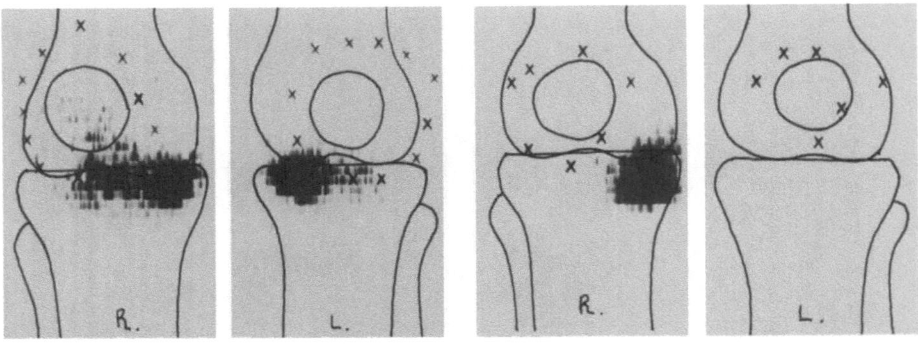

Figure 3. Seventy-year-old woman with right varus knee and symptomatic left valgus knee. Evident uptake on the medial side of the rigt knee and on the lateral side of the left knee. The uptake under the left tibial tuberosity indicates the healing process of a 1-month-old varus osteotomy. The patellofemoral joint disease, secondary to the valgus condition of the knee, is clearly shown by the high uptake

pain symptoms in the treated knee; sharp pains in the right knee, even at rest.

Case 3. Forty-five-year-old male with right varus knee, previously operated on for tibial valgus osteotomy. A residual varus is scintigraphically evidenced by uptake at the medial side of the knee.

Discussion

The analysis performed by us on 20 patients who had undergone valgus osteotomy of the knee shows that bone scintigraphy is a highly specific examination for the topographic diagnosis of residual overload lesions. This overload is medial in a varus knee and lateral in a valgus knee. Scintigraphy proved to be significant for precise localization. We therefore believe that bone scintigraphy with [^{99m}Tc]MDP could also be used for the diagnosis of axial deviations of the knee, especially when the clinical and radiographic pictures are typical. Instead, we suggest that radiography of the lower limbs under load only be performed later, to measure the degrees of deviation and select the surgical treatment.

It should be noted that medial or lateral condylar or patellofemoral, joint excess uptake in knees without neoplastic, inflammatory or traumatic pathologies occurs only under biomechanical conditions of imbalance.

References

Bauer GCH (1968) The use of radionuclides in orthopaedics: 4. Radionuclide scintimetry of the skeleton. J Bone Joint Surg [Am] 50:1681–1707

Jung A, Bisaz S, Fleisch H (1973) The binding of pyrophosphate and two diphosphonates by hydroxyapatite crystals. Calc Tissue Res 11:269–280

Kayen M, Silverton S, Rosenthall L (1975) Technetium 99m-pyrophosphate: studies in vivo and in vitro. J Nucl Med 16:40–45

Koshino T, Ranawat NS (1970) Effect of mechanical factors on bone metabolism in man. Strontium-85 scintimetry following osteotomy of the tibiae in gonarthrosis. Calc Tissue Res 4:159–160

Lull R (1983) Radionuclide evaluation of joint disease. Nucl Med Ann
Maquet PGJ (1976) Biomechanics of the knee. Springer, Berlin Heidelberg New York
Rosenthall L (1975) Technetium-99m pyrophosphate kinetics and imaging in metabolic bone disease. J Nucl Med 16:33–39
Rosenthall L (1976) Observations on the mechanism of 99m-Tc labelled phosphate complex uptake in metabolic bone disease. Semin Nucl Med 6:59–67
Subramanian G, McAfee JG, O'Mara R, Rosenstreich M, Mether A (1971) 99m-Tc polyphosphate PP46: a new radiopharmaceutical for skeletal imaging. J Nucl Med 12:399–400
Yano Y, McRae J, Vandyke DC, Anger HO (1973) Technetium 99m-labelled stannous ethane-1-hydroxy-1,1-diphosphonate: a new bone scanning agent. J Nucl Med 14:73–78

Knee-joint Replacements

Evolution of knee replacement at The London Hospital

M. A. R. Freeman

The London Hospital Whitechapel
London E1
England

The first prosthesis for the replacement of the knee used at The London Hospital was designed in 1969 and implanted in 1970. The prosthesis consisted of a cobalt-chrome component cemented to the distal femur which articulated as a roller in a trough with a high density polyethylene component cemented to the proximal tibia. The cruciate ligaments and the patella were resected. In 1971 the design was slightly modified to the Freeman/Swanson design and the patella was thereafter retained. The complications associated with this prosthesis were reported (1978) and will be briefly recapitulated. The modifications suggested by this experience were incorporated into the Freeman/Swanson prosthesis over the period between 1971 to 1976.

By 1976 the possibility had arisen of implanting a prosthesis without cement and accordingly the method of tibial fixation was modified to form the ICLH prosthesis. The results of cementless fixation of the tibial component were reported (1982): it was shown that the loosening rate and the symptomatic state of the knee without cement was no different to that obtained with cement. Since it was felt that cementless fixation offered certain advantages, the cementless procedure was applied over the years 1977 to 1980 to the other two components of the joint.

Experience with the ICLH prosthesis proved it to have two disadvantages: firstly the replaced patella subluxed laterally in 5 % of knees because there was no anterior midline groove in the anterior flange. Secondly flexion tended to be limited to about 90° because the articular surface of the tibia was too anterior, whilst the posterior lip of the component was too large. These defects were eliminated in the Freeman/Samuelson prosthesis which was first implanted in 1980. The results obtained using the Freeman/Samuelson prosthesis will be presented.

In certain circumstances, for example in revision surgery and in the presence of material bone defects it is desirable to use a metal backed tibial component and to attach both the tibial and femoral components to metal stems. Such implants are available in the Freeman/Samuelson system and their mode of use will be briefly discussed.

It is the authors view that the outcome of knee replacement is more closely dependent upon the operative procedure than upon the details of prostetic design. A successful operative procedure in turn depends upon appropriate instruments. Instrumentation was therefore provided for the Freeman/Swanson prosthesis. The instrumentation has fundamentally improved over the period 1970 to 1976 especially by the addition of a Tenser. In 1977, the instrumentation was co-ordinated into a set. This set proved satisfactory but had an unacceptably complicated appearance. Without altering in any way the principles of the procedure the instrumentation has now been simplified. The appearance and mode of use of the new instrumentation will be briefly discussed.

ICLH arthroplasty of the knee with cementless fixation of the tibial component: A 1–4 year experience

B. E. J. Albrektsson and P. Herberts

Departments of Orthopaedic Surgery, East & Sahlgren Hospitals
Göteborg
Sweden

Knee arthroplasties with non-cemented components have many potential advantages compared with arthroplasties in which cement is used. The results of clinical and radiographic follow-up for 1–4 years with cementless fixation of the ICLH tibial component are presented.

Material and methods

The study is prospective and longitudinal and 108 arthroplasties were performed on 94 patients from May 1978 through May 1982. The diagnosis was RA in 51 patients, primary OA in 41 patients, posttraumatic OA in 2 patients. There were 17 men and 77 women and the mean age for patients with OA was 70.5 years and with RA 57.5 years. Previous operations included osteotomy (6), synovectomy (24) and meniscectomy (3). The patients were evaluated subjectively and objectively in preoperative and postoperative follow ups every year. Radiographs were also taken including a skyline view of patella. Changes in the bone-polyethylene interface around the pegs and on the tibial plateau against the prosthesis were evaluated as well as changes indicating migration. In 6 knees cement was used to fill bone defects in tibia, all the other 102 tibial components were not cemented, while the femoral components were all cemented. Patella was replaced in 52 knees.

Results

Pain was the main indication for surgery and all patients were greatly improved with regard to pain. Only 3 patients had mild pain at rest 1 year postoperatively (2.8%). 2 patients had moderate and 27 mild pain when walking or moving the knee (28.7%). The main reason for this pain at motion was lateral patellar dislocation (25 partial and 20 complete). Preoperative valgus – varus deformity was present in 89 knees (82%), ranging from 40° of valgus to 30° of varus. Postoperatively at 6 months only 9 knees had any significant malalignment up to 10° of valgus or varus. Preoperatively 83% of the knees had flexion deformities ranging from 5-50°. Postoperatively no knee had a flexion deformity greater than 10°.

Early complications were observed in 22 patients (21%), 3 pulmonary embolisms, 1 myocardial infection, 5 transient peroneal nerve paralysis and 5 superficial wound infections. These early complications all resolved. 3 patients died from cardio-vascular disease 3-6 months postoperatively. Late complications were 1 delayed deep infection (after 14 months) and 4 mechanical loosenings. 5 patients (4,6%) were reoperated. Recurrent instability was severe in 2 knees and altogether 6 arthroplasties (5.7%) are failures. The radiographic study revealed tibial component settling in 25 knees (8 OA, 17 RA).

Discussion

The ICLH knee arthroplasty with cementless tibial component fixation gave good results symptomatically and mechanically in this short-term study. The main problem was lateral dislocation of the patella. Settling of the tibial component to some extent also occurred and it is not clear how this method of fixation will function in the long-term. The majority of the radiographic signs of settling have been identified first at 3 or 4-year follow-ups and in patients with progressive RA and poor bone quality.

Summary

108 knee arthroplasties were performed on 94 patients with fixation of the tibial component without cement. The study is prospective and the results of clinical and radiographic follow-up for 1-4 years are good or satisfactory in more than 90%. The radiographic examination, however, revealed changes in the position of the tibial component in 25 knees including 4 loosenings.

Cementless fixation of the Freeman-Samuelson total knee replacement including bone grafting and the use of stemmed components

K. M. Samuelson

Division of Orthopaedic Surgery, LDS Hospital
Salt Lake City, Utah
United States

Cementless fixation of the ICLH Knee, which was the immediate predecessor of the F-S knee, began in 1977. The effectiveness of cementless fixation of total knee components was demonstrated with that prosthesis.

Fully cementless implantation of all three components of a total knee has been performed by the author since 1979. The implantation of prototypes contined into 1980 when the current F-S was first implanted fully cementless. Follow-up on the first 132 knees now ranges from 6 to 36 months. 12 have been lost to follow-up for a variety of reasons thus leaving 110 functioning arthroplasties available for review. Prior to surgery all had moderate to severe pain. All were improved post-op, 57% had no pain and 36% had mild pain. Walking ability was improved in all except two patients in whom it remained unchanged. Range of motion improved in 49%, remained unchanged in 49%, and decreased in 2%. Average range of motion post-op was 110 degrees.

With the ICLH knee the author had a 9% incidence of patellar subluxation or dislocation. In the present F-S series there have been no cases of patellar subluxation, dislocation or fracture.

During the past three years bone grafts have been used increasingly to fill bony defects. The alternative treatments had been to either resect slightly more bone to get a smooth surface for cementless fixation or fill the defect with cement. With small defects bone grafts and the standard components can frequently be used. However, with larger defects it is necessary to use stemmed components to obtain adequate fixation and support for the prosthesis.

All patients with cementless knees, including those with bone grafts, have been allowed immediate full weight-bearing post-op.

McIntosh hemiarthroplasty: long-term results

M. S. Ali[1], *R. J. Crawford*[2] *and M. P. Robinson*[2]

[1] **Institute of Orthopaedics, Oswestry, R.H.A., United Kingdom**
[2] **Institute of Orthopaedics, Merseyside R.H.A., United Kingdom**

We present this paper on McIntosh hemiarthroplasty in two parts:

1. A surgical technique
2. Long-term results

The indications for McIntosh hemiarthroplasty are limited to patients who are sufficiently disabled with pain in the knee that does not respond to thorough conservative treatment and whose X-rays show *partial destruction* irrespective of the diagnosis.

In our view this prosthesis is not suitable if there is:

1. Disorganization of all the compartments
2. Loss of femoral curvature
3. Gross tibial plateau collapse
4. Massive subchondral cyst formation

Surgical technique

At first the original technique described by McIntosh was used. However, complications of wound healing led the senior author (M.P.R.) to develop a surgical technique that we shall describe. We have been unable to discover a description of this surgical technique in the literature.

For the operation the patient is placed supine on the table, under general anaesthesia and the tourniquet is applied. The table is tilted to 30 ° Trendelenberg with 30 ° knee flexion.

Approach

For the medial compartment a 10-cm oblique parapatellar incision is made starting at the level of the upper pole of the patella from a point *P* proximally to a point *D* distally about 2 cm medial to the tibial tubercle. The fascia, capsule and synovium are divided in the line of this incision and dissected off the medial tibial condyle as far as possible.

The joint is cleaned, the meniscus is removed and the femoral condylar osteophytes are resected.

Preparation of the plateau bed

The cuts to be made are marked on the tibial condyle as shown in Figure 1. Using a reciprocating saw the first cut is made just medial to the tibial eminence at an angle of 20 ° to the sagittal plane. Its depth depends upon the ex-

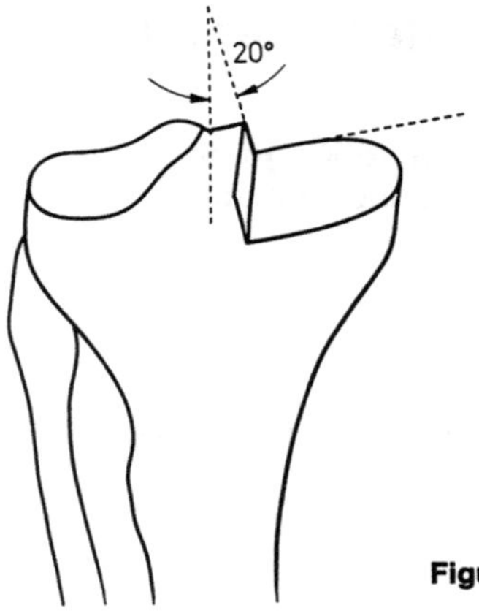

Figure 1. Preparation of tibial plateau

tent of bone destruction and deformity. The second cut is made at right angles to the first. The surface of the tibial plateau is excised preferably in one piece leaving a healthy cancellous bed for the prosthesis. Note the lateral slope of the bed which makes it more stable for the prosthesis, in particular on weight bearing. If the cut is horizontal the prosthesis tends to displace in this situation.

Selection of the prosthesis
A prosthesis is considered suitable if it matches the curve of the femoral condyle and achieves a neutral position of the leg as far as possible. It should be wide enough to fit tightly between the collateral ligament and the tibial eminence and deep enough to avoid tilting during flexion, as in Figure 2. The short prosthesis gets nipped between the tibial and femoral condyles. This does not happen if the prosthesis is deep enough as in this prosthesis, which is just right.

The wound is closed in layers on a suction drain with particular attention to tight closure of the capsule for stability of the prosthesis using monofilament nylon. Finally a Robert Jones bandage was applied. The approach for the lat-

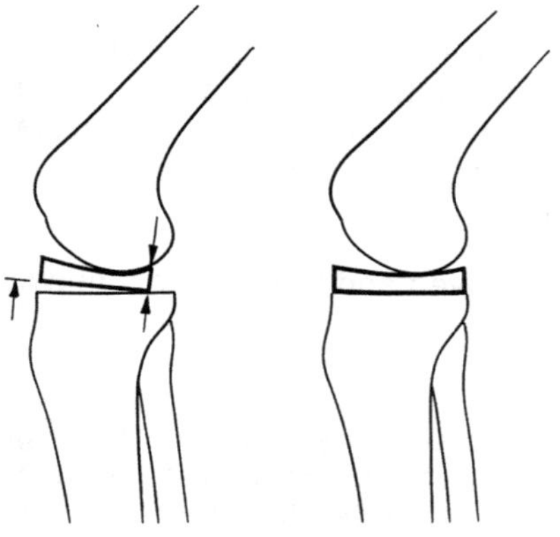

Figure 2. The selection of prosthesis

eral compartment is identical and two such incisions are made for biplateau replacement. When doing biplateau replacement it is advisable first to do the compartment which has greater laxity.

Postoperative plan
The patient is allowed up, weight bearing on a back splint and walking frame, on the 1st day after operation. On the 5th day the bandages are reduced and flexion commenced. The patient is discharged about 2 weeks following removal of sutures when near 90 ° of flexion has been achieved. Outpatient physiotherapy is continued for another few weeks. These are the ideal X-rays we would like to aim for, which of course are not always achieved.

Long-term results

Material and method
A total of 80 knees in 62 patients were operated on between 1967 and 1983. The surgical approach was changed in 1974 to the one described; since then 62 knees have been operated on. At follow-up 49 patients were examined and with 11 patients who had died the information was obtained from their notes, X-rays, next-of-kin and general practitioners. The follow-up information from two was inadequate. This leaves reasonably adequate follow-up information from 97% of cases. The follow-up period ranged between 1 and 12 years with a mean of 5 years.

The age at operation ranged between 41 and 90 years with a mean of 65 years.

Knee assessment
Three parameters were assessed, each divided into four grades (Table 1).

Table 1. Knee assessment

Assessment of pain	
Grade 0:	Severe pain, present all the time
Grade 1:	Moderate pain on minimal activity
Grade 2:	Minimum pain on normal activity for that age
Grade 3:	Ache
Grade 4:	No ache or pain
Assessment of overall functional capability	
Grade 0:	House bound
Grade 1:	Minimal with aids (can walk around the yard)
Grade 2:	Moderate with aids (can walk down to the local shop, i.e. 200 m)
Grade 3:	Moderate without aids (with aids can walk normally for that age group)
Grade 4:	Normal for the age group
Assessment of the range of knee motion	
Grade 0:	0°– 30°
Grade 1:	30°– 60°
Grade 2:	60°– 90°
Grade 3:	90°–120°
Grade 4:	120°–150°

Results

Pain

Nearly 45% had severe pain preoperatively while only 5% were in this category at the final follow-up. The graphs show a marked shift to the right, i.e. improvement. At the final follow up 84% improved their preoperative pain and this was long lasting. Eleven per cent remained unchanged and 5% were worse off. Of those who were worse off two have had total joint replacement elsewhere and one only had the operation 6 months ago. The remaining one had avulsion of the tibial tubercle 6 weeks after an old surgical procedure,

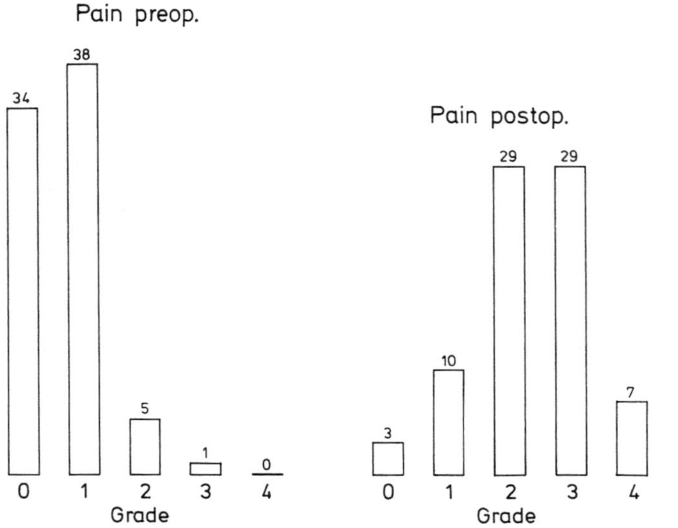

Figure 3. Assessment of pain

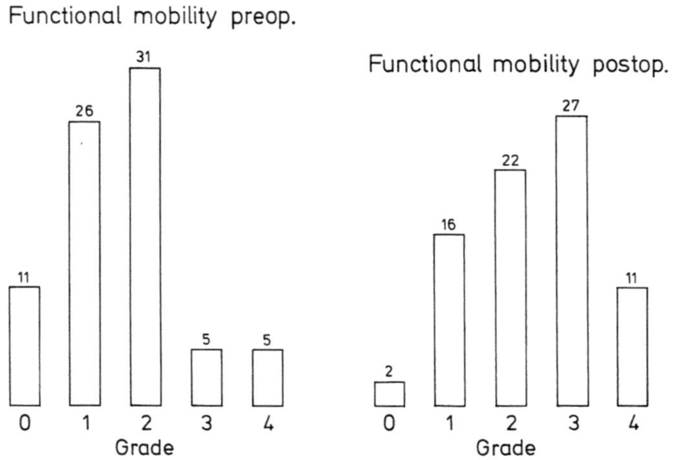

Figure 4. Assessment of functional mobility

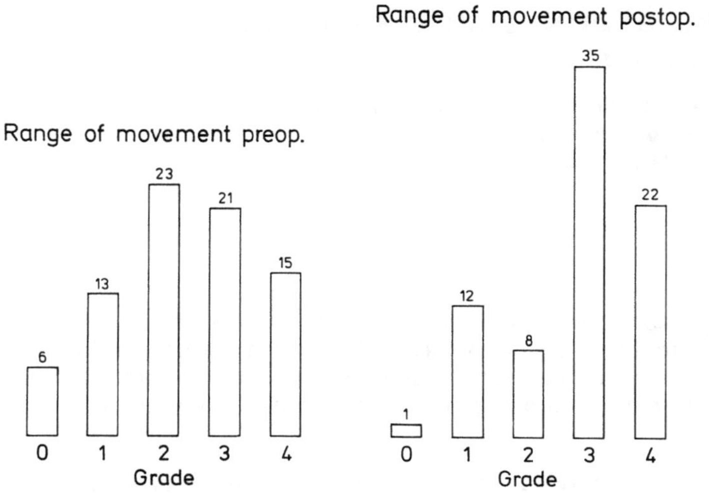

Figure 5. Assessment of range of motion

perhaps due to overenthusiastic physiotherapy. The prosthesis here dislocated and the knee was finally arthrodesed.

Overall functional capability
Figures 3 show a less impressive shift to the right; 55% improved, 35% remained unchanged and 10% were worse off.

Range of motion
Figures show little improvement compared with the above two parameters.

Conclusion
We therefore conclude that McIntosh plateau replacement is a very satisfactory procedure for partial destruction of the knee joint if the pain is sufficiently disabling to warrant surgery.

Biomechanical problems in knee prostheses

W. Braun, A. Rüter and H.-J. Graf

Klinik für Unfall- und Wiederherstellungschirurgie
Stenglinstr. 1, D-8900 Augsburg
Federal Republic of Germany

Introduction

While for many years the implantation of total hip prostheses has been a standard procedure in nearly every large clinic which performs orthopaedic surgery, the implantation of knee prostheses has not been accepted very widely. The main reason seems to be that the biomechanics of the knee are more complex.

The close relationship between the joint surface and the individual parts of the ligaments is particularly important for the movement of the knee linkage so that a change in one structure is not possible without affecting the function of the other. This is the reason for stress and durability problems of the hinged prostheses with fixed axes which are known and have been calculated.

On the other hand there are the so-called resurfacing prostheses with or without the cruciate gap. However, by resecting the eminentia the cruciate ligaments have to be sacrificed without replacing the function of the ligaments. Therefore experiments have been performed on cadaver knees to answer the question of whether this step has an influence on the mechanics of a resurfacing prosthesis.

Materials and methods

Based on the fundamental results of Menschik (1974, 1975) about the biomechanics of the knee linkage and the fact that, among other factors, the physiological motion is a very important condition for the long-lasting function of a knee prosthesis, the principal subject of our research has been the observation of the rolling and gliding motion and the final rotation of the knee in resurfacing prostheses. Our study was carried out on six cadaver knees without any disease or trauma.

RMC total knee prostheses (McCoy et al. 1980) were used which have a femoral, tibial and facultative usable patellar component. The tibial component is available with or without the cruciate gap.

After the preparation of the knee ligaments the femur was fixed in a goniometer. The points of articulation between the lateral femoral and tibial condyle were marked in extension. Then the motion of these points was observed by X-rays during flexion. This experiment was repeated after the dissection of both cruciate ligaments.

The same procedure was made with RMC prostheses. Then the proportion of distance covered by the marked points during the flexion motion was taken as a measure of the rate of gliding to rolling motion.

As a measure of stability of the knee in the sagittal plane, the release of the anterior and posterior tibial subluxation was taken. For this the change in distance between the femoral-tibial point of contact in flexion of 90 ° and the posterior edge of the tibia in a "Scheuba's apparatus" was used.

The final rotation was observed before and after dissection of the cruciate ligaments in normal and prosthetic knees and expressed by the change of angle between two Kirschner's wires fixed in the sagittal plane.

Results

The dissection of the cruciate ligaments in normal knees leads to a marked increase in gliding motion compared with the rolling motion during knee flexion of a factor of 1.3 (Figure 1). After implantation of the resurfacing prostheses the amount of gliding motion even with intact cruciate ligaments was increased approximately by a factor of 4. This, however, can only be seen up to a flexion of 90 °. Beyond 90 ° the rolling motion is favoured. Beyond 120 ° flexion there is only a tilting movement of the dorsal femoral condyle on the tibial plateau.

A similar sequence of movements is seen after the dissection of the cruciate ligaments, but with a much higher proportion of gliding in the first 90 ° flexion. Beyond 90 ° flexion the rolling of the femur on the tibial plateau was less prominent compared with the motion with intact cruciate ligaments, although after dissection of the anterior cruciate ligament the structure holding back the femoral condyle no longer existed (Figure 2).

When checking the stability of the sagittal plane by measuring the release of the anterior and posterior tibial subluxation, there was a remarkable instability after dissection of both cruciate ligaments. With intact ligaments a movement of the points of contact between tibial and femoral condyle under pres-

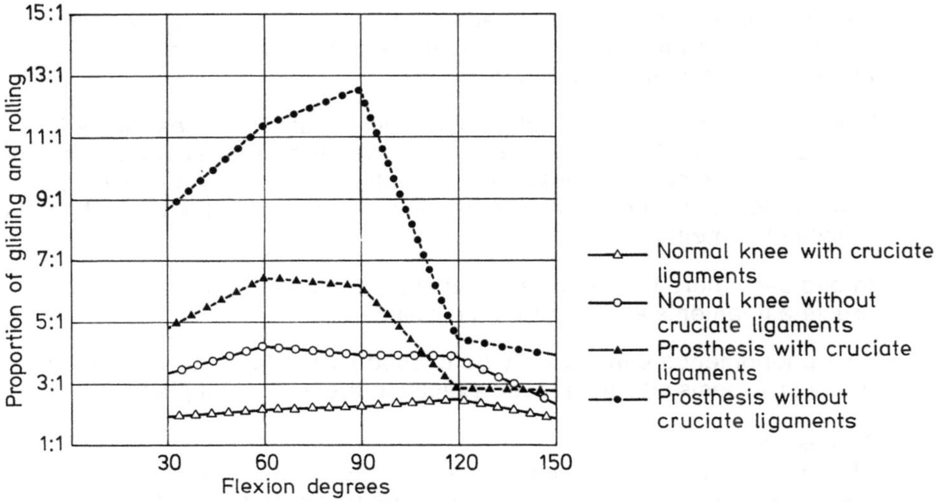

Figure 1. Proportion of flexing and rolling depending on flexion degrees

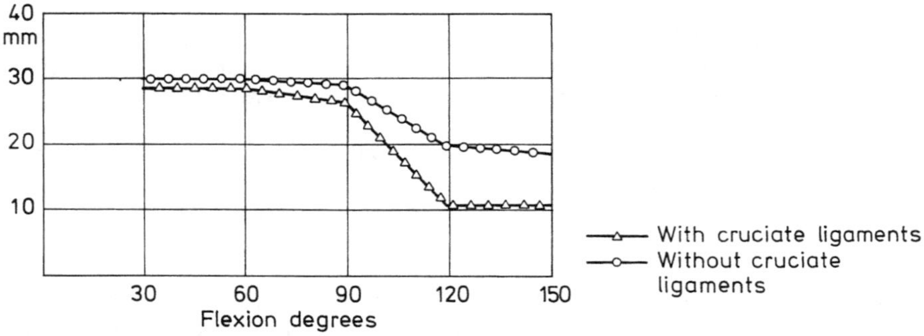

Figure 2. Prosthesis: distance between tibiofemoral articulation and dorsal tibial edge depending on flexion degrees

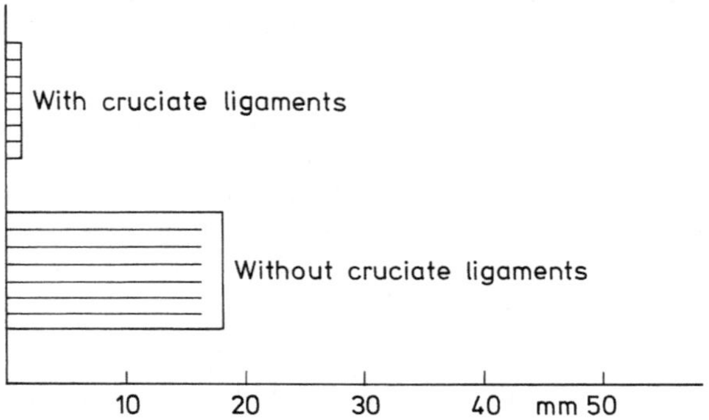

Figure 3. Prosthesis: average shifting of the tibia by ventral and dorsal subluxation with and without the cruciate ligaments

sure and tension of the tibial head could not be seen, whereas after dissection of the cruciate ligaments an average dorsal and anterior tibial subluxation of 18 mm was found (Figure 3).

The observation of the final rotation with our prosthetic knees showed no uniform behaviour: On normal knees the physiological final rotation of about 10 ° was observed. There was a significantly higher final rotation of up to 20 ° in the prosthetic knees, which was reduced to 10 ° after the dissection of the cruciate ligaments.

In one case there was no rotation at all, whereas after the separation of the cruciate ligaments an inner rotation resulted.

This phenomenon can possibly be caused by the fact that the implantation of the prosthesis was not placed exactly in the horizontal plane.

Discussion

The introduction of resurfacing prostheses has led to various advantages in knee prosthetic surgery, especially because they are not hinged, there is free rotation and there are better conditions in the retropatellar joint.

As our results show, the implantation of an RMC resurfacing prosthesis causes a change in the kinematics of the knee in a pathological way, even with intact cruciate ligaments. After dissection of the cruciate ligaments the pathological movements are further increased. Besides that, the noticeable instability of the prosthetic knees as a result of the loss of the cruciate ligaments was evident. In addition, the physiological final rotation could no longer be found; possibly an incorrect implantation in the horizontal plane may be the reason for a restricted rotation.

The results of our study enable the following useful statements about RMC total knee prostheses to be made and we think that they are true of all types of resurfacing prostheses:

1. Saving the cruciate ligaments is a very necessary requirement to maintain the physiological sequence of movements and to guarantee a long-lasting function.
2. By removing the cruciate ligaments in prosthetic knees a loss of stability occurs with a corresponding stress of the other knee ligaments.
3. It is important that both components of the prosthesis are placed exactly across each other in the horizontal plane in order to avoid pathological rotations in the knee which would cause a loosening of the prosthesis.

References

McCoy GF, et al. (1980) The Richards (RMC) knee replacement. Richards Manufacturing Company, Memphis
Menschik A (1974) Mechanik des Kniegelenkes: 1. Z Orthop 112:481–495
Menschik A (1975) Mechanik des Kniegelenkes: 2. Z Orthop 113:388–400

Biomechanics of knee prostheses

U. Munzinger and U. Wyss

Klinik Wilhelm Schulthess Zürich, Institut für physikalische Therapie
Neumünsterallee 3, CH-8008 Zürich
Switzerland

Introduction

The present study is based on our own investigations:

1. Dimensions of the femoral condyles (measurements in 70 cadaver femurs)
2. Strain gauge analysis on different GSB knee prostheses
3. Design of the tibial component with finite-element models
4. Extensive computer study based on standard clinical X-ray pictures (long-term evaluation of patients with knee arthroplasty)
5. Long-term computed tomographic evaluation with densitometry

Furthermore, a review of the literature published in the last 3 years is presented.

Dimensions of the femoral condyles

A total of 70 cadaver femurs were measured. The characteristic dimensions were not chosen with any particular knee prostheses in mind. The aim was to use a method whereby as many characteristic dimensions as possible could be determined from graphic recordings at a later time. The femoral condyles had to be measured in two directions to allow a three-dimensional evaluation. The method of recording the shape of the femoral condyles consisted in drawing the condyles at a scale of 2:1 by means of a pantograph.

A typical example of a recording of the frontal curvatures is shown in Figure 1. As all recordings are related to a coordinate system a three-dimensional reconstruction would be possible for prosthesis design.

An important part of each femoral condyle is made up of those areas where the greatest loads are set up during walking. Figure 2 shows how these areas were distributed on the sagittal recordings. The dimensions R 10 °/−10 ° and E describe the contact area during standing. The radii R 10 °/−10 ° and R 80 °/10 ° were fitted with a maximum deviation of 1 mm from the true curve.

Sections with different radii were chosen because they are easier to machine and control during production of an implant. However, they still represent the physiological curvature. Dimensions G and F were measured because they are important when a knee prosthesis is implanted with its stem extending into the femoral shaft. There is a close relationship between the size of the femoral condyles and the shaft diameter. An interesting finding is that the medial dimensions correlate more closely with the shaft diameter than do the lateral dimensions.

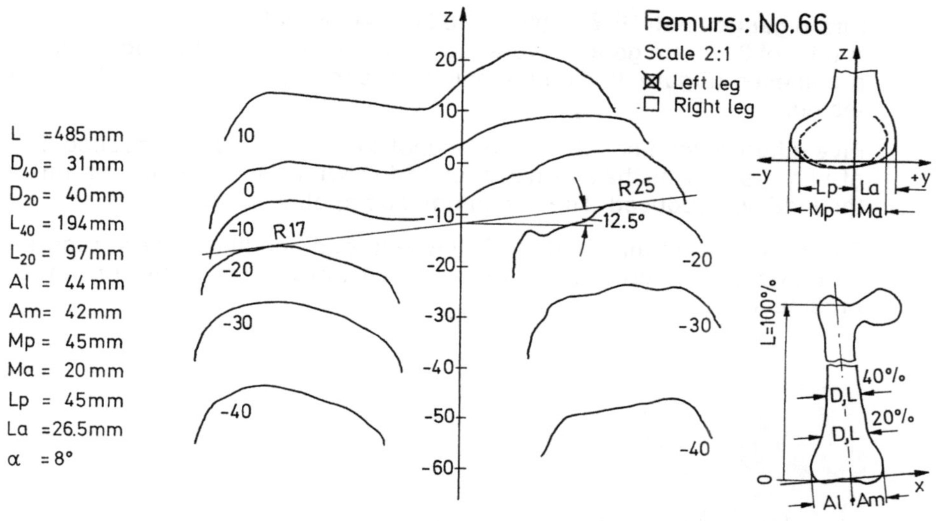

Figure 1. As all recordings are related to a coordinate system, a three-dimensional reconstruction is possible for prosthesis design. The measurements indicate a close relationship between size of femoral condyle and shaft diameter (*right* side of the graph)

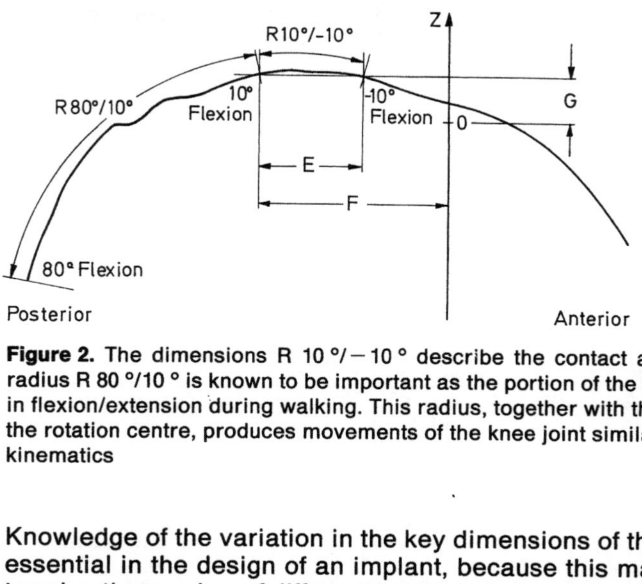

Figure 2. The dimensions R 10 °/−10 ° describe the contact area during standing. The radius R 80 °/10 ° is known to be important as the portion of the femoral condyles involved in flexion/extension during walking. This radius, together with the approximate location of the rotation centre, produces movements of the knee joint similar to those seen in normal kinematics

Knowledge of the variation in the key dimensions of the femoral condyles is essential in the design of an implant, because this makes it possible to determine the number of different implant sizes needed to serve 95% (or more) of the patient population. The orthopaedic surgeon should be able to decide on a specific size from standard radiographs before the operation. This can be done by measuring easily identifiable key dimensions on the radiographs if these dimensions dictate the correct implant size. A multiple regression analysis with the most important dimensions would reduce the number of relevant measurements.

Strain gauge analysis on different GSB knee prostheses

A total of 24 strain gauges were mounted on the femoral component of GSB prostheses (Figure 3). Components with and without femoral shields were tested.

Five different load conditions were analyzed. The load was applied in steps of 1 kN. As soon as the strain exceeded 450 N/mm^2 in one single strain gauge the load was reduced. The maximum load applied was 8 kN.

The maximum strains under *all* different load conditions were recorded in strain gauges 11 and 13 (Figure 4), which were in the posterior part of the prosthesis.

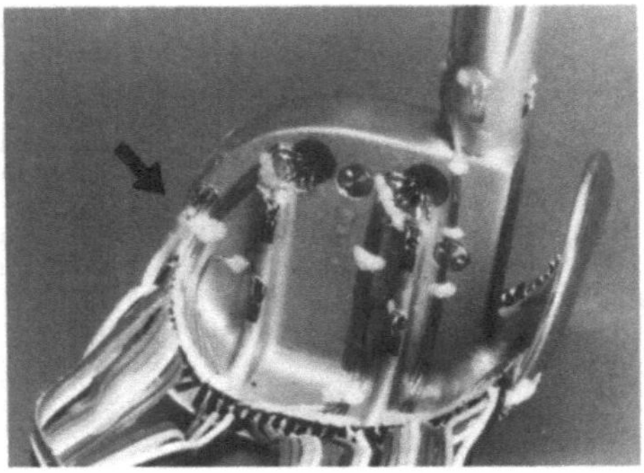

Figure 3. Strain gauge analysis of the femoral component: 24 strain gauges are mounted on the femoral component. Five different static load cases were analysed. The maximum stress is located posteriorly

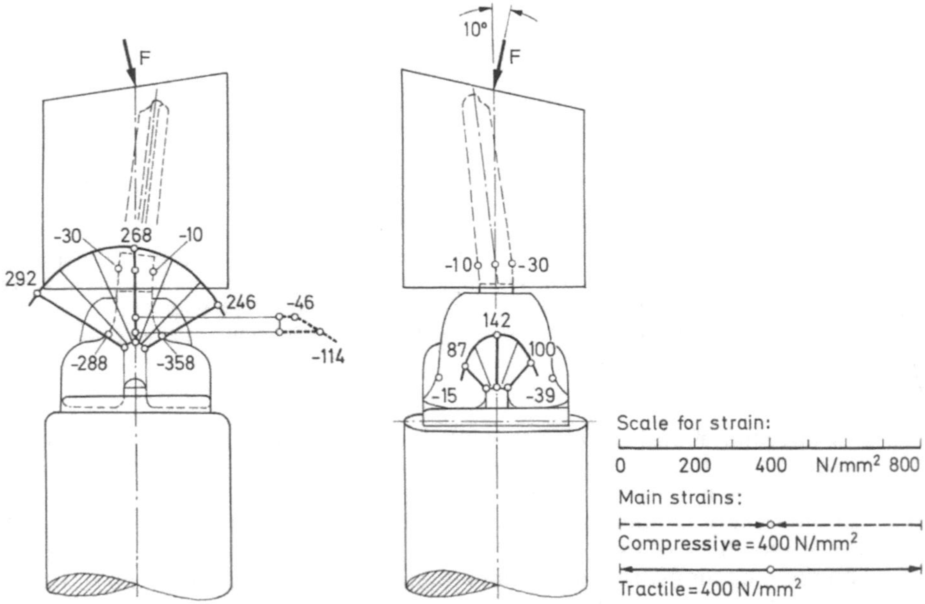

Figure 4. Load case with 5 kN (5 ° flexion and 10 ° varus): The greatest strains were measured in the posterior part (*left side* of the graph) with 292 N/mm^2. In the anterior part of the prosthesis (*right side* of the graph) the maximum strain measured was 142 N/mm^2

Comparison of femoral prostheses with and without femoral shields showed that the limit of 450 N/mm^2 was reached at half load in the prosthesis without femoral shield. The femoral shield has a considerable stabilizing effect on the whole of the femoral component.

Finite element analysis

Bartel et al. examined conventional and custom prosthetic tibial components by means of finite element analysis. Several loading configurations were tested, and the worst loading conditions were found to be those in which eccentric loads were placed on the margin of the tibial component. The results showed that the stresses on the cancellous bone beneath a conventional design prosthesis may be attenuated if a metal tray and a metal peg are used. A salvage design concept for revision in the presence of deficient cancellous bone was tested analytically and used successfully. This concept requires that some portion of the applied load be transferred directly to the tibial cortical shell. Stresses in the remaining cancellous bone were attenuated by the combination of a thickened metal tray and a metal support buttress.

Finite element analysis with GSB prostheses

Finite element models are idealizations of the actual bone implant composite (Figure 4). A structural model is generated by specifying the geometry and material properties of each region concerned (cortical bone, cancellous bone, cement, metal), the properties of the intervals between these regions, and the loads and restraints on the external surface of the structure. Finite element analysis solutions provide approximate values for the stresses at discrete points within each element in a chosen model. We studied seven load cases representing the most common in vivo loading conditions, with maximum load of 5000 N (Figure 5). Strains were measured in different sagittal planes and in transverse cuts.

Measurement of the load transmission with finite elements revealed that the compressive stress in the layer of cancellous bone immediately beneath the metal plateau was relatively low (maximal 5 N/mm^2), while the compressive stress at the extremity of the screw was up to 15 N/mm^2.

Four different tibial components were analysed (Figure 5):

1. Small plateau/long stem
2. Small plateau/short stem
3. Large plateau/long stem
4. Large plateau/short stem

The different loading cases are shown in Figure 5.

Conclusions

Loading case 1. Constraints in the prosthesis higher than the muscular forces. Maximal inflexion constraints in the symmetry planes.

Loading cases 2–4. Muscular forces higher than constraints in the prosthesis. Maximal inflexion constraints slightly shifted from the symmetry plane.

Loading case 5. Muscular forces and constraints in the prosthesis equal. Minimal inflexion constraints.

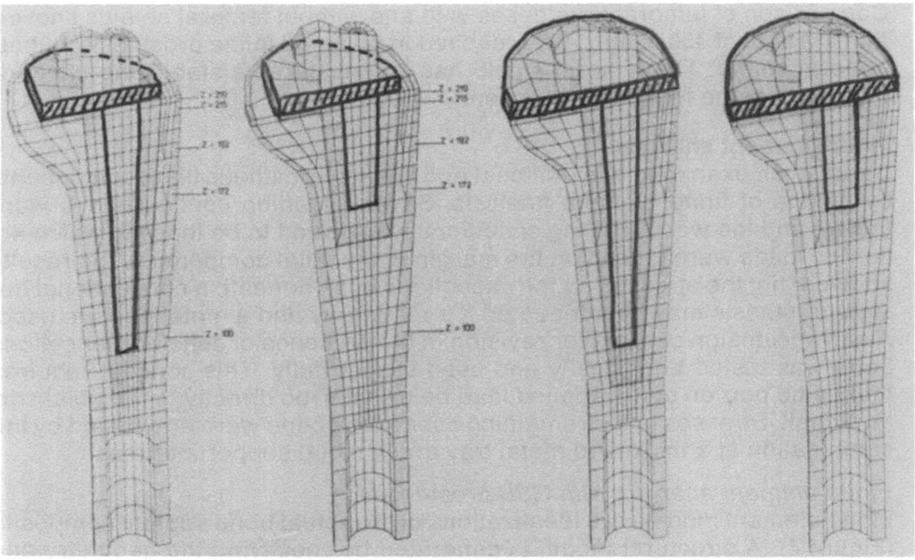

Figure 5. Four different tibial components were compared for fixation, two types with small plateau and long and short stem (*left side* of the graph), and two with large plateau and long and short stem (*right side* of the graph). Maximum strains in the tibial shaft of the prosthesis are lower in the short stem component (factor 0.40–0.71). The large plateau reduces the strains in the tibial shaft by a factor 0.69–0.83

Strains on the prosthesis

Effect of different stem lengths

Maximum strains on the tibial shaft of the prosthesis are lower in the short stem component. For the different load cases the reduction of the strains (fs) is as follows:

$$fs = \frac{\text{Short stem}}{\text{Long stem}}$$

Load case	1	1	3	4	5
fs	0.69	0.40	0.43	0.41	0.71

	F [N]	F_K [N]	α [°]	β [°]	Position F	F_T	F_B	F_S
1	5000	0	10	0	1	1000	600	1000
2	300	1700	10	5	3+4	1000	600	1000
3	300	1700	10	10	3+4	1000	600	1000
4	300	1700	10	15	3+4	1000	600	1000
5	300	1700	20	10	3+4	1000	600	1000

a α and β are valid for F and F_K

Figure 6a

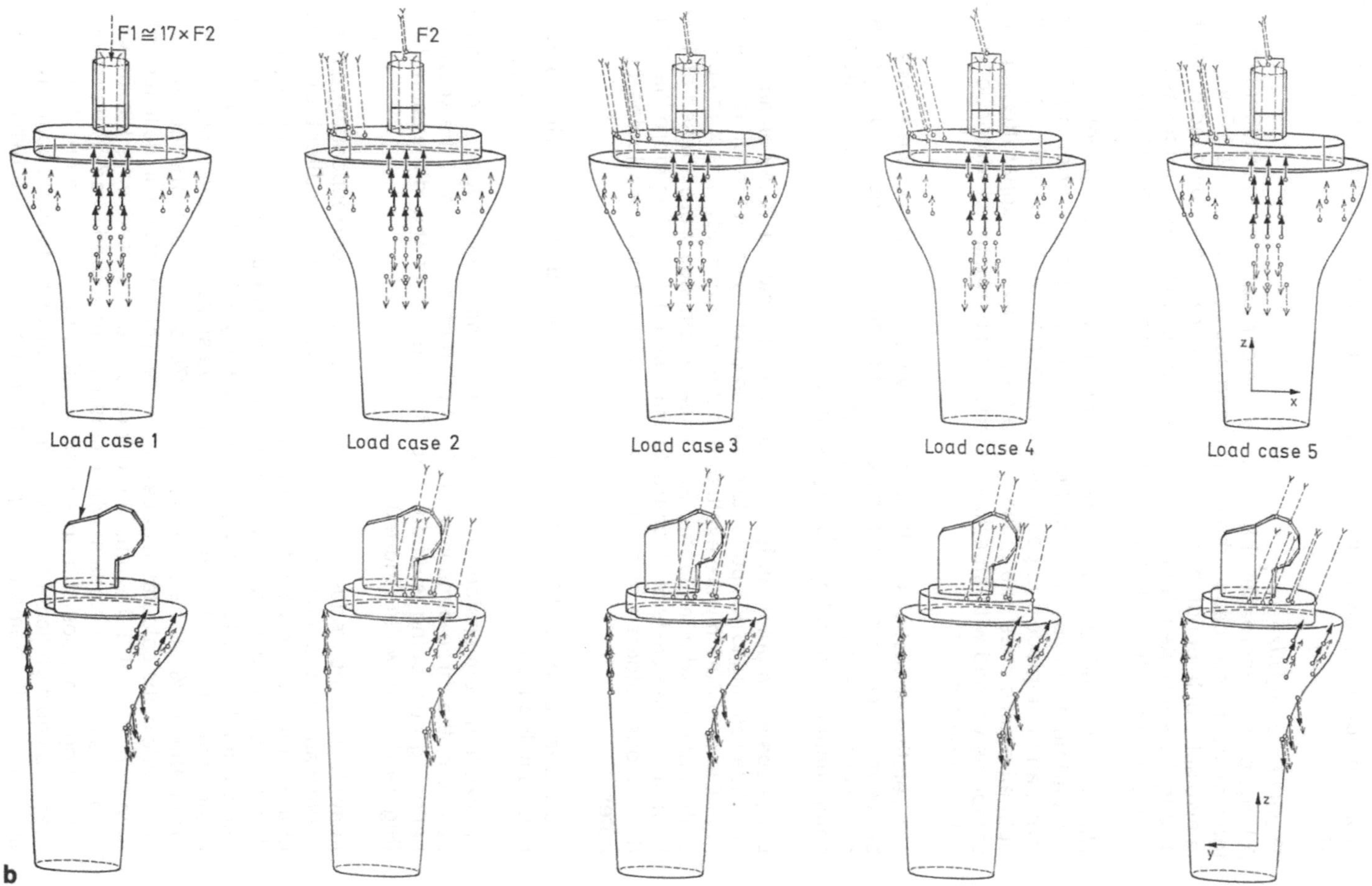

Figure 6. Five different load cases: The apparatus applied compressive load with anterior-posterior force and varus-valgus moment

Strains below the plateau are slightly higher in the short stem tibial component.

Effect of plateau size
A large plateau increases the strains in the cortical bone immediately below the plateau. In load case 1 the strains increase by a factor of 2.8. The plateau is also subject to bending forces. The strains are smaller by a factor of 0.69–0.83 in the short stem than in the long stem. Compression forces within the bone cement at the end of the stem do not change with the size of plateau.

Walker compared 12 tibial components for fixation. The components included compartmental ones jointed at the front, retaining the posterior cruciate ligament, and one-piece components with one, two, or three fixation posts; and both all-plastic ones and those with a metal tray. The apparatus applied a compressive load with anterior-posterior force, rotational torque, or varus-valgus moment.

The relative deflections, both compressive and distractive, were measured between the component and the bone. The least deflections occurred with one-piece metal-tray components with one or two posts. Compartmental components deflected by the largest amount.

Large-scale computer study based on standard clinical X-ray pictures
The data relating to 155 patients reviewed over 1 year at the Wilhelm Schulthess Clinic in Zürich were evaluated in the present study. The X-ray pictures of the patients with implanted GSB knee prostheses were studied at 1-year intervals on the basis of 45 characteristic dimensions. The more than 15000 dimensions gathered in the course of the study were evaluated by computer.

The measurements obtained from A–P and lateral X-ray photographs are plotted in Figure 7.

Thanks to the dimensions that refer to the bones only, a good impression is gained of the three-dimensional distribution of the bones of the knee in the patient group being studied. The distribution of the dimension AP 19 (Figure 7) is shown in Figure 8.

In addition to the frequency polygon (left graph), a corresponding gaussian curve was also plotted to allow optical assessment. The smaller the deviation of the frequency polygon from the gaussian curve, the safer it is to assume that the number of measurements is sufficiently large for a general analysis. The cumulative frequency is plotted on the right-hand side. The intersection of the mean value of 82.1 mm with the curve shows on the vertical axis of this graph that 52% of the total number of 378 dimensions are located on the "left" side of the calculated gaussian curve. The tolerance of the listed values is in the order of ± 0.5 mm. The reference values used were the known dimensions of the prosthesis, which could be measured exactly regardless of the radiographic position. In a postoperative followup of more than 5 years there was no significant change in the position of the femoral component, and sinking in of the femoral component was not measurable (which means it

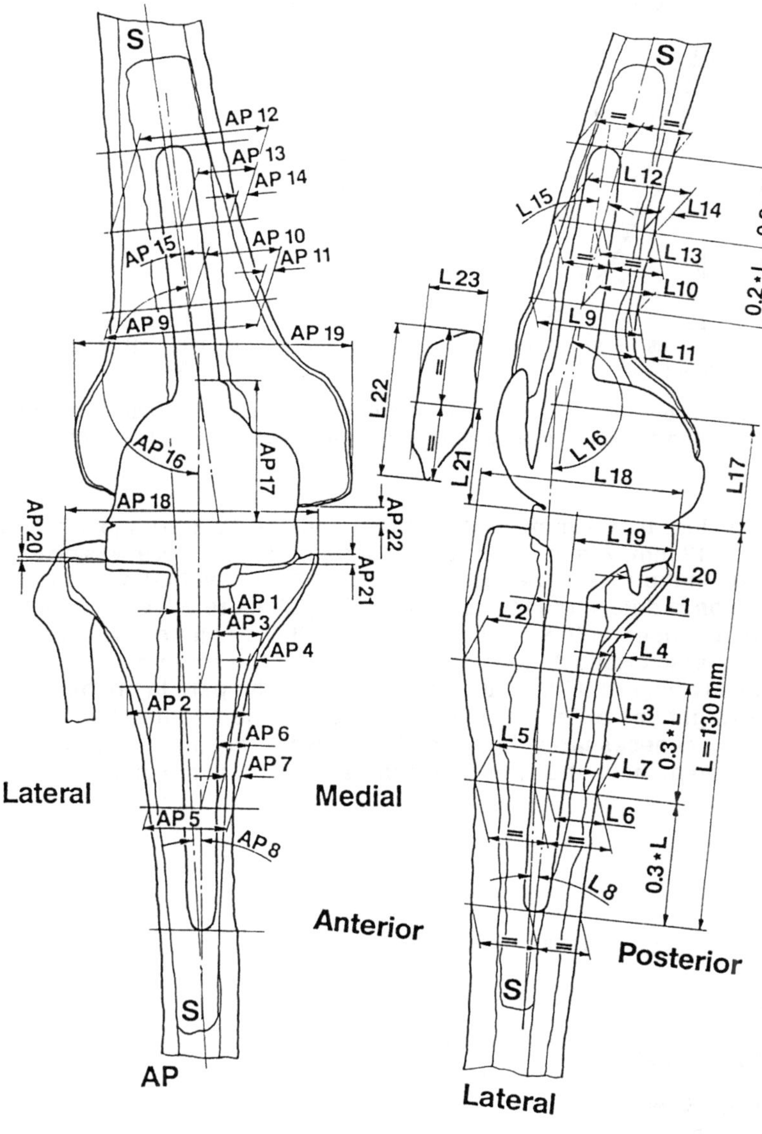

Figure 7. X-ray picture (A-P/lateral) with implanted GSB prosthesis: 45 characteristic dimensions are recorded. Positioning of the arthroplasty in femur and tibia is defined. Changes in the positions of the femoral and/or tibial components are measurable. Whereas sinking in of the tibial component is exactly measurable, changes in the axis (axis of the stem compared with femoral and tibial axis) are difficult to assess owing to inadequate X-ray technique

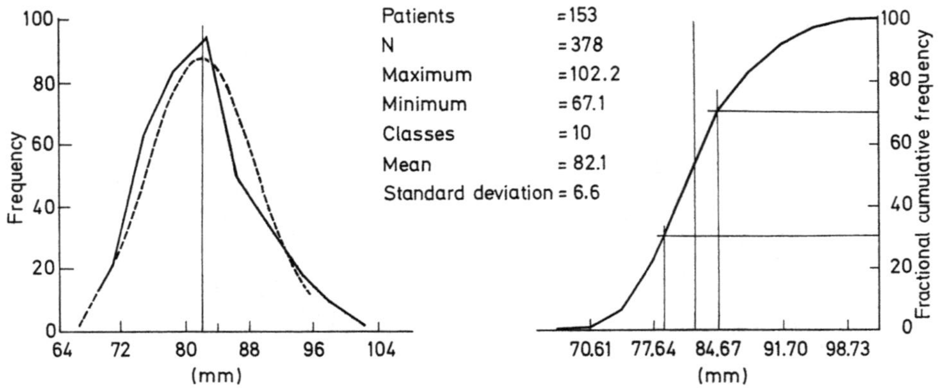

Figure 8. The distribution of the dimensions shown on a frequency polygon. A corresponding gaussian curve has also been plotted. The cumulative frequency is plotted on the *right*

must have been less than 2 mm). On the other hand, the tibial component had sunk in by up to 12 mm, with an average of 4.2 mm. Overall there was no significant change in the axis of the leg. A further object of evaluating the axial photographs was to determine the position of the patella relative to the prosthesis and the changes in the position of the patella over time (Cameron et al. 1982). The characteristic dimensions were fed into the computer and evaluated statistically. Figure 9 illustrates the position of the patella on the prosthesis. The straight line at the zero point represents the middle of the prosthesis, which is not necessarily the physiologically correct position of the patella. The starting point on the lines at 0 months represents the displacement

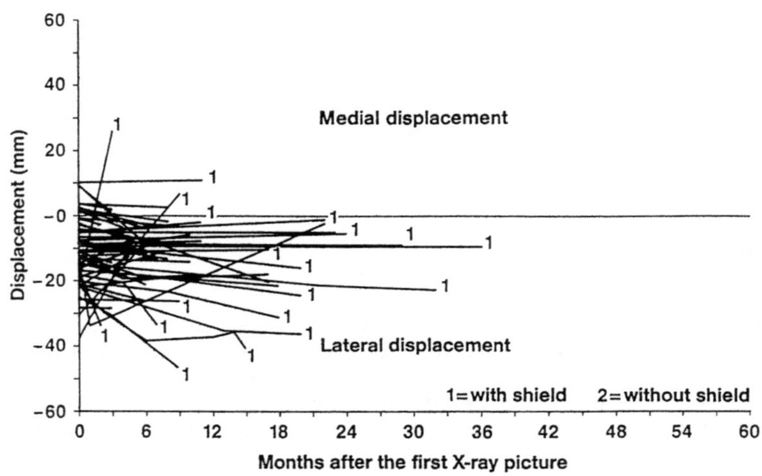

Figure 9. Evaluation of the axial photographs allowed determination of the position of the patella relative to the prosthesis and recognition of changes of this position in the years after the operation. Vertically medial and lateral displacements in millimeters are plotted. *0*, center of the femoral shield. There is a tendency for lateral shift of the patella

of the patella relative to the middle of the prosthesis. The lines connect the points with the displacement since the first axial X-ray. There was a significant relation between the axial position of the patella and operative technique. Obviously rotation of the tibial component must influence the position of the patella. This factor will be analysed in the CT study. Comparison of the operative techniques with medial and lateral approach to the patella revealed that the *lateral* approach gave a better alignment of the patella (average of 5.5 mm less lateral displacement, as measured to the midline of the femoral shield). The further advantages of the lateral approach to the knee joint are described in the section "*The Role of the GSB Prosthesis in Total Knee Replacement*".

Long-term computed-tomography evaluation with densitometry

The aim of the CT study is to obtain information about the bone quality and bone reaction with the implanted arthroplasty. A special CT system is used for bone densitometry. A series of 12 cross sections of the upper tibia is taken before the operation, 3, 6, and 12 months after the operation and at 1-year intervals subsequently. Since the cross-sectional area varies considerably from proximal to distal, it is a precise measurement that can be used to determine the level of the cuts each time. For each cut different parameters are calculated: Thickness of cortical bone, position of the stem of the tibial component, and attenuation coefficient (densitometry). In this way it is possible to give precise information about positioning of the tibial component and changes of the position of the tibial component relative to the bone (Figure 10). Indirectly, densitometry will show approximately the areas of load transfer.

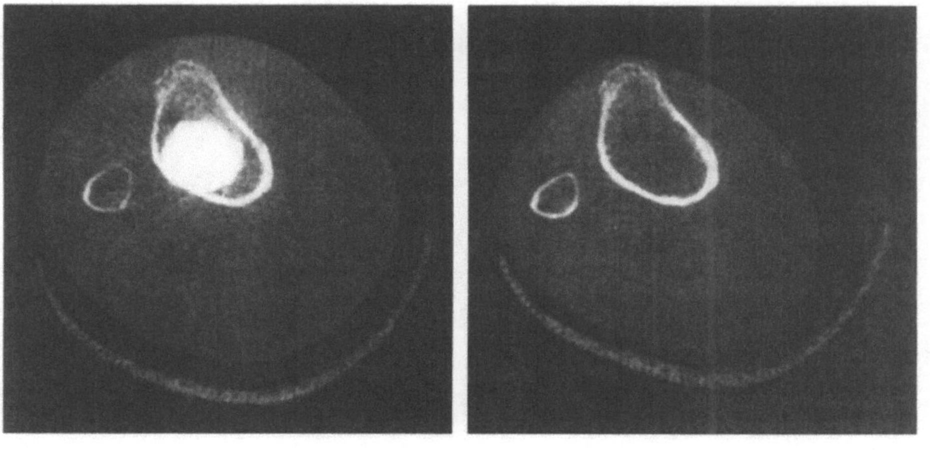

Figure 10. CT evaluation with densitometry: the position of the tibial component is recorded and changes in this position are measured. Densitometry allows assessment of bone quality

References

1. Bartel DL, et al. (1982) Performance of the tibial component in total knee replacement. J Bone Joint Surg [Am] 64:1026–1033
2. Cameron HU, Federkow DM (1982) The patella in total knee arthroplasty. Orthopedics and Related Research 165:197–199
3. Gschwend N (1981) Die GSB-Knieprothese – Prinzipielle Überlegungen und Ergebnisse. In: Jäger M, Hofer H, Häckel H (eds) Kniegelenksendoprothetik bei chronischer Polyarthritis – juvenile chronische Polyarthrosis. Huber, Berne (Aktuelle Probleme in Chirurgie und Orthopädie, vol 15)
4. Walker PS, et al. (1981) Fixation of tibial components of knee prostheses. J Bone Joint Surg [Am] 63:258–267
5. Wyss UP, Doerig M, Frey O, Gschwend N (1982) Dimensions of the femoral condyles. In: Huiskes R, et al. (eds) Biomechanics: principles and applications. Nijhoff, The Hague, pp 291–297

The GSB knee prosthesis
The original GSB model

U. Munzinger and N. Gschwend

Klinik Wilhelm Schulthess Zürich, Institut für physikalische Therapie
Neumünsterallee 3, CH-8008 Zürich
Switzerland

At the time of the development of the GSB knee prosthesis, more than 10 years ago, we were very much aware of the negative results of the pure hinge-type prosthesis, particularly the Shiers design.

The relatively short experience with the resurfacing type of prostheses had convinced us that this type of joint would not provide *both* an excellent range of movement *and* sufficient stability. In addition, severe ligament damage and deformity seemed to limit the number of cases in which a resurfacing prosthesis was indicated.

The GSB prosthesis was designed to incorporate the advantages of each of the above types of prosthesis without their disadvantages. As the axis of flexion is "wandering" rather than fixed, and the condylar surfaces are large, the kinematics of this joint do not deviate far from those of the normal knee. Minimal bone resection renders revision in the case of failure easier, and free play between the femoral and tibial components reduces the stress transferred to the intramedullary anchorage sites. The relatively simple operative technique and broad incision (Figure 1) allowing the correction of nearly any deformity permit even a relatively inexperienced surgeon to perform the procedure reliably.

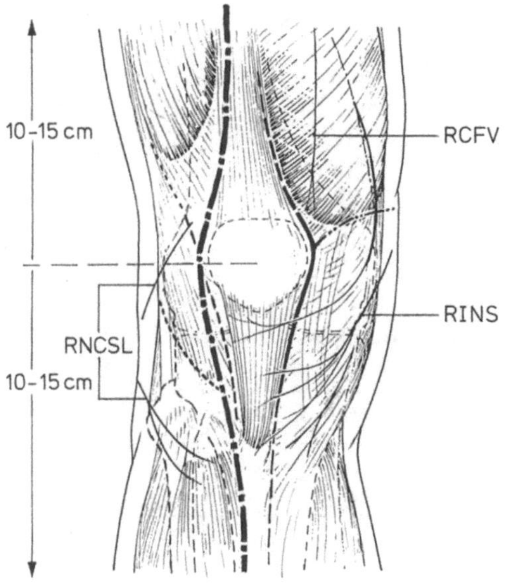

Figure 1. *Lateral* incision of the skin does not infere with its innervation. The *lateral* approach through the retinaculum has the following advantages: the proprioceptive fibres in the medial retinaculum are not dissected, and the function of the M. vastus medialis is not impaired; the patella is easier to centre in the neutral position; the blood flow of the patella is less badly disturbed (fewer patellar fractures?). *RCFV*, rami cutanei femoris ventrales; *RINS*, ramus infrapatellaris nervi sapheni; *RNCSL*, rami nervi cutanei surae lateralis

As a long-term follow-up study revealed nearly 2 years ago, the original model of the GSB prosthesis fulfilled our initial expectations (Tables 1–3).

The most impressive aspect of the results was the average gain in mobility, with a flexion of over 100 °, a very significant factor for the function of patients with bilateral arthrosis and rheumatoid arthritis. A loosening rate of only 2% at the 6-year follow-up was another advantage of the GSB knee prosthesis over the majority of other designs.

Table 1. Mobility

		Before operation	After operation	
Flexion:	Max.	130°	130°	
	Min.	20°	70°	
	Average	90°	104°	gain 28°
Flexion contracture:	Max.	70°	45°	
	Min.	0°	0°	
	Average	18°	4°	

Table 2. Walking distance before and after surgery in 48 patients operated on for rheumatoid arthritis and 52 operated on for arthrosis

Distance	Before		After	
	No.	%	No.	%
Rheumatoid arthritis				
1 km	1	2	20	42
−1 km	14	29.2	21	44
100 m	32	66.7	6	12
Wheelchair	1	2	1	2
Arthrosis				
	8	15.4	38	73
1 km	25	48.1	11	21
−1 km	19	36.5	3	6
100 m	–	–	–	–
Wheelchair	–	–	–	–

Table 3. Results recorded with GSB knee arthroplasty (follow-up longer than 5 years) ($n=118$)

Pain	Before operation			After operation		
Severe	80	68%	98%	6	4.5%	
Moderate	36	30%		22	18.5%	
Mild, occasional	2	2%		33	28%	76%
None	–	–		57	48%	

On the negative side was the relatively high percentage (23%) of patients who complained of patellofemoral symptoms, especially pain and difficulty in standing up and sitting down, and in going up and down stairs. The high rate of infection (13.5%) also required serious consideration. The great majority of infections occurred late, and in more than half there was definite evidence of a haematogenous aetiology. Was this due to the diminished circulation through the femoral condyle, because of the intramedullary anchorage – a necessary result of this type of stemmed prosthesis? Does axial deformity, with increased mechanical wear of the joint and resultant periarticular inflammation, play a role?

The reoperation rate (22%) was also clearly too high. These considerations led to further related investigations, and finally to modifications of the GSB prosthesis, the new model of which is characterized by:

1. Altered characteristics of the mechanical axis and contact zones. One important result of this is that the only contact in the prothesis now is metal on polyethylene.
2. An improvement of the sagittal kinematics of the joint, more closely approaching those of the normal knee, particularly in higher degrees of flexion when the femur moves a long way in the posterior direction. This has a beneficial effect on patellofemoral pressure.
3. Basic changes in the patellofemoral compartment with a patellar resurfacing prothesis and alterations in the patellar flange. The superior surface of the femoral component, originally flat, was modified to a slightly concave outline. Early attempts at patellar replacement, aiming to avoid cement fixation, relied upon implantation of the prothesis into a deep hole in the patella, which resulted in patellar fractures. The current design avoids this error (Figure 2).

The operative technique has been refined through the application of simplified instruments, and compared with condylar prostheses, the modified GSB knee prosthesis is easy for to insert even for a surgeon who does not perform such operations regularly.

Figures 4–7 provide information regarding the *results* in all cases operated on between 1980 and 1983. Below we shall examine whether there are significant differences between the 1-, 2- and 3-year results. It is notable that 13 different surgeons carried out the operations in question, and these included 9 trainees. This information appears to us to be a significant factor in the evaluation of a method. When a technique is so demanding that it requires the

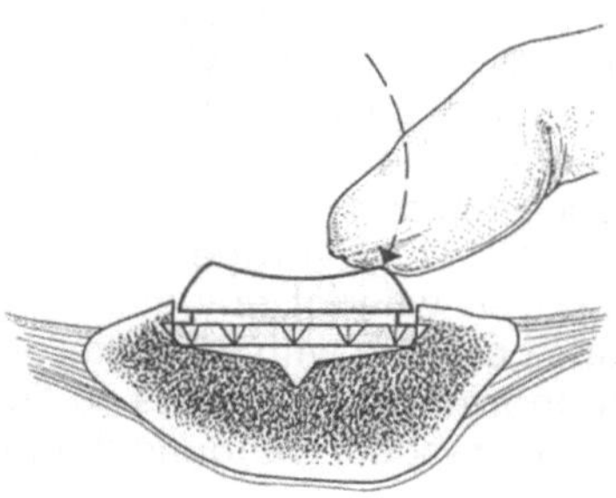

Figure 2. Cementless anchorage of the polyethylene inlay. The depth of the drilling has been reduced from 10 to 5 mm to minimize the risk of patellar fracture

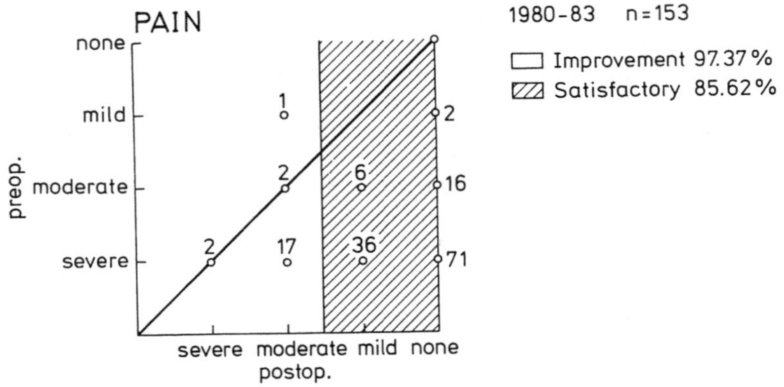

Figure 3. Reduction in pain was recorded in over 97% of patients who had received a GSB knee prosthesis. Nearly 50% of patients had severe pain preoperatively and were painfree after surgery

expertise of an operator with practically daily experience to obtain good results it should certainly not be propagated to an audience that includes surgeons whose experience extends to only 10 cases per year. It is precisely the technically demanding prostheses that are least accommodating, with clinical failure a highly predictable result of technical errors. In this connection it is necessary to consider whether the results obtained by a highly expert and specialized surgeon in personal series are relevant to, or attainable in the general orthopaedic community.

We reviewed the *results* in a series of 153 knees replaced with the current model of the GSB prostheses, with a follow-up of 1–3 years. In 75.54% of cases the indication for surgery was gonarthrosis, and in 24.46% rheumatoid arthritis. The arthrotic patients were older (72.43 ± 5.92 years) than the polyarthritic patients (59.4 ± 12.61). Most (82.01%) of the patients were female.

Pain was diminished in 97.37% of patients, and 85.62% were satisfied with this improvement, having only occasional pain or none at all. Only 2.61% noted no improvement and 0.65% were worse (Figure 3). *Walking ability* was improved in 88.28% of cases, and 87.58% of the patients were satisfied, being able to walk 1 km or more or for more than 30 min. Whereas preoperatively 83.01% of patients required one or two walking aids and four patients (2.61%) were confined to wheelchairs, after recovery from the operation 45.1% walked without aids and 38.56% required only one cane (Figure 4).

A particular advantage of this prosthesis is the large average gain in mobility. Postoperative active flexion averaged 107.73 ° (± 14.51), while passive flexion was 111.68 ° (± 16.12), with an extensor lag of only 3.97 ° (± 8.21). We note that this is a considerable advantage to our polyarthritic and to our bilaterally gonarthrotic patients, who experience difficulty in rising out of a chair if their knee flexion does not exceed 100 °. The average gain in the range of flexion-extension (13.67 °) was achieved without any sacrifice of joint stability, in contrast to some of the results obtained with condylar prostheses (Figure 5). In addition, formidable preoperative deformities could be corrected at surgery without difficulty, and in this respect we found that only

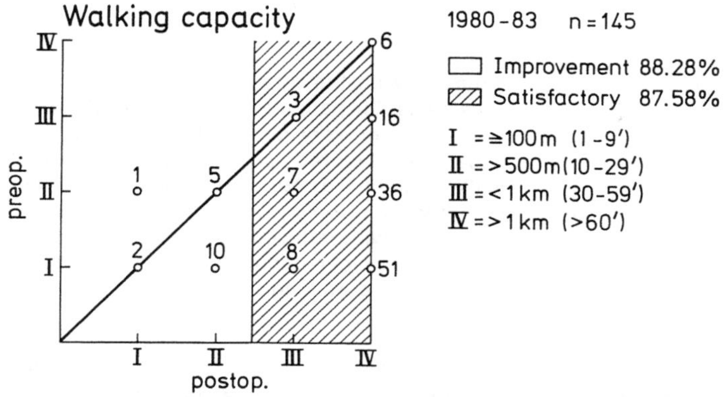

Figure 4. Walking ability of one-third of patients improved from category (grade, class) I (less than 100 m) to category IV (greater than 1 km) with a GSB knee prosthesis. Approximately 90% walk better than before their operations

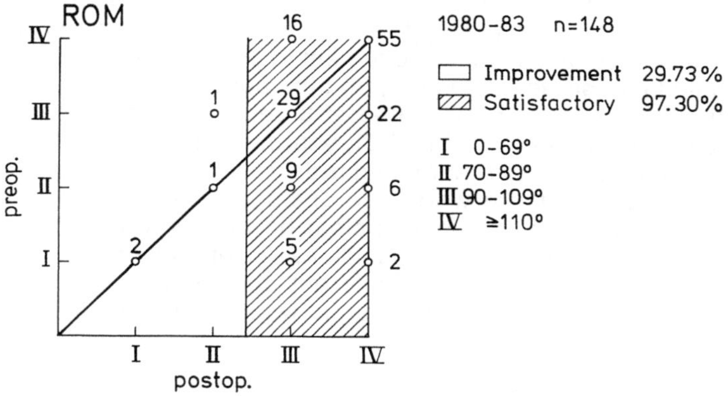

Figure 5. Range of motion. Approximately 30% of patients had an improvement in mobility with the GSB knee prosthesis; 97.3% have flexion of more than 90 °

1.59% of the knees operated on remained in a varus position postoperatively, whereas 56.03% were preoperatively deformed in varus. The results are displayed in Figure 6.

It has been nearly impossible to compare the results achieved with the various prostheses currently in use, to arrive at a meaningful evaluation of their merits and defects. The principal reason for this is the variability of the criteria utilized for evaluation and of the methods of presentation of the results. With this problem in view, Aubriot, Freeman and the authors of this article have undertaken to report the results in as homogeneous a manner as possible. It may well be possible to determine how much the results vary depending on the composition of the patient series. For example, the percentage of cases with rheumatoid arthritis in each series is certainly a decisive factor. Other factors not to be underestimated include the average age of the patients with gonarthrosis, and the severity of contralateral gonarthrosis and of coxarthrosis.

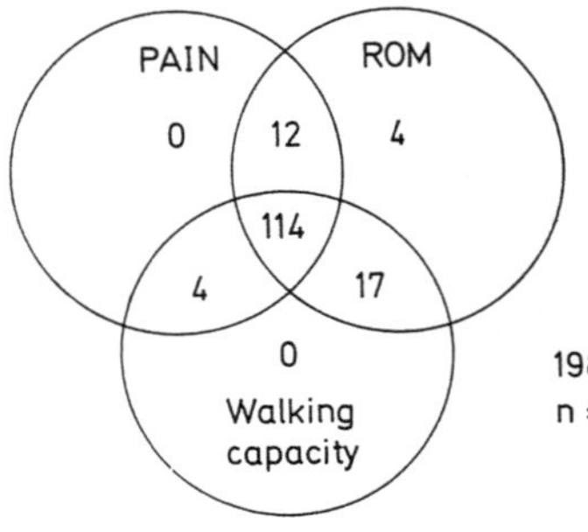

Figure 6. With the new model of the GSB knee prosthesis, 114 patients were found at follow-up to have good or very good results from all three aspects considered (pain, range of movement, walking ability). There were 17 patients who had a *restriction* in *both* walking ability and range of motion, 12 with reduced pain associated with restricted range of motion, and 4 with reduced pain and restricted walking ability

With reference to pain there is a significant difference between the results at 2 years (100% of patients improved over preoperative state) and at 3 years (91.67%). In studying the progression of the patients' symptoms we see that their evaluation of their symptoms is not static. How are we to interpret the fact that "only" 79.36% of the patients had "no or only minor pain" 1 year after surgery, while in the 2-year group the corresponding figure was 88.89%, and that at 3 years, 91.67%? It is conceivable that progressive adaptation of soft tissues may cause improvement to be experienced after 1 or 2 years. It should be observed, however, that the percentage of rheumatoid arthritis patients in the group evaluated at 3 years after surgery was 41.94%, with an average age of 52.18 ($\pm$15.41) years, whereas in the 1-year group only 19.31% of patients had rheumatoid arthritis, with an average age of 60.09 ($\pm$10.64) years, and there were also analogous differences (e.g., age, bilaterality) in the arthrosis group. It is clear how hesitant we must be when using data as a basis for important decisions. In retrospect, the difference in mobility of the knee among the different prostheses is less pronounced than expected, but the difference in walking ability is rather greater.

Every surgical method must be evaluated in the light of its complications. If the complications are specific and severe and are not amenable to correction through changes in the design and implementation of the method, then its continued use must be called in question.

Among the many possible complications, the most significant are those that place the patient's life at risk or lead to failure of the implant, such as infection and loosening. In the last 3 years we have had no deaths attributable to the surgery in our series of 153 GSB knee prostheses. Systematic anticoagulation and early mobilization no doubt play a significant role in this connection.

Loosening of the prosthesis was seldom seen with the original GSB model, even after very long follow-up. None has yet been seen in the current series.

Infection still occurs too frequently, accounting for 1 case in the 3-year series and 1 in the 1-year series, a total of 2 of 153 cases. In one case, incision and drainage have led (at least temporarily) to a good result, and in the other case it was necessary to remove the prosthesis and arthrodese the knee, which consolidated successfully. The patella is the commonest problem, with

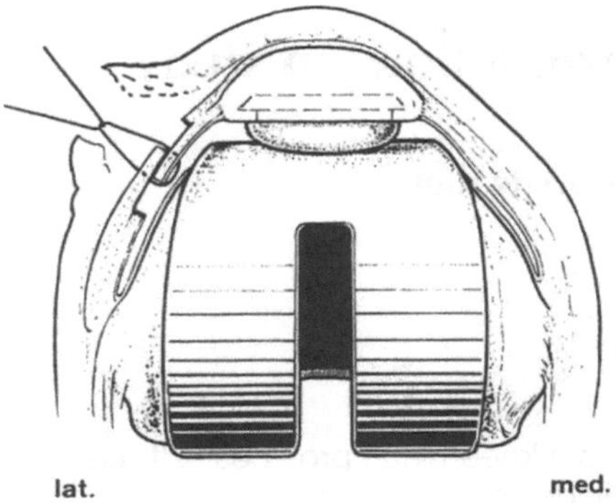

Figure 7. Before closure of the wound the patellar tracking is analysed. Usually lengthening of the lateral retinaculum is necessary. If the suture of the lateral retinaculum is inadequate patellar tracking is not impaired (no subluxation)

16.99% subluxations, 13.72% luxations and 6.54% patellar fractures. Clear improvement has been noted since we began to approach the knee routinely through a lateral parapatellar incision to lengthen the lateral retinaculum (Figure 7) and avoid any weakening of the vastus medialis (Figure 1). With a new uncemented patellar prosthesis (Figure 2), which requires a much smaller bony resection, patellar fracture has become rare. We believe that the newly developed trough in the patellar surface of the femoral flange is an additional improvement.

The 7.83% reoperation rate is undoubtedly too high, although 4.5% required only patellar revision.

Evaluation of the assembled results reveals that 114 of 151 patients (75.49%) experienced an improvement in all essential parameters, and 21.85% in at least two parameters. It is notable that the patients' and the surgeons' assessment of the results were in close agreement: very good results comprised 73.86% (patient assessment) or 72.55% (surgeon assessment) of cases, while good results were found in 15.09% (patient assessment) or 26.99% (surgeon assessment) of cases. With approximately 89% good and very good results, the success rate of this procedure nearly reaches the long-sought 90% goal, and even approaches the rate achieved in total hip arthroplasty (Figure 4).

In conclusion, on the basis of our experience as reported here, what are the indications and contraindications for the GSB knee prostheses? The basic indication is the painful destroyed knee, which strongly reduces walking capacity and is neither amenable to conservative management nor likely to respond to joint-sparing surgery such as osteotomy. Knee replacement arthroplasty is vastly preferable to arthrodesis for every diagnosis, with the exception of the sequelae of sepsis. Deformity and instability of nearly any proportion pose no condraindication.

Moreover, the GSB is particularly suited to the surgeon whose annual number of prosthetic knee operations is limited, and in whose hands the technically demanding condylar prostheses are known to be liable to more complications. As a revision or salvage prosthesis after failure of nonconstrained condylar prostheses, the GSB special prosthesis is also available.

The Blauth knee – A long-term follow-up study

J. Hassenpflug

Department of Orthopaedic Surgery, University Kiel
D-2300 Kiel
Federal Republic of Germany

The Blauth Knee Prosthesis is constructed as a knee-hinge prosthesis. It has been implanted since 1972 without any changes in design. In a prospective multicentre-study the knee joints were regularly controlled. We report on the experience on 420 knee-prostheses implanted at 4 participating hospitals. In more than 75% the prostheses could be controlled clinically and roentgenographically. The average period of follow-up was more than 3 years (range 1 – 11 years). In contrast to the bad results obtained with knee-hinge prostheses reported in the literature we noticed only very few serious complications: Loosening of the prosthesis (n = 2), infections (n = 9). Pain symptoms were recorded preoperatively and were compared qualitatively and quantitatively with those after treatment. After surgery more than 85 % of the patients had no or only slight pain. 10 % of the patients complained about retropatellar pain. Correction of leg axis was always achieved.

Long-term evaluation of knee endoprostheses by actuarial analysis

A. Siegel and K. Heinert

Endo-Klinik
Holstenstraße 2, D-2000 Hamburg 50
Federal Republic of Germany

Introduction

Our experience with total knee replacements is based on 4900 cases operated on in our clinic within the plast 14 years. The best way to study the efficacy of a prosthetic implant is by long-term surveillance in the human body under normal load-bearing conditions. Objective analyses of large series are best obtained by the construction of life tables whereby prostheses still in situ are designated as "survivals" and loose prostheses are treated as "deaths". This method is being increasingly accepted in comparing the efficacy of different total hip implants [2, 7].

Materials and method

The purpose of this study was to assess and compare the clinical results by actuarial methods of two total knee replacement designs with a medium-term follow-up period. A definite number of patients are followed entering the series at different times, i.e. at the time of operation. At follow-up the survival time (firmly fixed prosthesis) or the time to failure (onset of the complication requiring a second operation) is determined for each patient. As we are dealing with homogeneous groups of patients, life tables and survival functions may be used to describe the distribution of survival times.

The advantage of this ongoing method is that by the use of the individual data gained at the last follow-up plus additional updated information the probable survival times for the prosthesis can be determined.

The statistical significance of differences in the time of survival for two or more homogeneous groups of patients is tested by rank tests. Such evaluations are necessary to compare different treatment regimens. The influences that factors like the patient's age and the diagnosis have on the survival times within the same group can be assessed. Such knowledge is of great clinical importance for determining the indications for surgery and for informing the individual patient about risk and expectations accompanying a certain procedure.

The survival curves depict graphically the cumulative annual survival function. The study presented here relates to follow-up investigations made in 1981 on a total of 1679 patients operated on between 1969 and 1978.

Depending on the indication for surgical intervention two different knee systems were used:

1. Non-constrained St. Georg sledge prosthesis in 945 patients with intact ligaments [3, 5, 9] (Figure 1)

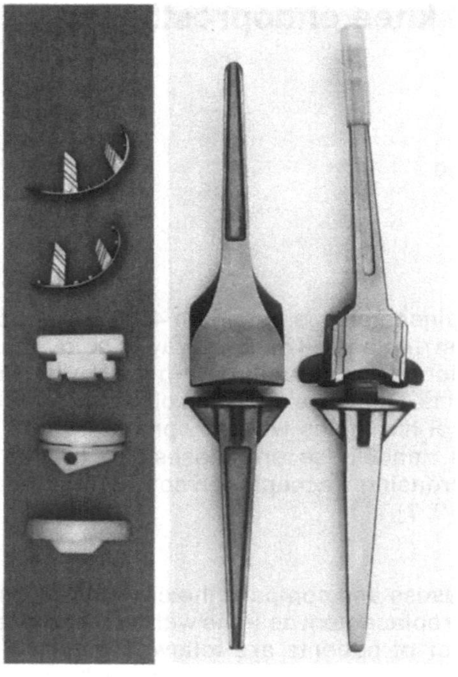

Figure 1. St. Georg sledge prosthesis and total hinge, first and second generation

2. Fully constrained St. Georg total hinge prosthesis in patients with deficient knee ligaments [first generation 226 and of the second generation 508 (total 734), as of 1976, were used] [1, 5] (Figure 1)

Thus a total of 1679 prostheses were used for the two systems.

Results

Of 945 sledge prostheses 822 were functioning in situ at the time of follow-up. The type and number of complications are shown in Table 1. Of 734 total

Table 1. Frequency and type of complications 1969–1978 (year of follow-up 1981) with sledge prostheses, model St. Georg ($N=945$)

Type of complications		Unicondylar medial ($N=366$)	Unicondylar lateral ($N=72$)	Bicondylar ($N=507$)
Mechanical loosening	Femoral component	–	–	–
	Tibial component	16	4	16
	Both components	2	–	–
Fracture of the metal sledge		1	–	1
Operative-technical errors		4	1	7
Ligamentous deficiencies		15	3	30
Contralateral osteoarthritis		10	5	–
Infection		–	1	5
Sudeck's disease		–	–	2

Table 2. Frequency and type of complications 1969–1978 (year of follow-up 1981) with total hinge prostheses, model St. Georg ($N=734$)

Type of complications		1969–1975 1st generation ($N=226$)		1976–1978 2nd generation ($N=508$)	
Mechanical loosenings	Femoral component	3		2	
	Tibial component	–	13	2	14
	Both components	10		10	
Fracture of the femur at the proximal end of the prosthesis			5		3
Infection			5		6

hinge prostheses 688 were firmly fixed at follow-up. The rate of failure was reduced by half in the second-generation St. Georg total hinge prosthesis. The type and number of complications are shown in Table 2.

The survival curves indicate the reason and time of failure. The following graphs depict our experience with infection, aseptic loosening and failure rates of non-constrained versus fully, constrained prostheses.

As seen in Figure 2 infections occurred during the first 6 years at a constant rate in patients operated on with the sledge prosthesis. By comparison, infections in patients operated on with the total hinge prosthesis occurred more frequently, and the majority of these within the first 3 postoperative years.

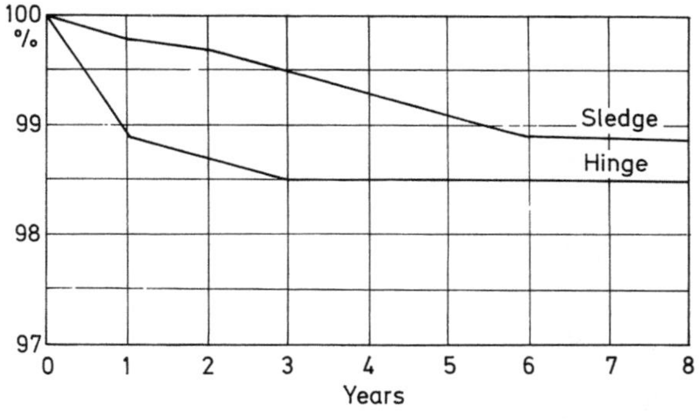

Figure 2. Deep infection in knee endoprostheses

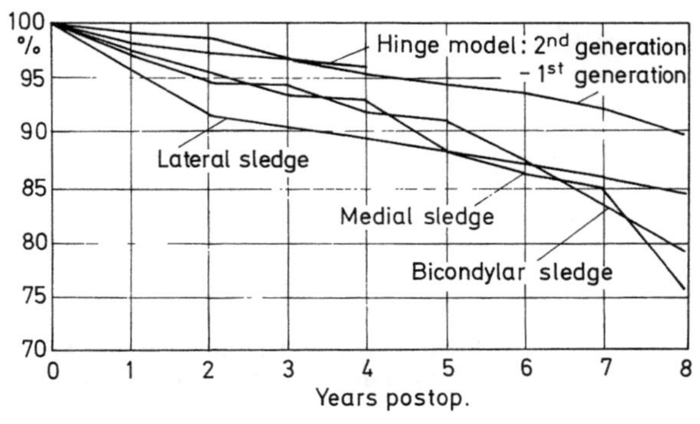

Figure 3. Failure rates (survival curves) of different knee prosthesis (mechanical loosening)

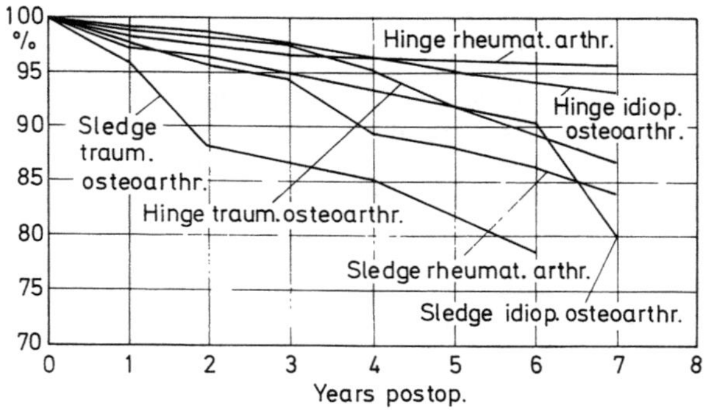

Figure 4. Failure rates (survival curves) of sledge and hinge prostheses according to the diagnosis

As seen in Figure 3, mechanical loosenings occurred continuously over an 8-year postoperative course.

With extended follow-up the sledges show a higher rate of failure when compared with the total hinge prosthesis. The difference is statistically significant. This increased failure rate in the non-constrained group may be attributed to failure of the ligamentous support with time (Figure 4).

Conclusions

The results obtained are encouraging and induced us to stick to our chosen path. As a result of the study we now pay even greater attention to the sta-

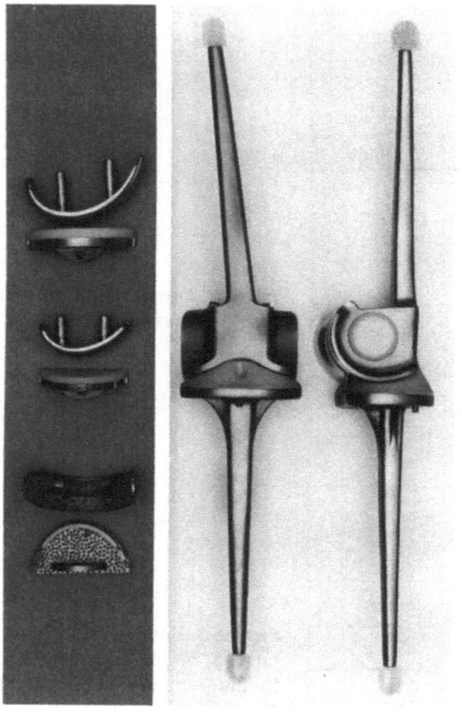

Figure 5. Sledge prosthesis and tibial rotating knee prosthesis (TRKP) Endo model

bility of the ligamentous support. A failure rate due to ligamentous insufficiency is therefore expected to decrease in the future. In order to improve the mechanical instructional properties of the tibial component the polyethylene was seated on a metal tray and its femoral surface adjusted to the anatomy. In 1976 the hinge prosthesis was improved by a design change (second generation). With our latest model, the tibial rotating knee prosthesis (TRKP) Endo model we expect a further reduction of failure rates. Since 1980 this has been implanted in 200 knees. Its efficacy is also being evaluated by the use of life tables and survival curves. Our experiences with the TRKP to date correspond with the experimental basis and theoretical expectations on which this new design was developed [4, 6] (Figure 5).

The method presented in this paper should encourage other workers to undertake similar studies assessing different types of knee prosthesis inserted by using uniform-indication operative technique and a sufficiently large number of patients.

References

1. Buchholz HW, Engelbrecht E (1973) Die intracondyläre total Kniegelenksendoprothese Modell „St. Georg". Chirurg 44:373
2. Dobbs HS (1980) Survivorship of total hip replacements. J Bone Joint Surg [Br] 62:168–173
3. Engelbrecht E (1972) Die operativen Behandlungsmöglichkeiten bei der Kniegelenksarthrose. Hamburger Ärztebl 26:346
4. Engelbrecht E (1984) Die Rotationsendprothese des Kniegelenks. Springer, Berlin Heidelberg New York Tokyo
5. Engelbrecht E, Siegel A, Röttger J, Buchholz HW (1976) Statistics of total knee replacement: Partial and total knee replacement design "St. Georg". Clin Orthop 120:54
6. Engelbrecht E, Nieder E, Strickle E, Keller A (1981) Intracondyläre Kniegelenksprothese mit Rotationsmöglichkeit – Endo Modell. Chirurg 52:368
7. Heinert K (1982) Langzeitergebnisse von Hüftendoprothesen nach einer durchschnittlichen Verlaufszeit von mehr als 10 Jahren. Statistische Auswertung von 2293 Fällen. Dissertation, Faculty of Medicine, Hamburg
8. Röttger J, Heinert K (1984) Die Knieendoprothesensysteme „St. Georg". Beobachtungen und Ergebnisse nach 10 Jahren Erfahrung mit über 3700 Operationen. Z Orthop
9. Siegel A (1974) Experiences with the sledge prosthesis ("St. Georg" design). In: The knee joint. Excerpta Medica, Amsterdam

The Guépar II hinged knee prosthesis

J. H. Aubriot and the Guépar Group

Department of Orthopaedic Surgery, Centre Hospitaler Régional
Caen
France

It may seem surprising, in 1984, to propose a review of hinged knee prostheses, a review which would be more appropriate to an historical study of this branch of surgery. Although, in my current practice, this type of prosthesis is employed in only less than 10% of total knee replacements, it seems useful to discuss it.

The aim of this review is twofold:

- To analyse the progress achieved in the field of hinged prostheses by the use of the Guépar II model as compared with the original Guépar I, discussed in 1970 by the group I represent here
- To discuss the place of such a prosthesis in current prosthetic surgery of the knee

In the group studied on two occasions, in 1979 and 1982, we have observed the long-term results with our first hinged Guépar I prostheses with follow-ups of 5–10 years.

The weak points of our first model are plainly apparent.

- Patellar disalignment (27%), a cause of instability and pain explaining many of the mediocre functional results
- An increased incidence (16%) of aseptic femoro-tibial loosening, not paralleled by clinical intolerance, which required reoperation in less than 10% of cases
- An increased incidence (8%) of deep infection, the surgical treatment of which has often proved difficult and unreliable, as only half the attempts at arthrodesis have resulted in bony fusion
- The frequent observation at reoperation of metallic debris arising from wear on the hinge axis

We had not waited for a 10-year follow-up to take note of these problems; since 1977 we have incorporated the following modifications and created the Guépar II prosthesis, which differs from the first model in the following points:

1. Broader epiphyseal base-plates.
2. Thicker and, especially, longer diaphyseal stems (20 cm in the femur, 19 cm in the tibia) to provide better anchorage and lessen the risks of malposition. Further, the inclination of the femoral diaphyseal axis to the mechanical axis of the knee has been reduced to 5 °.

3. Deeper groove in the trochlear shield and virtually routine use of a patellar disc for better stabilization of the patella and elimination of painful contact phenomena between an eburnated patella and a metallic trochlea.
4. Use of polyethylene bearings between the hinge axis and the tibial component with suppression of movements of the axis around the femur.

With a much shorter follow-up than for our first model, we have studied the problems and results with 112 prostheses in our group, i.e., in a multicentre study.

The patient material of the study is interesting insofar as it shows the nature of this series as regards patient selection for this operation:

- The average age was high (77 years), 80% of the operations being performed in patients over the age of 70: the oldest subject was 96.
- A high proportion of the knees (almost 50%) had already been treated surgically, mostly (30%) with some sort of prosthesis. As many as four previous operations had been performed in some cases.
- Arthrosis was the predominant aetiology (75%), which may account for the high average age.

These three factors probably largely explain the morbidity of the operation in this series.

Our chief problem is still the frequency of general operative complications, which resulted in a 6% death rate. This subject alone deserves a separate discussion. I mention only that when I do still use a hinged prosthesis, I now release the tourniquet before cementing. I no longer use a plug, nor do I introduce the cement with a syringe; in other respects, all anaesthetic precautions are taken.

Most of the intraoperative mechanical complications occurred during reoperation on knees with existing prostheses. These fractures, or false passages, do not give a good radiological appearance. They delay weight-bearing and rehabilitation; but all those in our series consolidated, and none promoted eventual loosening.

I do not wish to embark on a tedious discussion of postoperative and late complications; three points deserve emphasis.

1. We still have a serious incidence of deep infections (8%), which may be due to the bulk of the prosthesis and the persistence of dead spaces. Compared with semiconstrained or nonconstrained prostheses, it must be said that the treatment of these deep infections remains difficult, though in some cases, paradoxically, they are well tolerated and do not not require reoperation.
   Some minimal treatments (excision, antibiotic therapy) have permitted stabilization with a moderate functional result. The classical approach of arthrodesis is no guarantee of a good result, not so much because of infection but from failure of bony fusion.
   In two cases where the prosthesis was changed, the procedure is still too recent for the outcome to be assessed; the second is a success as far as

infection is concerned but flexion is limited to 50 °. One case only has required early amputation, owing to the severity of associated skin problems.

2. Thanks to the grooving of the trochlea and the use of a poylethylene patellar disc, our incidence of lateral subluxations of the patella is very low (5%), and these are always moderate and well-tolerated even when the patella was luxated preoperatively.
3. We seem no longer to encounter aseptic femoro-tibial loosening; we have observed only one case of painful aseptic loosening responsible for a bad result; we did not reoperate because the general condition was poor.

This satisfactory outcome as regards maintenance of fixation, without fracture of the diaphyseal stems, seems due to the modifications we have introduced, which allow almost uniformly good alignment of the prosthesis in the frontal and sagittal planes, provide good diaphyseal anchorage with only 10% of margination, and are not found at reoperation to be associated with metallic debris from wear of the hinge axis on the bearing.

The study of the functional results, with a follow-up of 1–6 years, relates to only 84 knees for which all complications are considered. We have adopted a four-point scale for each of our criteria.

Now we shall analyse the results in more detail from the aspects of pain and mobility.

The results for pain give an overall idea of the outcome and progress in each case compared with the preoperative status. The 3% with pain are accounted for by two cases of infection and by the single case of aseptic loosening.

The results for the range of flexion are highly consistent: in virtually half the knees there is a range of 110 ° or more, and the knees with a range of less than 90 ° are those which were stiff initially or in which complications occurred (mainly infective). Residual fixed flexion of more than 10 ° was exceptional. Stability of these knees is uniformly good, since we seem to have solved the patellar problem.

In assessing the overall resuit, the members of our group did not wish to use a scoring system, preferring minimum levels of performance based on the essential criteria of pain, mobility and stability.

The outcome for walking is more difficult to incorporate and arises only insofar as the prosthesis is responsible for limitation of walking.

I suggest to the committee of our society that we study proposals for a common method of application of criteria for our future meetings. I have presented our own results according to a system which may be open to improvement, but which seems to correspond fairly well to the reality expressed by the patient as regards his or her functional performance.

These figures – only 74% good or excellent results – are not entirely satisfactory. A study of the causes of the mediocre and poor results clearly reflects the complications and problems I have mentioned: infections; advanced age in the patients, who have often had several previous operations; prostheses inserted at an advanced stage of the disease, which has already restricted mobility. Because of these conditions, although only 3% of the knees in our series were painful enough to constitute a handicap, I find it difficult to compare these figures with the results currently reported for other types of prostheses.

I should like to deal rapidly here with the indications accepted for the hinged prosthesis in our practice, after recalling the advantages of this prosthesis:

- Ease of insertion with a good anatomical result
- Immediate stability
- Minimal patellar problems
- Femoro-tibial loosening exceptional

I have to say that, personally, during the last 2 years I have used this hinged prosthesis in only 9% of all arthroplasties. I mainly employ the total condylar prosthesis, and the overall functional results are assessed on the same criteria. The improvement is very clear, since there are fewer complications in knees which presented simpler problems at the outset. But even so, the functional outcome was not altogether satisfactory and we have now, in the Guépar Group, perfected a semi-constrained, asymmetrical prosthesis which retains the posterior cruciate ligament and the possibility of rotary movement. The initial results are very encouraging, but I believe that there is still a legitimate place for a hinged prosthesis like the Guépar II, since we seem to have solved the problems presented by our first model:

- Painful patellar subluxation
- Femoro-tibial loosening, debris from metallic wear of the hinge axis

I retain four types of indications:

- Certain situations requiring renewal of hinged prostheses. In certain cases it is nevertheless possible to envisage a movement away from the hinged prosthesis to a semi-constrained insert.
- Rheumatoid arthritis when gross deformity of the knee is combined with marked osteoporosis.
- Certain abnormalities of the knee associated with gross anatomical derangement at the hip, for example when resection of the femoral head and neck in cases where total hip replacement is not justified for various reasons has repercussions on the knee.
- The very rare tabetic arthropathies: With this pathology, in order to prevent loosening it seems necessary to ensure good diaphyseal anchorages.

A final indication, which is not really part of this discussion but which leads one to reflect on the excellent functional possibilities offered by hinged prostheses, is the presence of bony tumours of the lower end of the femur necessitating bony resection.

Even in our own practice, the hinged Guépar II prosthesis is rarely used, but it is an arthroplasty which should not be entirely forgotten since it is useful in difficult cases where it is often important to operate rapidly and to obtain a good anatomical result without problems.

To improve the results, what is required is not a new design of prosthesis, since the functional outcome in uncomplicated cases is satisfactory, but reduction to the minimum of the two main complications, operative cardiac arrest and deep infection, while realizing that this "last-resort" prosthesis is often used for patients who are in extremity after previous operations.

The posterior stabilized total condylar prosthesis: A 2- to 5-year follow-up study of 50 severely deformed knees

P. Aglietti, R. Buzzi and A. Pisaneschi

First Orthopaedic Clinic of the University of Florence
Italy

The total condylar prosthesis designed at the Hospital for Special Surgery, New York, in 1973 was modified in 1978 by the addition of a tibial polyethylene spine and a transverse femoral cam to provide the function of the posterior cruciate ligament. The results with the total condylar I have been shown to be very satisfactory with a follow-up of 3–5 years [1, 4], but specific areas of deficiency [5] were identified. Posterior subluxation was sometimes noted as a consequence of inadequate fit in flexion; the range of motion was 95 ° on average and normal function, defined as unlimited walking, stair climbing and transfer activities without aids, was present in 22% of the cases. This represented an improvement over previous experiences [3] but was still far from ideal.

The interaction of the intercondylar spine with the posterior cam was thought to provide posterior stability, to increase the range of motion and to improve the lever arm of the quadriceps mechanism, without any adverse effect on the tibial component fixation.

The present study was undertaken to assess whether these goals were met in our first 50 posteriorly stabilized total condylar prostheses.

Material and methods
From January 1979 to December 1981 we operated on 54 knees in 44 patients (the operation was bilateral in 10 patients). The average age was 65 years and the patients were predominantly female.

The preoperative diagnoses were osteoarthritis in 35, rheumatoid arthritis in 18 and osteonecrosis in 1. Several patients had had a previous surgical operation on the knee, mainly tibial osteotomies (5) and synovectomies (6).

Thirty-two knees had a varus deformity (15 ° on average), 11 knees had a valgus alignment (23 ° on average) and in 11 patients the predominant deformity was flexion contracture (37 ° on average). Furthermore 11 knees were stiff and 3 completely ankylosed.

The operation was performed through a mildine approach [2]: most of the knees required an extensive release to achieve adequate balance between medial and lateral soft tissues but, provided this was carefully accomplished, it was possible fully to correct every deformity without the need of a constrained prosthesis. In the stiff knees the inverted incision of Coonse and Adams was most helpful in achieving immediate and extensive exposure. For severe flexion contractures a posterior capsulotomy was performed.

Bone deficiency which could not be compensated for by the standard technique was a frequent finding, especially on the medial side of the tibial plateau in the varus knees. The necessary build-up was obtained preferably either with cement reinforced with mesh and screws or with a bone graft fixed with screws.

General complications were infrequent (5%), and of no consequence for the patient. Local complications were more frequent (15%), mainly delayed wound healing, which was treated by a slowing down range of motion exercises.

All the patients were revised personally by one of the authors and evaluated using the Hospital for Special Surgery Knee Rating System which allots 100 points to the normal knee. Results were categorized as follows: excellent (85–100 points), good (70–84), fair (60–69) and poor (less than 60).

Results

Follow-up was achieved in 50 patients, and it was 36 months on average (min., 24; max., 58 months).

The knee score significantly increased from a low 36 to a high 85 at follow-up on average. Results were excellent in 34, good in 11, fair in 5 and poor in none.

The fair results were due to loosening of both femoral and tibial components in one case, to suspected infection in one case and to lateral laxity after a lateral release in a valgus knee in another. A rheumatoid patient had a bilateral knee prosthesis for bilateral ankylosis in flexion, and improved to the level of a fair result to her satisfaction. In the last knee with a fair result the problems arose from the patella catching during extension.

Normal function was obtained in 56% of the cases, the rest all being improved.

Maximum flexion was 101 ° on average, ranging from 80 ° to 120 °.

The ideal alignment (5 °–15 ° of valgus) was achieved in 78% of the cases, and the errors were commoner in the placement of the femoral than of the tibial component.

Radiolucent lines were studied according to the zones method. Overall significant radiolucent lines (complete, progressive or more than 2 mm wide) were seen on both components in the same knee, the fair result suspected of infection around a tibial component in an otherwise symptomless 68-year-old woman.

Conclusions

Excellent or good results were achieved in 90% of these severely deformed knees. We found an increased number of patellar problems compared with our previous experience with the total condylar I. This can almost completely be solved by careful attention to patellar tracking and more extensive use of the lateral release.

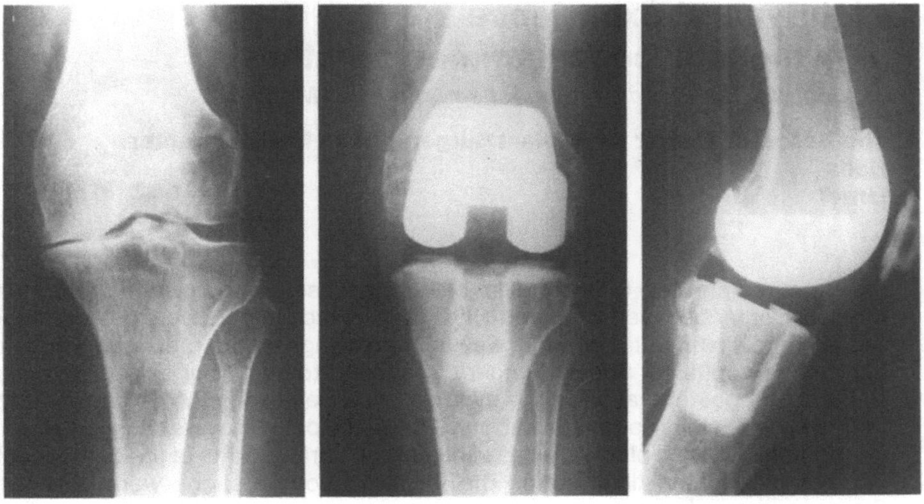

a b c

Figure 1. **a** Medial gonarthrosis in a 66-year-old woman. **b, c** Good alignment and absence of lucent lines in the anteroposterior and lateral view after a 5-year follow-up period

Improved instrumentation is now available for a more accurate component position; the correct limb alignment is of critical importance and this can be better achieved with the new tenser.

Posterior cruciate excision is necessary in most of these severely deformed knees in order fully to correct the deformity.

Posterior cruciate substitution is a good forward step, and it has proved useful in avoiding posterior subluxation, increasing the range of motion and improving function.

No increased fixation problems have been noted so far: 96% of the tibial components showed no signs of loosening in this series (Figure 1).

References

1. Aglietti P, Rinonapoli (1986) Total condylar knee replacement: a five-year follow-up study of thirty-three knees. Clin Orthop 186:(in press)
2. Insall JN (1984) Surgery of the knee. Churchill Livingstone, New York
3. Insall JN, Ranawat CS, Aglietti P, Shine J (1976) A comparison of four models of total knee-replacement prostheses. J Bone Joint Surg [Am] 58:754
4. Insall JN, Scott M, Ranawat CS (1979) The total condylar knee prosthesis: a report of two hundred and twenty cases. J Bone Joint Surg [Am] 61:173
5. Insall JN, Lachiewicz PF, Burstein AH (1982) The posterior stabilized condylar prosthesis: a modification of the total condylar design. J Bone Joint Surg [Am] 64:1317
6. Insall JN, Hood RW, Flawn LB, Sullivan DJ (1983) The total condylar knee prosthesis in gonarthrosis. J Bone Joint Surg [Am] 65:619

Eight years' experience with the total condylar knee prosthesis

M. Soundry, M. Iusim, A. Menachem and D. G. Mendes

The Research Center for Implant Surgery, Haifa Medical Center
Haifa
Israel

One hundred and two total condylar knee prostheses were inserted at the Haifa Medical Center between 1975 and 1982. 80% of the patients were osteoarthritic. The average hospital stay was four weeks. The average preoperative score according to the Hospital for Special Surgery was found to be 43 points and increased to 89 points postoperatively. The average postoperative R.O.M. was 90° which interfered with stairs negotiation ability. 97% of the patients were satisfied. Roentgenographically, radiolucency was seen around various parts of the components but not around the tibial stem. The following complications were observed: 3 supracondylar fractures successfully treated conservatively, 2 recurrent dislocations of patella treated surgically, 1 patellar fracture, 2 cases of loosening and 1 low grade infection.

We would like to submit that in our hands the prosthesis was successful both objectively and subjectively in more than 90% of the patients, but was noted to have limited flexion.

Total knee replacement: comparison of Attenborough, total condylar and kinematic knee

K. Hardinger, B. Livingstone, J. C. Murphy and M. Shatwell

Centre for Hip Surgery, Wrightington Hospital, Wigan, Lancs
Wigan
England

Between 23rd January 1978 and 7th January 1982, 141 Attenborough knee replacements were performed at Wrightington Hospital of which 106 were primary procedures.

Between 5th July 1979 and 7th June 1982, 553 total Condylar knee replacements were performed of which 497 were primary procedures.

Between 22nd September 1980 and 30th June 1983 124 Kinematic knee replacements were performed of which 113 were primary procedures.

Review of these cases would indicate that there is:

an unacceptable complication rate with the patella in the Attenborough knee prosthesis and a high incidence of tibial loosening.

tibial loosening in the total condylar knee replacement has been diminished with the use of the metal tray.

Improvement in function and degree of flexion between total Condylar knee replacement and Kinematic knee replacement are compared.

The outcome of the infected knee arthroplasty

D. P. Johnson and G. C. Bannister

Department of Orthopaedic Surgery, Bristol Royal Infirmary
Bristol
United Kingdom

Infection of arthroplasty of the knee is a major problem. The incidence of deep infection in the majority of published series is between 2% and 7%. Little is known of the outcome of the various treatments used. This analysis was undertaken to define the natural history and outcome of the infected arthroplasty of the knee.

In order to collect adequate numbers of cases and follow-up a retrospective analysis of a consecutive series of 471 knee prostheses which had a minimum of 1 year follow-up was performed. The operations were performed for 328 patients and consisted of 431 primary operations and 40 revisions.

There was a variety of prostheses used, both hinged and non-hinged. The operations were all performed in a conventional turbulent flow operating theatre with cement fixation and using antibiotic prophylaxis. In the earlier cases this consisted of cephradine though the later cases received cefuroxime 750 mg preoperatively and repeated intramuscularly 8 h and 16 h postoperatively.

It was apparent during the study that some infections followed a benign course while others resulted in failure of the arthroplasty. In an effort to define the character of the infection, we have divided them into two categories: superficial infection and deep infection involving the prosthesis. Superficial infection was defined as clinical evidence of extracapsular inflammation and a positive wound culture. Deep infection was defined as clinical evidence of deep inflammation, positive wound culture and identification either by surgery or sinogram of extension of the infection to the prosthesis.

The leucocyte cell count was found not to be of significant diagnostic help.

Of the 471 cases reviewed 23 cases of superficial infection and 25 cases of deep infection were identified. The incidence of superficial infection in the 431 primary operations was 5% whereas in the 40 revision operations it was 2%. The incidence of deep infection in the primary operations was 4% whereas in revision surgery it was four times as great at 15%.

There were two significant predisposing factors to deep infection identified: the presence of rheumatoid arthritis and the pre-existing presence of superficial infection.

All patients with superficial wound infection obtained pain-free gait within 5 months. Of the 25 cases of deep infection 14 occurred in the perioperative period and 11 occurred after initial primary wound healing.

There was objective evidence by an initial negative exploration or sinogram that 7 of the 14 early deep infections had progressed from an initial superficial infection, whereas the origin of the remainder was less well defined. Of the 11 cases of late deep infection two cases had a bacteriologically proven source of haematogenous spread of infection to a previously healthy prosthesis. One was a beta haemolytic streptococcal sore throat and the other case was a *Staphylococcus aureus* urinary tract infection during a transurethral resection of the prostate.

The organisms cultured were predominantly *Staphylococcus aureus*, though *Staphylococcus albus*, streptococci, Gram-negative bacilli and diptheroids were also isolated.

In the 25 cases of deep infection long-term antibiotic treatment was initially used in all cases for a mean duration of 1.3 years, during which time the symptoms of only two patients were eradicated. Therefore long-term antibiotic treatment in deep infection was only effective in 8% of cases.

Other treatment included excision of sinus tracts, which was undertaken in four cases; in each case the sinus recurred. Debridement of the joint was attempted 27 times, but it was always unsuccessful in eradicating the symptoms of infection. Free split skin grafts were undertaken in two cases in an attempt to provide skin cover for an exposed prosthesis. In both cases the graft failed to survive. However, gastrocnemius musculocutaneous flaps were undertaken in three cases. These were successful in two cases in providing permanent skin cover. One case was unsuccessful due to a failure to eradicate the infection prior to grafting.

Exchange arthroplasty was unsuccessful in the two attempted cases. Subsequently one underwent arthrodesis successfully and one underwent amputation.

Arthrodesis was attempted in a total of 12 cases, two of which required subsequent bone grafting. Bony ankylosis was obtained in 6 cases, after a mean duration of 10 months of immobilization, although more importantly pain-free gait was obtained in 11 of the 12 cases, often when fibrous ankylosis was present. A painful fibrous ankylosis only occurred in one case.

The outcome of the 25 cases of deep infection of knee arthroplasty resulted in arthrodesis being undertaken in 12 cases. Long-term antibiotic treatment, though initially carried out in all cases, was the only form of treatment in nine cases, and amputation was performed in four patients, although all four amputees subsequently walked with prostheses. The nine cases treated by long-term antibiotics resulted in eradication of symptoms in two cases, while seven continued to be symptomatic. Most had copious purulent discharges, many were painful and one patient requires an electrical device to assist him into and out of bed.

When interviewed the patients valued a pain-free knee more than joint movement or a pleasing cosmetic result. Pain-free gait has been attained in only 17 of the 25 deeply infected arthroplasties.

In conclusion, deep infection in a knee arthroplasty is eradicated by long-term antibiotics alone in only 8% of cases, whereas arthrodesis provided the pain-free gait which these unfortunate patients desire in 92%.

Acknowledgment. The authors wish to thank Mr. A. H. C. Ratliff and the surgeons of Winford Orthopaedic Hospital, Bristol, for their assistance.

A policy for knee replacement

R. A. J. Baily and C. E. Ackroyd

University of Bristol
Bristol
England

Arthritis of the knee presents a variety of problems which each require differing solutions. The Bristol Knee Group have been engaged for the past ten years in the evaluation of certain designs of knee prostheses in the attempt to formulate a policy for knee replacement based on rational principles and on carefully monitored results.

Material and methods

All patients undergoing knee replacement by members of the knee group since 1974 have been fully documented and have been followed up at intervals of six months, one year, and then yearly. 120 knees treated with the Sheehan prosthesis and 90 knees treated with the St. Georg Sledge prosthesis, used as a unicompartment replacement on either the medial or lateral side, are available for analysis together with a smaller number of knees with the Kinematic prosthesis, which will have a shorter follow up period but will be included to illustrate present practice.

Results

Overall results for the Sheehan prosthesis (original design) show that although 85% results are satisfactory after two years, this percentage drops to 56% after a mean four year follow up (range 2-10 years). The causes of deterioration appear to be wear of the central stud and sinkage of the components. The Kinematic knee shows 92% satisfactory results but this is a maximum two year follow up. The St. Georg prosthesis followed up for a similar period to the Sheehan shows virtually no tendency to deterioration and the level of satisfactory results remains at 86%. Relief of pain and improvement of walking ability had been consistent with this prosthesis but improvement in the range of movement has been less apparent.

Conclusions

The Sheehan prosthesis, at least in its original form, appears to deteriorate with time in a proportion of patients so that the long term results are not as good as those reported in other series using different prostheses. The Hamburg St. Georg Sledge prosthesis used as a unicompartmental device in gonarthrosis has been consistently successful in properly selected patients. The Kinematic prosthesis shows promise as a standard treatment for more advanced arthritis of the knee.

The PCA total knee prosthesis

K. A. Krackow and D. S. Hungerford

Division of Arthritis Surgery, The Johns Hopkins University
Department of Orthopaedic Surgery at the Good Samaritan Hospital
Baltimore, Maryland
USA

The Porous Coated Anatomic "Total Knee replacement, implanted with the use of the Universal Total Knee Instruments" was designed to reproduce physiologic, anatomic alignment of the lower extremity and to resurface the femoral, tibial, and patellar aspects of the knee permitting normal kinematic motion patterns. This relatively unconstrained prosthesis models the normal medial and lateral asymmetries of the knee to allow physiologic rolling and sliding during flexion, near normal passive axial rotation, and further active axial rotation of a normal degree.

A total of 414 PCA total knee arthroplasties have been performed at the Division of Arthritis Surgery of the Johns Hopkins Orthopaedic Department at the Good Samaritan Hospital, Baltimore, Maryland, U.S.A., from January, 1980 through December, 1983. Of these prostheses, 119 were implanted between January 1, 1980 and December 31, 1981, providing a minimum two year follow-up for this review. Only six of these cases have been lost to follow-up, three due to death unrelated to surgery and three due to moves necessitating follow-up elsewhere. Thus, results of 113 knees have been analysed. In addition, the assumptions of anatomic alignment about the knee, anatomic consideration of prosthetic design, and specifics of surgical technique are shown.

Thirty six of 113 prostheses were implanted in patients with rheumatoid arthritis. The average age was 60 years (range 20-78), with an average follow-up of 37 months (range 24-48). Eleven of 36 were implanted without cement, and 25 of 36 with cement. Good and excellent results occurred in 10 of 11 uncemented cases with 1 of 11 having a fair result due to quadriceps lag. Twenty of 25 cemented knees achieved good and excellent results, and there were five of 25 poor results, due to persistent flexion contracture and limitation in range of motion — these in very severely involved patients, most of whom were non-ambulatory pre-operatively. However, pain relief was good or excellent in all of this sub-group.

Seventy one of 113 prostheses were implanted in patients with osteoarthrosis. [average age = 73 (range 39-95); average follow-up = 34 months (24-48)]; 26 of 71 were implanted without cement, and 45 of 71 with cement. The results of cemented and uncemented cases were proportionately comparable: 65 of 71 (91.5%) experienced good to excellent results, four of 71 (5.6%) a fair result, and two of 71 (2.8%) a poor result. The poor results were cemented knees with persistent pain and limited ranges of motion without evidence of infection or loosening.

Six of 113 prostheses were implanted in patients with avascular necrosis; two out of six with cement, and four of six without cement, [mean age = 42 (26-79), and mean follow-up of 35 months (24-48)]. All six were rated good or excellent.

Eight of 414 (1.9%) patients had further surgery for: two cases of infection, three cases of displaced patellar buttons, before a design modification, two cases to reduce the size of the implanted femoral component from medium to small, and one case of early failure due to poor cement technique involving a tibial component.

Currently, approximately 85% of our components are implanted without cement, because the results in our uncemented cases appear as good, if not better, than in our cemented ones. This two to four year early experience is encouraging, especially in regard to cementless fixation, and justifies continued use of this approach to total knee arthroplasty.

Rehabilitation

Injection-induced quadriceps contractures in children – the advantage of a proximal release

A. Jackson, P. Hutton and J. L. Pozo

Great Ormond Street, Children's Hospital
London
Great Britain

The clinical presentation and management of seventeen children with progressive quadriceps contractures is presented. All of the children suffered a severe illness within the first few weeks of life and received intramuscular thigh injections. Two distinct operative procedures were used in the treatment of these injection induced contractures. One group was treated by a distally placed quadricepsplasty, and the second by a proximal release. The advantages of a proximal release are discussed.

Material and methods

In seventeen children a total of 31 quadriceps contractures were reviewed. 12 were treated conservatively (Group 1) 10 by a distal quadricepsplasty (Group 2) and 9 by a proximal release (Group 3). The average post-operative follow-up in group 2 was 10.5 years and in group 3 2.3 years. The essential presenting symptom was that of a painless limitation of knee flexion. A thigh dimple was present in all cases. In the cases reviewed the contractures were associated with genu reçurvatum, tibial torsion, patella alta, hypoplasia of the patella and fragmentation of the inferior pole of the patella.

Results

None of the conservatively treated group (Group 1) showed an increase in the range of knee movement at follow-up. Six of the contractures had deteriorated – In Group 2 and Group 3 all cases had a significant increase in the range of knee movement post-operatively which was maintained at follow-up. The most significant finding was that in seven of the ten cases treated by a distal quadricepsplasty an extension lag was noted at follow-up. The extension lag varied between 5 degrees in four knees, 10 degrees in one knee and 20 degrees in two knees. None of the nine cases treated by a proximal release at the site of the skin dimple (Group 3) showed an extension lag at follow-up.

Summary

The advantage of a proximal release over a distally placed quadriceps plasty in the treatment of injection induced quadriceps contractures in children is demonstrated. The surgical technique will be discussed, and the effect of these contractures on the patella demonstrated.

Refraining from postoperative immobilization in the treatment of knee instabilities

E. O. Münch and J. M. Schmidt

Orthopaedic University Hospital Munich
8000 München
Federal Republic of Germany

The question of whether to treat knee instabilities post operatively by immobilization or early functional mobilization was solved at our hospital in favour of immediate mobilization.

After operative treatment of fresh and old anteromedial instabilities grade II we deploy the following regimen: Placement in a posterior plaster of Paris splint and active physical therapy from the 4th postoperative day between 30 and 60 degrees, increasing the range of motion up to the 6th week to 90 degrees knee flexion. Full extension is blocked after procedures on the anterior cruciate ligament up to the 12th week. During post-operative treatment the use of electric stimulation of the vastus medialis muscle and the ischio-crural muscles is employed.

For fresh and old anteromedial knee instabilities grade III we use an adjustable splint immediately postoperatively with an excentric joint axis. After the 4th postoperative day passive mobilization on an electric splint is begun. Physical therapy is then done on an outpatient basis including isometric exercises, active range of motion exercises limited by the splint and PNF. The range of motion is gradually increased with the splint, blocking full extension up to the 12th postoperative week. During this time, electric stimulation is employed additionally. Further measures after the 12th week comprise improvement of coordination, endurance power and mobility with the final aim of full athletic rehabilition.

An attempt to objectively evaluate TNS as pain relief after knee surgery

I. Arvidsson, G. Borg, E. Eriksson and E. Knutsson

Section of Trauma, Dept of Surgery, Clinical Neurophysiology Lab. Karolinska Hospital and Dept of Psychology, Stockholm University Stockholm Sweden

Transcutaneous nerve stimulation (TNS) is widely used for pain treatment and has been recommended as an adjunct in the rehabilitation after knee surgery in order to reduce the need for postoperative morphine.

Material and methods

A small battery operated TNS unit that the patient can monitor himself (Tenzcare[R]) was tested on 13 patients that had been operated with reconstruction of the anterior cruciate ligament with the use of the patellar tendon. The patients were operated under epidural anaesthesia and the epidural catheter was left in place and kept open with repeated injections of minute amounts of phys saline. Sterile electrodes for TNS treatment were applied after skin suture. The morning after surgery ordinary EMG and integrated EMG from the quadriceps of the operated leg was recorded and a subjective grading of the amount of pain during attempts to contract the quadriceps according to the so called Borg-scale was obtained. After this placebo-TNS was given during a period of 15' and the same experiments were then recorded. TNS was then given for a period of 15' and the experiments repeated. Finally an injection of a dilute solution of local anaesthetic (20 cc of 0.25% lidocaine) was given into the epidural catheter. This dose has been found to give only sensory block and no motor anaesthesia in earlier studies. 30' later ordinary and integrated EMG were obtained and a psychologic grading of the pain on muscle contraction was obtained.

Results

The results of a typical experiment are shown in figure below. Initially most patients had great problems retrieving their quadriceps function due to severe pain. After placebo TNS integrated EMG improved some 7% but the psychological pain increased on an average 10%. After real TNS the psychological pain grading diminished 27% on an average (range 10-83%) and integrated EMG improved 183%. These differences are statistically significant. After the epidural injection finally the psychological pain grading diminished 86% (range 55-100%) and the integrated EMG improved on an average 745%.

Discussion

TNS evidently can diminish the very severe pain after a reconstruction of the anterior cruciate ligament. Since this is regarded one of our most painful procedures, this proves that TNS is an alternative in the postoperative pain treatment. Epidural reinjections of local anaesthesia are more effective undoubtedly but have proven difficult to administer to a larger number of newly operated patients due to need for reinjections every 2 hour. The small TNS unit can be monitored by the patient himself. In the immediate postoperative period it may need to be combined with some intramuscular morphine but after 24-36 hours it has proven to be sufficient.

Summary
A small patient monitored battery operated TNS unit was tested in the postoperative period after ant. cruciate reconstruction. It was able to diminish pain and improve muscle function and thus reduce the need for other analgesics.

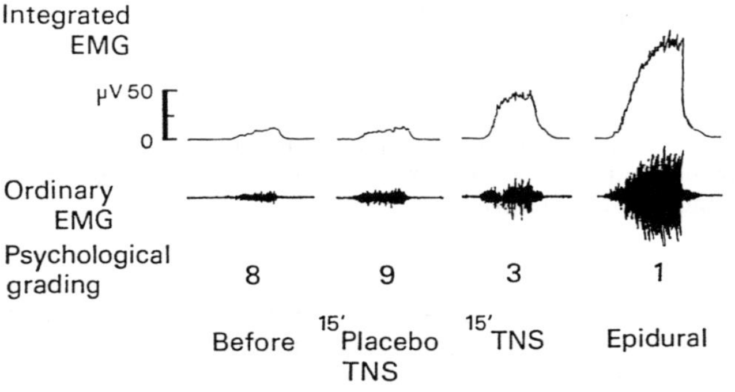

Rehabilitation after lesions of the knee joint – experiences made in 2019 athletes (1962–1983)

J. Weber

Zentralinstitut des Sportmed. Dienstes
August-Bebel-Straße 12, 8216 Kreischa
German Democratic Republic

The object of the rehabilitation treatment of athletes is the recovery of the ability of training and of participation in sports contests as prompt and as perfect as possible.

In this we see a difference to the "normal" rehabilitation, for it is not only the question of reusing a joint, but of reobtaining the tolerance of outstanding physical charges.

A sports medical rehabilitation has to fulfil the following tasks:

1. Conservation and recovery of the general athletic traning status in order to prevent a relieving syndrome.
2. Recovery of the stability and of the flexibility of the injured extremity.
3. The general state and the tolerance of local charges of the knee joint must allow the re-starting of the specific sports training.

In sports traumatology lesions of the knee joint occur very frequently. The recovery has to be done under daily clinical control, in order to prevent a disharmony between the real charge tolerance and the actual charges due to daily physiotherapeutic treatment and training. For this reason we are measuring the skin temperature two times per day. Furthermore we are using sports medical and methodical tests at the beginning, in the course, and at the end of a rehabilitation period for monitoring the results of our efforts. In this context emphasis is laid on dynamographic measurements of the muscular force of the lower leg extension. Concerning the physiotherapeutic treatment electrotherapy is of major importance. The physical charge we are applying as rehabilitation training is divided into two phases: to begin without any physical charge of the injured extremity, we are afterwards step by step involving the injured knee joint.
The type, the intensity and the duration of the applied physical charges are pointed out depending on a given diagnosis and the course of the rehabilitation. Special attention is paid to the recovery of atrophied muscles.

Experiences gathered so far on rehabilitation results of meniscectomies, ligament lesions and lesions of the cartilage imposed various recommendations concerning a general or a specific re-charge after a lesion.

Is the rehabilitation after knee ligament surgery effective enough?

J. Lysholm, Y. Tegner, M. Odensten, M. Nordin and J. Gillquist

Department of Orthopaedic Surgery, University Hospital
S-581 85 Linköping
Sweden

Rehabilitation after knee ligament surgery is long and demanding. Many studies suggest that several patients never resume normal muscle function in the operated leg.

Method
25 patients, all men (mean age 25.0 ± 6.2 years), group I were examined 12-29 months (mean 19.3 months) after treatment of a knee injury. All had completed a standardized rehabilitation programme during 1 year and showed a stable knee at the follow-up. Isokinetic muscle strength in quadriceps and hamstring muscles was determined. A functional test including one leg jump and running in a figure of eight (40 m) was done. The time for running in the turn and straight ahead was registered separately. A functional knee scoring scale evaluation was also done (Lysholm & Gillquist 1982). For comparison the same examination was done in 67 healthy male soccer players (mean age 23.5 ± 4.5. years; group II) and in 26 men with sympatomatic old anterior cruciate tears (mean age 26.8 ± 6.8 years; group III).

Results
Patients in group I and group III needed significantly longer time for running in the bends than healthy soccer players (4.17 ± 0.73 and 4.12 ± 0.82 compared to 3.42 ± 0.35, $p < 0.001$). There was no significant difference between the groups in running straight ahead. Group I patients showed the same result as the healthy soccer players (group II) in the jump test, but group III patients showed significantly worse jumping ability ($p < 0.001$). Likewise, no significant difference in muscle strain between groups I and II was found, but group III showed less than normal quadriceps strength (86% of healthy leg). The mean score was 94.4 ± 5.2 points in group I and 81.1 ± 4.8 points in group III ($p < 0.001$).

Conclusion: The results suggest that muscle rehabilitation was adequate. The results in the figure-of-eight may be an early sign of an insufficient ligament repair indicating a risk for increasing instability in the future, although the joint still 1-2 years after the injury was stable.

The effect of a strength training programme on function in patients with cruciate injuries

Y. Tegner, J. Lysholm and J. Gillquist

Sports and Trauma Research Group, Department of Orthopaedic Surgery, University Hospital
S-581 85 Linköping
Sweden

Introduction

Treatment of old cruciate injuries is aimed at elimination of functional instability, for example, the giving way of the knee. The feeling of giving way is the major feature of the disability that follows anterior cruciate injury. There are two approaches to treatment. One is to eliminate the static instability by means of extra- or intra-articular reconstruction. The other is to train compensatory functions such as muscle strength. Very little is known about the effect of a strength training programme not aimed at eliminating static instability in the affected knee. Many surgeons maintain that strength training is effective in some patients, but few have presented any substantial evidence. Noyes and associates recently showed that about 30% of patients with anterior cruciate injury will respond favourably to a rehabilitation programme and modification of activity.

Material

Sixty-nine patients – 53 men and 16 women – with significant instability problems were treated by a 3-month strength training programme. Fifty had sustained injury to the anterior cruciate and 13 to the posterior, and 6 patients had injuries to both. At least 1 month before starting training all patients underwent arthroscopy in order to establish the full extent of injury and to treat meniscus lesions that could interfere with the training.

Evaluation system

An objective and reproducible method for evaluation is imperative in order to obtain a correct picture of the effects of different treatments. The system used in this study has previously been shown to give a reliable assessment of the disability. It consists of four different parts.

1. A knee function score to grade symptoms in sport and daily activities on a 100-point scale. A score above 84 points is considered good and a score below 65 points poor.

2. An activity grading scale with 11 levels, where 10 represents an elite soccer player, 7 an elite jogger and 0 a patient on sick leave or receiving a disability pension because of the knee problem.

3. A performance test where the knee is put to strain in sport-like situations. After warm-up on an ergometer cycle the following are performed:

a) A one-leg hop. Three attempts are made and the quotient between the best results for the injured and uninjured legs is used.
b) Running in a figure-of-eight in two laps, each 20 metres long.
c) Running up and down a 25-step spiral staircase, once.

d) Running up and down a 55-metre-long indoor slope, once. There is a 180 ° turn halfway up the slope.

4. Measurements of strength using a Cybex II isokinetic dynamometer. Strength is measured isokinetically at 30 ° and 180 °/s, and isometrically at 60 ° knee flexion. The peak torque values for the hamstrings and quadriceps are used. The relative strength is expressed as the quotient between the injured and uninjured legs.

All patients were examined in this way before and after the training period. Strength was measured each month in order to follow the effects of training. Twelve patients were also evaluated with Lysholm's knee function score, activity grading and strength measurements 2 years later.

Results

One patient did not complete the training programme because her knee gave way so frequently that reconstruction was necessary. After training another 14 patients (20%) considered their functional disability so great that they asked for an operation.

Knee score

The mean preoperative score was 73 ± 15 points. A significant increase to 83 ± 15 took place during training. At the start 17 patients were graded as excellent or good and 27 as poor. After training a significant improvement ($P < 0.001$) was noted: 38 patients were classified as excellent or good and only 9 as poor (Table 1). No reduction was seen in patients followed up 2 years later.

Table 1. Score classification at the start (69 patients) and at the end of the training period (68 patients)

Score classification	Start	End
Excellent/good	17	38
Fair	25	21
Poor	27	9

Activity level

The median activity level before training was 2, which corresponds to inability to carry out any type of heavy work or sports. The activity level increased significantly ($P < 0.001$) during the training period. Over the following 2 years a further increase occurred in a few patients. The rest remained at the same level.

Strength measurements

There were significant increases in all strength measurements ($P < 0.001$). Quadriceps strength at 30 °/s increased by more than 20%. However, only the hamstring strength returned to normal (Figure 1). In 48 patients (70%) the relative quadriceps strength was below 0.85 at the start. During training the quotient increased to above 0.85 in 32 patients (67%). Only 18 patients (26%)

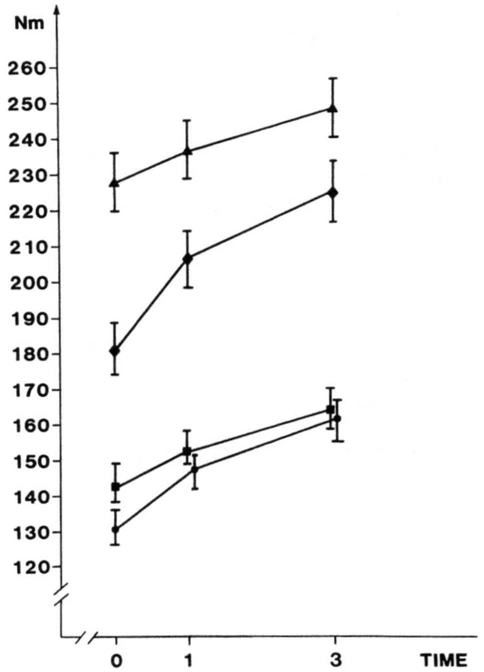

Figure 1. Strength development during the training period. ▲ indicates quadriceps strength of the uninjured leg; ◆ indicates quadriceps strength of the injured leg; ■ indicates hamstring strength of the uninjured leg; and ● indicates hamstring strength of the injured leg

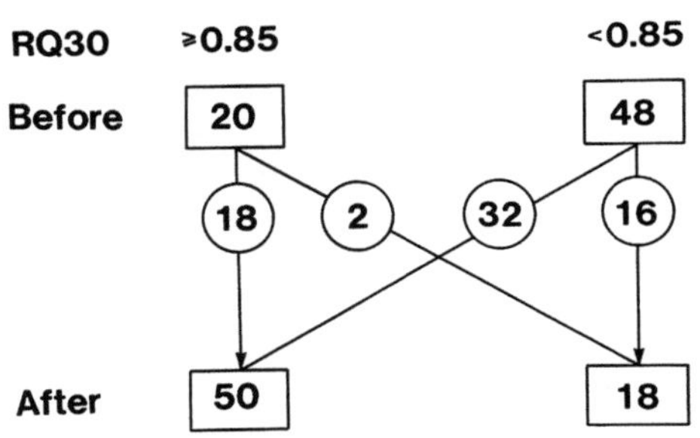

Figure 2. Relative quadriceps strength at 30 °/s (RQ30) for the 68 patients that completed the training programme

Table 2. Results in performance tests. Running times are given in seconds. The quotients refer to injured/uninjured knees

	Before	After
Figure of eight	12.2	11.7
Hop quotient	0.88	0.93
Staircase	10.3	9.4
Slope	21.0	20.0

showed a relative strength of less than 0.85 after training ($P<0.001$; Figure 2). Patients followed up after 2 years had maintained their strength even though no strength training had actually been prescribed.

Performance test

The test results were significantly better after training. The patients ran the figure-of-eight, the staircase and the slope faster, and they hopped a longer distance ($P<0.001$; Table 2). Patients with a relative quadriceps strength above 0.85 achieved better test results than those with a lower relative quadriceps strength.

Conclusions

Increasing thigh muscle strength improves knee function. Symptomatic relief can be obtained without surgery in many patients, and we recommend a period of strength training before considering operation.

It seems that once strength has been regained, good knee function will persist over a long period of time.

Tumours

Treatment of osteosarcoma in the knee joint region

H.-J. Oestern, H. Tscherne and P. Weinel

Unfallchirurgische Klinik und Kinderklinik, Abt. Onkologie der Medizinischen Hochschule
3000 Hannover
Federal Republic of Germany

The treatment of osteosarcoma especially in children has changed over the years from amputation to limb salvage.

Material and methods:
In the tumour centre of Hanover Medical School we operated on 8 patients during the last 3 years with osteosarcoma of the distal femur or tibia head. The following **diagnostic procedures** were performed in all patients:
1. X-rays in 2 planes of the whole femur and tibia and radio-scans.
2. CT-Scan and angiography of the femur and tibia to determine the extent of the tumour.
3. CT-Scan of the lung to recognize lung metastases.

Treatment: All patients were treated in the following manner:
1. Biopsy
2. Polychemotherapy for 12 to 18 weeks
3. Definitive operation

The following definitive operations were performed:
1. Amputations (n=2)
2. Resection-arthrodesis (Enneking) (n=5) employing an intramedullary rod and autogenous segmental cortical grafts obtained from the same extremity
3. Prosthetic replacement (n=1)

Results:
1. Pulmonary metastases developed in 3 patients (1 with amputation, 1 with prosthetic replacement, 1 with resection arthrodesis). In the last patient a resection of pulmonary metastases was performed. This patient died 2 years after the first operation.
2. Out of the 8 patients 2 died of pulmonary metastases.
3. Bone healing of the resection arthrodesis was achieved on average 9 months after the first operation. In 3 patients secondary cancellous bone grafting was necessary.

Summary:
The indication for resection-arthrodesis in osteosarcoma is a tumour with an uninvolved tissue between the lesion and the neurovascular bundle in a young patient to get a stable painless leg. Any compromise between complete tumour resection and limb salvage is contraindicated, because it involves unwarranted risk of recurrence.

Massive replacement for tumours of the knee

H. B. S. Kemp

Royal National Orthopaedic Hospital, Brockley Hill, Stanmore
Middlesex HA7 4LP
United Kingdom

Amputation is a mutilating operation, particularly for the adolescent, in whom the physical and psychological effect is immeasurable. Prior to the introduction of endoprosthetic replacements it was, apart from radiotherapy, essentially the only available method of treatment of tumours, particularly of the lower limb; for, in general, the most frequent sites for the occurrence of primary bone tumours in the appendicular skeleton are in the proximal and distal femur and the proximal tibia. Due to the pioneering work of Prof. John Scales and his colleagues in the Department of Biomedical Engineering at the Royal National Orthopaedic Hospital, it has now become possible to save many of the limbs which formerly would have been treated either by amputation or by radiotherapy. The objectives are: to relieve pain and improve function without a greater risk to life than with amputation; to preserve the whole or part of the limb and to enable, in certain cases, the patient with a limited expectation of life to have an improved quality of life with normal ambulation.

In 1949, the late Sir Herbert Seddon performed the first replacement of the upper femur. In 1954, the late Jackson Burrows performed the first replacement of the knee joint for an osteoclastoma in a young woman.

The prosthesis could be regarded as primitive in design but it was the forerunner of the modern prosthesis used today. It functioned satisfactorily until 1975, when eventually it failed due to metal fatigue. It was replaced by a contemporary prosthesis and the patient continues to lead an active family life.

Since that time, replacements have been made of the knee joint for a variety of tumours. There have been 93 osteosarcomas, 22 chondrosarcomas, 13 fibrosarcomas, 16 parosteal sarcomas, 43 osteoclastomas and 17 others.

When the patient is first referred, assuming that a biopsy has not been taken, the lesion, where possible, is biopsied through a paramedian incision, which can then be excised when a definitive procedure is performed. The patient is subjected to all the routine investigations, which include isotope scanning, CT scanning and, if the lesion is thought to be malignant, CT scanning of the lungs. Patients with malignant disease are normally subjected to at least two courses of cytotoxic therapy prior to replacement surgery.

Major prostheses are individually designed and custom built. For this, both clinical and measurement radiographs are required, the former for accurate identification and delineation of the lesion, the latter to provide the measurements on which the dimensions of the prosthesis will be based. The measurement radiographs can only be achieved by using a stationary grid. True AP and lateral views of the whole bone as well as of the contralateral side are required. In the lower limb, unless the patient's condition precludes it, full-length standing radiographs of both limbs should be taken on one film to ensure that the geometry of the limb is restored. A radiopaque centimetre scale 100 cm long is placed alongside the limb and in the same plane as the bone which is to be replaced. In this way the necessary accurate measurements can be achieved, providing the limb and scale are parallel to the film. Modular construction is not considered to be cost effective and limits the development of improved prostheses.

The amount of bone to be replaced either proximally or distally to the tumour is decided upon on the basis of these radiographs and the scans and, when there is any doubt, on the basis of the core biopsies of the diaphysis.

A typical prosthesis consists of an anodized titanium alloy stem shaped to fit the femur or tibia. This is shrunk fitted and riveted to the titanium shaft, which in turn is cemented to a standard knee unit. The component for normal bone consists of the appropriate portion of a Stanmore hinged knee prosthesis. Massive bone replacements incorporating a knee joint total 174 distal femurs and knees, 56 proximal tibias and knees, 10 total femurs and knees and 2 distal femurs and proximal tibias with a knee.

The surgical procedure does not essentially differ from the standard approach that is generally used to insert a knee replacement, apart from the need to extend the incision either proximally or distally to allow for adequate resection of the tumour. The knee joint is exposed and disarticulated. If the tumour is too large to permit this, the diaphysis is divided at the predetermined level and the tumour primarily resected.

Tumours of the distal femur do not generally present any major problem except in those instances where the neurovascular bundle is involved. Generally, these structures can be dealt with appropriately, though obviously the patient's prior consent must always be obtained for amputation.

Care should be taken to ligate the posterior geniculate artery as this can cause secondary haemorrhage. Resecting the tibia can be more difficult technically. First the site of division of the popliteal artery needs to be identified and, wherever possible, the anterior tibial artery preserved. If the proximal fibula can also be preserved, it is sufficient to retract the common peroneal nerve. If it is necessary to remove the proximal fibula, the nerve and its associated muscles are carefully resected subperiostally, distally, from the bone.

Muscles that are detached in the process of a massive resection normally gain attachment to the fibrous sleeve that develops around the prosthesis. The one exception is the patellar tendon. Consequently, when the tibia is resected, provision has to be made for its reattachment. A transverse hole is made through the tibial component in the course of manufacture, so that, at operation, it is possible to thread a polyester-knitted ribbon through this hole and the tendon can then be stitched to this ribbon. The site of resection is carefully measured to the lower pole of the patella and the patella is then positioned with the correct degree of tension. Failure to do this will lead to quadriceps lag or restrict the knee flexion postoperatively.

Because a major prosthetic replacement of the knee is essentially subcutaneous, the primary objective is to achieve skin healing. During this period, the patient is restricted to isometric quadriceps exercises. However, once healing has been obtained, the knee is actively mobilized, and it is not unusual for the patient to be fully ambulant and discharged from hospital in 3–6 weeks.

Two examples of patients who have had knee replacements are, first, a 52-year-old woman who had no recollection of how long the swelling had been present. The lesion was an osteoclastoma and the technetium scan showed an interesting feature, namely, that the tumour was totally necrotic. Because of the size of the tumour, CT scans were carefully examined, but only by using a contrast scan was it possible to show that the neurovascular bundle was not involved. Because of its size, the tumour was primarily resected and only then could the prosthesis be inserted.

The second patient, a 24-year-old woman, presented with what subsequently was shown to be an aneurysmal bone cyst. She had been aware of a swelling for some 6 years. The tumour had undergone pathological fractures and there were secondary changes in the distal femur. Because of these changes, the prosthesis included both tibial and femoral extensions. Neither of these patients subsequently achieved a range of more than 70 ° knee flexion, but in other respects they led relatively normal lives.

Obviously not all cases are successful, and out of a total of 204 patients, five sustained fractures of the prosthesis, though in fairness to the biomedical engineers, these occurred in the earlier stages of development. Three patients had aseptic loosening of the prosthesis, two had fractures of related bone and eight have become subsequently infected, of whom five had had previous radiotherapy.

As I mentioned earlier, the most promising recent advances have been made in the management of malignant tumours, in particular, osteogenic sarcomas. Whereas the earlier cytotoxic regimen did not appear markedly to improve the prognosis, the present high-dosage methotrexate programmes suggest that a higher survival rate will be obtained. We had only operated on 35 such cases prior to 1982, whereas more than 100 such patients have now had prosthetic replacements.

Of the follow-up of the 35 patients treated to the end of 1981, only 13, i.e., 30%, were alive 2 years later. Nineteen were dead and two had been lost to follow-up, having returned to their own countries. The recent figures suggest that our results will be more satisfactory. It should be pointed out, however, that even for those patients who have unfortunately died, their quality of life was enhanced and they did not have to tolerate a limb that was painful and scarred due to radiotherapy or, what is worse as far as the adolescent is concerned, to be subjected to amputation.

An example of an osteogenic sarcoma was seen in a 17-year-old girl who presented with a classically painful swelling of the distal femur. The radiographs show the typical early changes of an osteogenic sarcoma. Prior to surgery she had two courses of chemotherapy. This led to a very considerable contraction of the soft tissue involvement that was seen in the CT scans and the treatment produced marked sclerosis of the tumour. As a result it was possible to resect this lesion and replace it with a prosthesis. The patient continues to make satisfactory progress 18 months later.

Over the past 8 years, 25 growing prostheses have been inserted for tumours of the knee joint. Twenty-one of these prostheses have an intramedullary stem sliding in a polyethylene sleeve set into the unaffected bone to accommodate its natural growth. Fourteen have a mechanism in the femoral component to produce growth by periodic lengthening of the prosthetic shaft.

The original growing prosthesis was unsatisfactory in that extension was obtained by a screw thread which commonly became clogged by fibrous tissue.

The present design consists of a femoral titanium alloy shaft which is cemented at operation into a modified Stanmore knee unit. The femoral shaft has a sliding member which is prevented from rotation. This carries an intramedullary stem which is cemented into the femur. Inside the stem unit is a piston which is driven distally by the addition of tungsten carbide ball bearings, increasing the length of the prosthesis. On the tibial side the shaft is tapped, after a template has been placed on the tibial plateau, and, an ultra high molecular weight polyethylene sleeve is screwed into the marrow cavity, so that it lies immediately distal to the growth plate. The titanium alloy tibial component consists of a tray which is then recessed into the plateau of the tibia and the shaft of the component is seated in the polyethylene sleeve. No cement is used, and, in consequence, growth of the diaphyseal plate automatically extends the component. The femoral casement can be opened through a small incision at yearly intervals and ball bearings fed in to extend the femoral component.

In conclusion, if traditional ways have to be abandoned we should remember that every tradition was once an innovation. Massive replacements are now being carried out with increasing frequency for bone tumours. There is little doubt at the present time that this is possibly the most satisfactory treatment we can offer the patients affected.

Synovial chondromatosis of the knee: a clinical and histopathological study of 13 cases

C. Fabbriciani and E. de Santis

Clinica Ortopedica Università Cattolica Sacro Cuore
Roma
Italia

Introduction

Synovial chondromatosis is a rare condition that mostly affects the knee and is characterized by a process of cartilaginous metaplasia of the connective elements of the subintimal layer of the synovium. We have employed the term "chondromatosis", but in the literature many different terms are used ("joint chondroma", "synovial chondroma", and particularly "osteochondromatosis", which is the term most frequently employed). However, ossification is only an evolutionary stage following the formation of new cartilaginous tissue.

It must be emphasized that synovial condromatosis is a primary condition of the synovial membrane and that it must be clearly distinguished from those conditions in which the presence of loose bodies is observed, such as arthrosis, arthritis and osteochondrial fractures. Indeed, the mere presence of loose bodies, independent of their number, cannot be a diagnostic criterion.

For the selection of our material we adopted the following strict criteria:

1. Cartilaginous metaplasia was in progress at a number of foci and was surgically and histologically demonstrated

2. At first examination no significant arthrosic modifications of the involved joint were evident

3. There were always a number of loose bodies present

In agreement with Jaffe (1958), we think that one cannot speak of true chondromatosis in the absence of an intrasynovial chondrogenesis and when there are no evident signs of arthrosis.

According to Milgram's description (1977 a, b) one must also distinguish three different stages of the condition that comply with the evolutional process criteria: a first active synovial stage without production of loose bodies (Figure 2); a second stage with formation of loose bodies (Figures 3–5) and a third stage in which loose bodies are present but the synovium is in a state of quiescence.

Material

On the basis of the above-mentioned criteria we selected 13 cases of synovial chondromatosis of the knee from 131 cases operated on for intra-articular

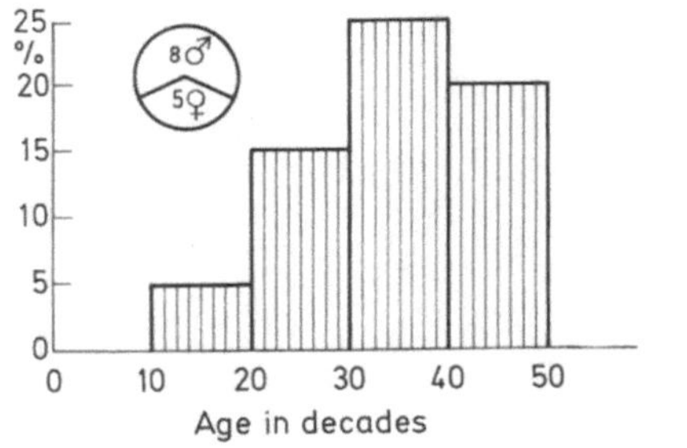

Figure 1. Synovial chrondromatosis of the knee (13 cases)

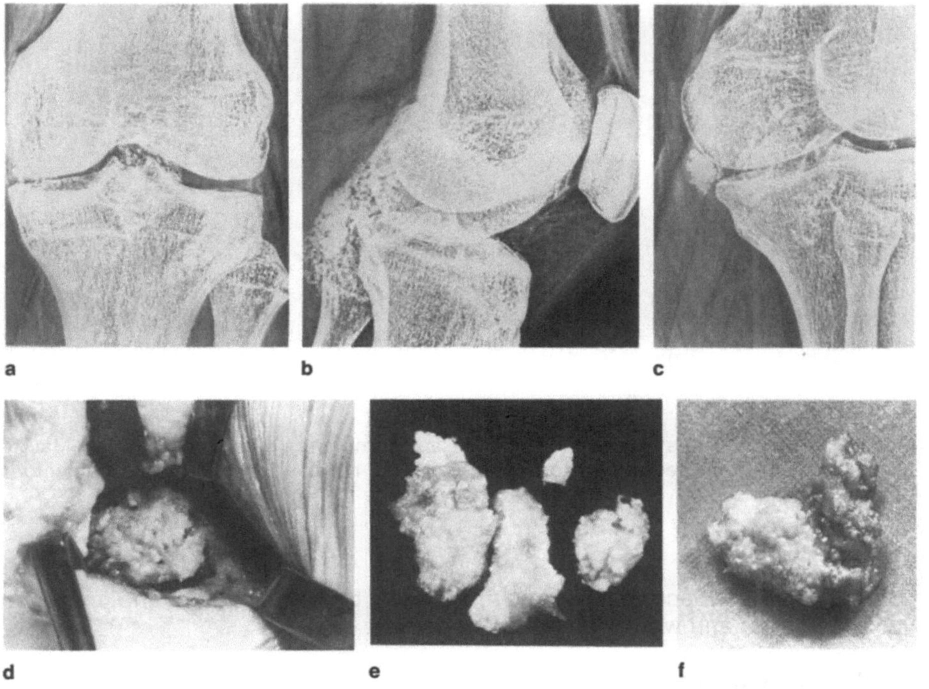

Figure 2. a–c Posterior localization of synovial chondromatosis of the knee. The X-ray shows numerous calcifications, both in the medial and in the lateral side of the knee. Intrasynovial proliferation associated with calcifications and ossifications, in the absence of loose bodies, is peculiar to this localization. **d** Observation at surgery. **e, f** Specimens

loose bodies over a period of 16 years. They included 8 males and 5 females, ranging in age from 16 to 51 years with a maximum incidence between 30 and 50 years. We saw no cases beyond this age limit (Figure 1).

X-Ray

In all our cases the X-ray picture was positive and showed secondary calcification and ossification processes. Nevertheless, in the early forms the picture can be totally negative: in such cases arthrography and arthroscopy can be very useful for diagnostic purposes. In most cases chondromatous areas are visible in the X-ray picture as multiple radiopaque areas often with mul-

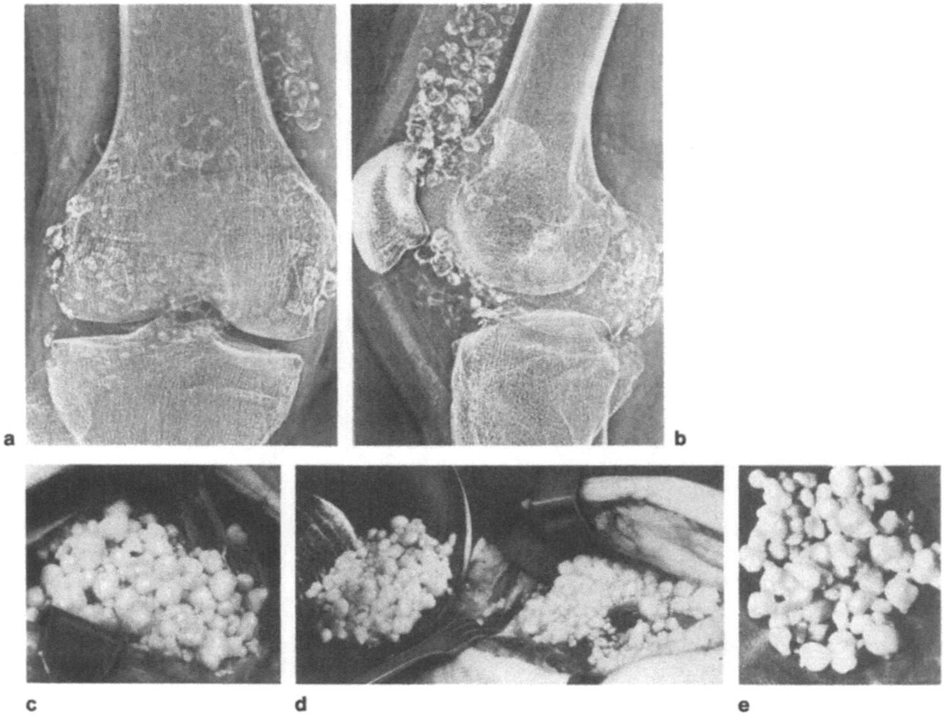

Figure 3. a, b. Typical synovial chondromatosis with numerous loose bodies. c, d Macroscopic aspect at surgery. e Posterior loose bodies removed through retroligamentous arthrotomy

tilobar outlines. Secondary forms are usually characterized by the presence of a few large and well-ossified loose bodies.

Pathological aspects

Synovial chondromatosis is characterized by a very variable number of foci of chondroid metaplasia of the synovium; at times they are so numerous as to form lumps. In less overt cases only palpation reveals more consistent areas, corresponding to developing cartilaginous bodies within the synovium. In these primitive intramural structures intermediate stages can be identified that result in the formation of nodules that are sessile on the synovium or are connected to it by a thin pedicle (Figure 4b). Usually cartilaginous metaplastic processes only affect some areas, and it is rare for the synovial membrane to be totally involved. The synovium of the non-affected areas is hypertrophic and congested.

The microscopic image shows one or more foci of cartilaginous metaplasia within the stroma of the synovial membrane below the intima. Even in those nodules that are nearest to the synovial surface there is always a continuous cell lining that surrounds them in the joint cavity. In smaller formations it is

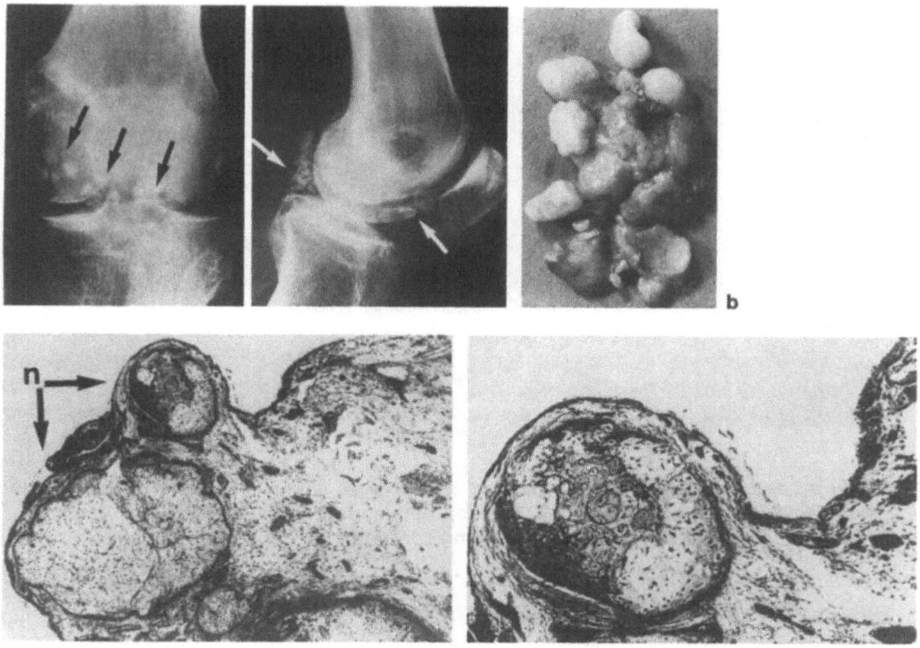

a b

c d

Figure 4. a Observation of anterior and posterior localization of synovial chrondomatosis of the knee. **b** The synovial membrane is removed and different phases of cartilaginous metaplasia are shown (*arrows*). **c, d** Cartilaginous bodies inside the synovial membrane *n*

sometimes possible to detect the transformation process of connective cells into cartilage cells. Larger nodules have a lobular structure; they are made up of hyaline cartilage whose cartilaginous cells are often clustered in isogeneic groups within a rich basic substance.

In the more mature osteocartilaginous bodies three layers are present: an external one made up of fibrous tissue and residues of the synovial membrane, an intermediate cartilaginous layer and an internal bony layer (Figure 5c). Ossification that takes place according to the enchondroidal model can also be observed in those bodies that are no longer connected to the synovial membrane. It usually occurs late in the primary forms whilst it occurs early and more frequently in secondary forms. In some cases areas were observed with giant cartilage cells with cellular polymorphism and nuclear hyperchromia, evidence of a marked proliferative activity. If seen in different sites, such histological findings might suggest a diagnosis of chondrosarcoma, whilst they are frequently present in the primary form of synovial chondromatosis (Murphy et al. 1962). When present, these histological features are an important criterion for distinguishing primary from secondary forms (Figure 6).

On the other hand, although the possibility is mentioned in the literature of chondrosarcomata secondary to pre-existent synovial chondromatosis

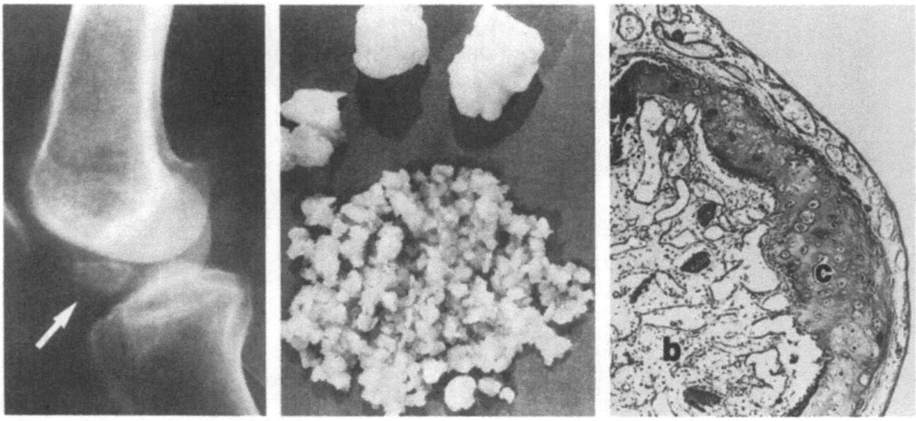

a b c

Figure 5a–c. Synovial chrondromatosis of the knee. **a** The X-ray shows only big loose bodies. **b** At surgery numerous little cartilaginous bodies invisible at X-ray can be recognized. **c** Histological section showing cartilaginous body (*c*) and bone (*b*)

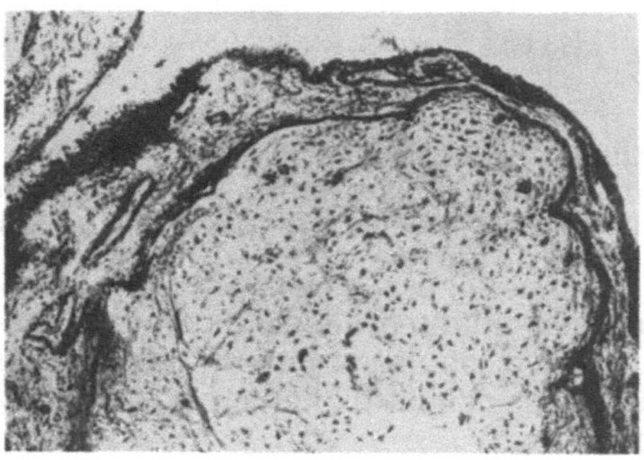

Figure 6. Histological findings in synovial chondromatosis of the knee: giant cartilage cells with cellular polymorphism and nuclear hyperchromia

(Reinmann and Kienböck 1931; Goldman and Liechtenstein 1964; King et al. 1967; Dunn et al. 1974; Milgran and Addison 1976), this has to be explored with the greatest caution. Of 276 chondrosarcomata observed at the Mayo Clinic, none had a synovial origin (Murphy et al. 1966). These data raise doubts as to the true existence of such an origin.

Treatment

The synovial chondromatosis of the knee can be treated only surgically. The operation consists of the removal of the loose bodies and should not be performed as a sole procedure – as advised by some authors (Wilmoth 1941; McIvor and King 1962; Jeffreys 1967) – but is to be associated with the removal of parts of the synovial membrane involved in the cartilage metaplastic process. The foci of chondroid metaplasia – which were always present in our observations – must be detected and excised by means of a partial synoviectomy (performed in nine of our cases). In four cases where large areas of synovium were involved a total synoviectomy was necessary. In two cases a double route of access was required, both anterior and posterior, to remove all the floating bodies.

Results

The results of the surgical management of our cases – with a follow-up of between 2.1 and 14.3 years – were generally good. There was only one recurrence 2 years after a partial synoviectomy and in this case a further synoviectomy had to be performed. The recovery of the knee function was satisfactory although a slight limitation of flexion was always observed. In only two cases was there a marked impairment of flexion that did not exceed 115°.

Conclusions

Synovial chondromatosis is a chronic progressive disease usually in the knee, whose aetiology is unknown. It must be distinguished from other conditions producing loose bodies in the knee joint on the basis of strict histological and radiological criteria. Management is solely surgical and consists in removal of the floating bodies and a more or less extensive synoviectomy, according to the extent and size of the cartilage metaplasia. In our 13 cases of synovial chondromatosis of the knee the recurrence rate was low (1 case). A malignant development of the newly formed tissue is extremely improbable.

References

1. Burny F, Coutelier L, Hinsenkamp M, Nicod C (1976) Ostéochondromatose. Etude clinique, microradiographique et biomécanique. Acta Orthop Belg 42:301–317
2. Christensen JH, Poulsen JO (1975) Synovial chondromatosis. Acta Orthop Scand 46:919–925
3. De Santis E, Fabbriciani C, De Fazi G (1981) Condromatosi sinoviale articolare. Arch Putti Chir Organi Mov 31:253–259
4. Dunn E, McGavran MH, Nelson P, Gaeer RB (1974) Synovial chondrosarcoma. J Bone Joint Surg [Am] 56:811–813
5. Fisher AGT (1921) A study of loose bodies composed of cartilage and bone occurring in joints, with special reference to their pathology and etiology. Br J Surg 8:493–523
6. Goldman RL, Lichtenstein L (1964) Synovial chondrosarcoma. Cancer 17:1233–1240
7. Jaffe HL (1958) Tumours and tumorous conditions of the bones and joints. Lea and Febiger, Philadelphia
8. Jeffreys TE (1967) Synovial chondromatosis. J Bone Joint Surg [Br] 49:530–534
9. Jones HT (1924) Loose bodies formation in synovial osteochondromatosis. J Bone Joint Surg 6:407–458
10. King JW, Spjut HJ, Fechner RE, Vanderpool DW (1967) Synovial chondrosarcoma of the knee joint. J Bone Joint Surg [Am] 49:1389–1396
11. McIvor RR, King D (1962) Osteochondromatosis of the hip joint. J Bone Joint Surg [Am] 44:87–97
12. Milgram JW (1977 a) Synovial osteochondromatosis. A histopathological study of thirty cases. J Bone Joint Surg [Am] 59:792–801
13. Milgram JW (1977 b) The classification of loose bodies in human joints. Clin Orthop 24:282–291
14. Murphy FP, Dahlin DC, Sullivan CR (1962) Articular synovial chondromatosis. J Bone Joint Surg [Am] 44:77–86
15. Reinman H, Kienböck R (1931) Über Gelenks-Osteochondromatose mit Sarkombildung. Röntgenpraxis 3:942–944
16. Villacin AB, Brigham LN, Bullough PG (1979) Primary and secondary synovial chondrometaplasia. Histopathologic and clinicoradiologic differences. Hum Pathol 10:439–451
17. Wilmoth CL (1941) Osteochondromatosis. J Bone Joint Surg [Am] 23:367–374

Synovectomy in cases of pigmented villo-nodular synovitis of the knee. A follow-up study

V. Tsemanis, C. Constantinides and J. Galanis

Asclepion Hospital
Athens
Greece

Pigmented villo-nodular synovitis, in its diffuse or localised form, is still a rare disease of unknown etiology, which affects mostly the knee joint. Its differential diagnosis is not easy and its prognosis should be guarded. In this paper an analysis is tried of 17 cases of the diffuse form of the disease, that were treated in the last 15 years at the Asclepion Hospital, Athens, Greece.

Material and methods

A follow-up study was carried out on a total of 37 cases of operated knees registered as P.V.S. and 11 of its localized form (referred to sometimes as benign synoviomas as well). Only the diffuse cases were considered. We were able to trace and reexamine 17 patients in the follow-up, all suffering from unilateral disease and all operated (open arthrotomy). The mean follow-up was 6.4 years. There were 12 women and 15 men. Mean age 36. The oldest was 69 and the youngest a 3 years old baby girl. Nearly 2/3 had a paracentesis before the operation, which revealed light coloured bloody fluid. There was a history of vague trauma in 1/3 of the cases. Only 3 cases had been arthroscoped before the operation – which was usually an extensive thorough synovectomy. Four patients were re-operated and a second synovectomy was carried out.

Results

The clinical results were graded as very good in 9 cases, fair in 5 and poor in 3, in reference to continuing pain, stiffness, and gradual bony involvement. One of the poor cases went into a fusion of the knee, and another one is considered for a TNR. In 1/3 we have experienced residual swelling of the knee joint which subsequently synovitis with moderate results. Steroids were used in two cases to control recurrent synovitis with moderate results. Out of the original 17 cases, 4 had minimal to significant bone involvement mainly of the tibia. These 4 cases, as expected, did less well than the others.

Discussion and conclusion

A retrospective study of 17 cases of diffuse PVS affecting the knee joint has been carried out. After carefully going through the literature, we have concluded that a) diffuse P.V.S. – as distinct to the localized form of the disease, is still a disease of unknown etiology, b) synovectomy of the knee, even repeated synovectomies, has not been provided with the results we should have liked but – so far – it is the only possible treatment and c) when bone is involved serious therapeutic problems arise. It is suggested that a) diagnostic arthroscopy should be tried at an early stage of the disease, as well needle biopsy and paracentesis, b) if our findings are positive an arthrotomy – synovectomy should be carried out at once, and c) our prognosis should be guarded for a long time.

Subject Index

MIX
Papier aus verantwortungsvollen Quellen
Paper from responsible sources
FSC® C105338

If you have any concerns about our products,
you can contact us on
ProductSafety@springernature.com

In case Publisher is established outside the EU,
the EU authorized representative is:
Springer Nature Customer Service Center GmbH
Europaplatz 3, 69115 Heidelberg, Germany

Printed by Libri Plureos GmbH
in Hamburg, Germany